Colorectal Cancer: Diagnostic and Therapeutic Advances

Colorectal Cancer: Diagnostic and Therapeutic Advances

Edited by Jane Mayer

hayle
medical

New York

Hayle Medical,
750 Third Avenue, 9th Floor,
New York, NY 10017, USA

Visit us on the World Wide Web at:
www.haylemedical.com

ISBN: 978-1-63241-874-6

Cataloging-in-Publication Data

Colorectal cancer : diagnostic and therapeutic advances / edited by Jane Mayer.
   p. cm.
Includes bibliographical references and index.
ISBN 978-1-63241-874-6
1. Colon (Anatomy)--Cancer. 2. Rectum--Cancer. 3. Colon (Anatomy)--Cancer--Diagnosis.
4. Colon (Anatomy)--Cancer--Treatment. 5. Rectum--Cancer--Diagnosis.
6. Rectum--Cancer--Treatment. I. Mayer, Jane.
RC280.C6 C65 2020
616.994 347--dc23

Table of Contents

Preface

Over the recent decade, advancements and applications have progressed exponentially. This has led to the increased interest in this field and projects are being conducted to enhance knowledge. The main objective of this book is to present some of the critical challenges and provide insights into possible solutions. This book will answer the varied questions that arise in the field and also provide an increased scope for furthering studies.

Colorectal cancer or bowel cancer refers to the development of cancer in the colon or rectum of the gastrointestinal tract. It is the third most common form of cancer. The most common form of colon cancer is adenocarcinoma. Colorectal cancer can occur with age and lifestyle choices. A small number of cases can occur due to underlying genetic factors. Screening is recommended from the age of 50 to 75 as it can be effective in preventing cancer deaths. Colonoscopy and sigmoidoscopy can effectively test for the presence of the cancer, while its spread can be determined through imaging techniques. The cellular characteristics of the tumor can be found from the analysis of tissue taken from a surgery or biopsy. For individuals with localized colorectal cancer, the preferred treatment is complete surgical removal, through an open laparotomy or laparoscopic surgery, followed by a colostomy. Chemotherapy may also be used prior to the surgery to shrink the growth. Colorectal cancer can recur, especially in the liver and lungs. This book presents the diagnostic and therapeutic advances in colorectal cancer in the most comprehensible language. Different approaches, evaluations, methodologies and advanced studies on colorectal cancer have been included herein. As the field of oncology is emerging at a fast pace, this book will help the readers to better understand the latest research and therapeutic advances.

I hope that this book, with its visionary approach, will be a valuable addition and will promote interest among readers. Each of the authors has provided their extraordinary competence in their specific fields by providing different perspectives as they come from diverse nations and regions. I thank them for their contributions.

Editor

Colonoscopy — Indications and Contraindications

Jigar Bhagatwala, Arpit Singhal, Summer Aldrugh,
Muhammed Sherid, Humberto Sifuentes and
Subbaramiah Sridhar

Abstract

This chapter discusses some of the major indications and contraindications for colonoscopy. Advances in colonoscopic techniques have expanded the role of colonoscopy beyond conventional screening, surveillance, and diagnosis to various complex therapeutic and interventional utilities. Several guidelines with new information are being published and updated regularly in the field of colonoscopy and are currently used in clinical practice. However, there is still a lack of well-designed randomized clinical trials investigating the role of colonoscopy in early diagnosis and treatment of various conditions and its impact on long-term survival and disease status. Nevertheless, retrospective observational studies and a few randomized clinical trials abundantly supply data supporting the role of colonoscopy in the diagnosis and management of colonic pathologies in the absence of comparable alternatives.

Keywords: Colonoscopy, Indication, Contraindication, Screening, Surveillance, Diagnostic, Therapeutic

1. Introduction

In the 1960s, Drs. William Wolff and Hiromi Shinya developed a way to probe the full length of the colon using a tube with electronic sensors [1]. Since its inception, colonoscopy has become a very popular method for screening of colorectal cancers and for treating a variety of conditions of the lower gastrointestinal tract. The decision to perform colonoscopy should take into account the indication and contraindication for the procedure, the risks of the procedure, and the cost. A key quality measure of colonoscopy is the indication for the procedure, because as high as 20-50% of colonoscopies are performed for inappropriate indications [2]. Performing colonoscopy for inappropriate indications not only exposes patients to procedure-related complications such as bowel perforation, bleeding, infection, and cardiovascular events, but also increases on the health-care-related cost. Therefore, several societies including the American Society of Gastrointestinal Endoscopy (ASGE) and the European Panel on the Appropriateness of Gastrointestinal Endoscopy (EPAGE), have established guidelines for appropriate use of colonoscopy. In this chapter, we aim to outline the common indications and contraindications for performing colonoscopy and detail the evidence supporting the facts.

2. Indications for colonoscopy (table 1)

2.1. Lower gastrointestinal (GI) bleeding

Lower GI bleeding may occur in the form of occult bleeding, melena, scant intermittent hematochezia, or severe hematochezia [3]. Lower GI bleeding from any cause requires colonoscopy either urgently or routinely. Patients with occult GI bleeding require colonoscopy to exclude malignant or adenomatous etiologies. Patients who are not good candidates for colonoscopy can be evaluated using CT colonography [4]. In patients presenting with melena, upper GI endoscopy is performed first to identify any upper GI causes. If the upper GI endoscopy does not reveal a source of bleeding, colonoscopy is then indicated to identify any colonic source. Intermittent scant hematochezia can be diagnosed by anoscopy with/without sigmoidoscopy for low-lying lesions in the anus, rectum, and sigmoid in patients who are younger than 40. However, colonoscopy may still be required if a definitive source cannot be identified. On the other hand, colonoscopy is the recommended procedure for patients with intermittent hematochezia who have one of the following risk factors: age >50, family history of colon cancer, or other alarming symptoms such as weight loss, anemia, and change in bowel habits [5, 6]. Overall, colonoscopy has been reported to have a higher yield than other modalities such as proctosigmoidoscopy, single-contrast barium studies, or combined flexible sigmoidoscopy and double-contrast barium enema for diagnosis of lower GI bleeding. In case of severe hematochezia, hemodynamic stability determines the diagnostic and therapeutic approach [7-9]. In hemodynamically stable patients, urgent (within 8-24 h) colonoscopy is recommended [10-13]. In critically ill patients, upper endoscopy is indicated first followed by colonoscopy after excluding the upper GI tract as the source of bleeding [14]. The therapeutic indications of colonoscopy for the treatment of lower GI bleeding are discussed separately in this chapter.

Indications for colonoscopy:
1.Lower GI bleeding
2.Screening and surveillance of colorectal polyps and cancers: a. Colon cancer b. Surveillance after polypectomy c. Colorectal cancer post-resection surveillance d. Inflammatory bowel diseases
3.Acute and chronic diarrhea
4.Therapeutic indications for colonoscopy: a. Excision and ablation of lesions b. Treatment of lower GI bleeding c. Colonic decompression d. Dilation of colonic stenosis e. Foreign body removal
5.Miscellaneous indications: a. Abnormal radiological examinations b. Isolated unexplained abdominal pain c. Chronic constipation d. Preoperative and intraoperative localization of colonic lesions

Table 1. Indications for colonoscopy

2.2. Screening and surveillance of colorectal polyps and cancers

2.2.1. Colon cancer

According to the World Health Organization report in 2012, colorectal cancer (CRC) is the third most common cancer in men (746,000 cases, 10% of the total) and the second in women (614,000 cases, 9.2% of the total) worldwide. In 2014, the American Cancer Society predicted that about 136,830 people would be diagnosed with colorectal cancer in the United States, and about 50,310 people were predicted to die of the disease. Recent studies show declining in the CRC incidence and mortality rates, which have been attributed to the awareness of the risk factors and reduced exposure to them, the effect of early detection and prevention through polypectomy, and improved treatment [15]. The recommendations for screening colonoscopies are divided based on the known risk factor profile: 1) screening in the average-risk population and 2) screening in patients with a family history of colon cancer.

In the average-risk patient, current American, European, and Asian guidelines recommend beginning CRC screening with colonoscopy at the age of 50 years and every 10 years thereafter regardless of the gender. However, the American College of Gastroenterology recommends that the screening colonoscopy begin at the age of 45 years in African Americans [16, 17]. Published evidence favoring the effectiveness of colonoscopy in reducing mortality from CRC by routine colonoscopy is insufficient because of a lack of randomized controlled trials and the limited consensus in guidelines on the appropriateness of colonoscopy. However, a few studies have modeled and predicted the impact of screening colonoscopy on CRC incidence and mortality using various transition models in hypothetical average-risk individuals aged 50 years. These studies have found that initial screening colonoscopy and repeat colonoscopy every 10 years might reduce CRC incidence by 58% and the reduction in CRC mortality is approximately 64% [18, 19]. In the average-risk individuals, yearly fecal occult blood testing (FOBT) and flexible sigmoidoscopy (FSIG) every 3 years are also accepted methods of screening for CRC. A follow-up colonoscopy, however, is warranted to completely visualize the entire length of the colon for patients with positive FOBT results or FSIG findings of adenoma in the distal colon [20-23].

Family history of CRC is a major risk factor for CRC. It has been estimated that the first-degree relatives of CRC patients have two- to threefold increased risk of dying from CRC, and the risk is inversely associated with the age of diagnosis of the affected family member [24]. Patients with a single first-degree relative with CRC or advanced adenoma (adenoma ≥1 cm in size, with high-grade dysplasia, or villous elements) diagnosed at age ≥60 years are recommended to undergo routine CRC screening same as an average-risk individual beginning at age 50 years. On the other hand, patients with a single first-degree relative with CRC or advanced adenoma diagnosed at age <60 years, or two first-degree relatives with CRC or advanced adenomas should receive colonoscopy every 5 years beginning at age 40, or 10 years earlier than the age at diagnosis of the youngest affected relative, whichever comes first [16]. The data supporting these recommendations emerge from the retrospective studies rather than the randomized control trials [25, 26].

Patients with a family history of hereditary nonpolyposis colorectal cancer (HNPCC), an autosomal dominant disease, are recommended to start the CRC screening at the age of 20-25 years or 10 years prior to the earliest age of HNPCC diagnosis in the patient's family member, whichever comes first. The recommended interval for colonoscopy is every 1-2 years until age 40, then annually thereafter [27-30]. This condition, in particular, has two-thirds of adenomas occurring on the right side and warrants colonoscopy for complete colonic surveillance [31]. Indications for performing colonoscopy in individuals with a history of familial adenomatous polyposis (FAP) are guideline-dependent after genetic testing returns positive. FSIG and colonoscopy have not been compared head-to-head regarding their effectiveness and reducing mortality in patients with FAP in the clinical trials and, as such, either FSIG or colonoscopy annually is recommended, starting at the age of 10-12 years [16]. A colonoscopy is deemed necessary when polyps are detected on FSIG and a decision to perform polypectomy is made.

2.2.2. Surveillance after polypectomy

Post-polypectomy surveillance constitutes 20% of the performed colonoscopies, thereby constituting a large share in the amount of health care expenditure [32, 33]. Adhering to the indications for the repeat colonoscopy for the surveillance of CRC after the first colonoscopy, therefore, is very important as earlier colonoscopy can increase the risks to the patient and add to the health care cost whereas delaying the surveillance can also increase the risks by increasing the chances of missed interval cancers. Various observational studies report a 2-5%

risk of an advanced neoplasia 5-10 years after a negative colonoscopy, a risk that is comparable to the risk of advanced colonic neoplasia in the average-risk patients undergoing their first colonoscopy [34-39]. Moreover, the risk of developing CRC 10 years after a negative colonoscopy is reported to be significantly lower (adjusted OR 0.26) [36, 40], supporting the current recommendation of repeat colonoscopy every 10 years in the average-risk general population.

Although the detection and removal of polyp(s) can offer a significant reduction in the mortality of CRC, the development of interval cancers, i.e., the cancers occurring after the initial colonoscopy with polypectomy, appears to be the highest in the first 3-5 years. In 2012, the United States Multi-Society Task Force (USMSTF) published a revision of the 2006 guidelines on post-polypectomy surveillance and divided recommendations based on the presence of polyp(s) (hyperplastic vs. adenomatous), the number and the size of adenomatous polyp(s), villous component and high-grade dysplasia in the polyp, and the presence of serrated lesions or serrated polyposis syndrome (>20 serrated polyps of any size throughout the colon) at baseline colonoscopy. In 2013, the European Society of Gastrointestinal Endoscopy (ESGE) published its post-polypectomy surveillance guidelines, stratifying risk into: low risk (1-2 adenomas <1 cm), intermediate risk (3-4 small adenomas or one >1 cm), and high risk (>5 small adenomas or >3 adenomas with at least one >1 cm) based on the first colonoscopy. According to the USMSTF guideline, it is indicated that patients with 1-2 tubular adenomas <1 cm have a repeat colonoscopy in 10 years; whereas patients with a high-risk adenoma (defined as adenoma with villous histology, high-grade dysplasia, adenoma>10 mm, or three or more adenomas) are recommended to have surveillance interval of 3 years. According to the ESGE guideline, the high-risk group should undergo surveillance at 1 year, the intermediate-risk group at 3-yearly intervals until two consecutive examinations are negative, and the low-risk group requires no surveillance colonoscopy or 5-yearly colonoscopy until one negative examination after which surveillance can be discontinued. The evidence supporting the indications in the arena of surveillance for the serrated polyp is insufficient. According to the USMSTF guideline, sessile serrated polyp(s) <1 cm with no dysplasia should be considered low risk and can be followed at a 5-year interval. However, sessile serrated polyp(s) ≥1 cm or sessile serrated polyp with dysplasia or serrated adenoma should undergo surveillance at 3 years and serrated polyposis syndrome should be surveyed annually. The ESGE recommends that patients with serrated polyps <10 mm in size without dysplasia should be classified as low risk, whereas patients with large serrated polyps (≥10 mm) or those with dysplasia as high risk and undergo surveillance accordingly. Patients with ≥5 serrated polyps proximal to the sigmoid, of which ≥2 are sized ≥10mm, or with ≥20 serrated polyps of any size are classified as serrated polyposis and should be referred for genetic testing.

2.2.3. CRC post-resection surveillance

There are no clear survival benefits for performing colonoscopy in patients who have had colon cancer resection. However, a majority of the groups and societies such as American Cancer Society (ACS), and a joint American Cancer Society/US Multi-Society Task Force on Colorectal Cancer, Cancer Care Ontario [41-44], recommend post CRC resection surveillance. An indication to perform colonoscopy in these patients will help detect metachronous CRCs and polyps as well as anastomotic recurrences of the initial primary cancer at a stage that would allow further treatment. Currently, a follow-up colonoscopy is indicated at 1 year after the surgical removal of CRC. If no new cancer or polyp(s) is identified, a colonoscopy is repeated at 3 years and at 5 years if the findings are negative for interval development of cancer. An exception to this indication is HNPCC, which requires colonoscopic surveillance every 1-2 years regardless of the surgical resection of the cancer.

2.2.4. Inflammatory bowel diseases and other colitis

The indications for colonoscopy in inflammatory bowel disease (IBD), namely ulcerative colitis (UC) and Crohn's disease (CD) fall under a large spectrum. Colonoscopic diagnosis and differentiation between the UC and CD, assessment of the extent and severity of disease activity, treatment effectiveness, surveillance of malignancies, and endoscopic treatment, such as stricture dilation, are all within the scope of colonoscopy and its indications in IBD. Currently, American, European, and other international societies and guideline-defining bodies recommend endoscopic visualization of the entire colon for the initial diagnosis of IBD and other colitis [45-48]. The clinical presentation and laboratory data characterizing both diseases may overlap but endoscopic visualization of the mucosa of the rectum, colon, and terminal ileum, and the extent of the disease involvement may help differentiate the disease processes. Moreover, colonoscopy offers the opportunity to perform biopsy, which is the major advantage of colonoscopy. Unless contraindicated because of severe colitis or possible toxic megacolon, a full colonoscopy with intubation of the terminal ileum should be performed during the initial evaluation of patients with a clinical presentation suggestive of IBD. Ileoscopy is superior for the diagnosis of CD of the terminal ileum when compared with radiological methods, especially for mild lesions [49, 50]. During the colonoscopic examination, biopsy samples should be obtained both from areas affected by the disease and from unaffected areas. After initiating therapy, a smaller number of biopsy samples may be necessary to confirm the diagnosis. In postsurgical follow-up, biopsies of the neoterminal ileum are indicated when disease recurrence is suspected. In patients who have undergone ileal pouch-anal anastomosis, biopsies of the afferent limb are indicated when Crohn's disease is suspected [46]. Other forms of colitis, such as drug-induced, infectious, vascular, and radiation colitis also present in a similar pattern and require colonoscopy at baseline for the diagnosis and the assessment of severity.

Patients with IBD have an increased risk of CRC compared to those without IBD [51-55]. In fact, CRC accounts for one-sixth of ulcerative colitis-related deaths [56]. There is a lack of randomized control studies demonstrating the effectiveness of colonoscopy in improving survival in the IBD patients from CRC. However, numerous observational studies have reported that colonoscopic surveillance of CRC in IBD offers early detection of cancers and improves CRC-related survival in IBD patients [57, 58]. In a retrospective study of 6,823 patients with IBD in US tertiary referral hospitals followed-up for at least 3 years, the incidence of CRC among patients without a recent colonoscopy was 2.7% which was significantly higher than among patients with a recent colonoscopy (1.6%) [59]. Additionally, a colonoscopy within 6-36 months before diagnosis was associated with a 64% reduction in mortality rate [59].

According to most guidelines, colonoscopies are indicated for CRC screening starting at 8-10 years from initiation of IBD-related symptoms [48, 53, 60-62]. The National Institute for Health and Clinical Excellence (NICE) London 2011 guideline, however, recommends only offering colonoscopic surveillance to patients with Crohn's colitis involving more than 1 segment of the colon or left-sided or more extensive UC, but not isolated ulcerative proctitis. Most guidelines recommend yearly follow-up colonoscopy for high-risk patients (those with primary sclerosing cholangitis, extensive colitis, active endoscopic or histologic inflammation, a family history of CRC in a first-degree relative before 50 years of age, personal history of dysplasia, presence of strictures on colonoscopy, and, possibly, gender), and every 2-5 years for those without major risk factors.

2.3. Acute and chronic diarrhea

Patients presenting with acute diarrhea should undergo initial evaluation with stool studies. If blood and stool cultures are inconclusive, or if symptoms persist or worsen despite empiric therapy, then colonoscopy is indicated due to its high diagnostic yield [63]. For most patients with chronic diarrhea, patients with suspected acute diffuse *Clostridium Difficile* colitis, pregnant patients, patients with predominantly left-sided symptoms (tenesmus/urgency) and patients with multiple morbidities, a flexible sigmoidoscopy can be used for the initial evaluation. Even if patients have macroscopically normal-appearing mucosa, biopsies must be obtained to exclude microscopic diseases. If flexible sigmoidoscopy yields inconclusive results, if diarrhea persists, or if there is suspicion of inflammatory bowel disease (IBD) or cancer, then colonoscopy should be the next investigative study.

Histology is an integral component of colonoscopic evaluation of chronic diarrhea because several diseases, such as microscopic colitis, eosinophilic colitis, amyloidosis, and IBD, may appear normal on endoscopy but are abnormal on microscopy. In patients undergoing colonoscopy for chronic diarrhea, IBD or colitis is the most likely disease to be detected [64]. Microscopic colitis can be lymphocytic or collagenous and is characterized by nonbloody, watery diarrhea. On endoscopy, microscopic colitis can be missed because of patchy colonic involvement. Even if mucosa appears normal endoscopically, multiple biopsies from both sides of the colon are necessary to avoid missing microscopic colitis [65]. If there is suspicion of inflammatory diarrhea, then a biopsy of the terminal ileum is helpful in the diagnosis. However, a biopsy of the terminal ileum has the highest diagnostic yield in patients with known or suspected Crohn's disease, terminal ileal abnormalities on imaging, or endoscopic findings of ulcers, ileitis, or erosions [66].

Colonoscopy is not routinely used to evaluate acute diarrhea because it is commonly due to infectious etiology. If stool tests are negative and/or if diarrhea persists, then endoscopy is indicated. An additional important exception is the case of an immunocompromised patient. In a patient with diarrhea with HIV, organ or bone marrow transplant, or on immunosuppressive medications, a colonoscopy with biopsy is necessary to exclude CMV colitis and graft versus host disease (GVHD). In such cases, colonoscopic evaluation of diarrhea has higher sensitivity and cost-effectiveness than FSIG [67]. Patients who undergo stem cell transplant often present with diarrhea in the initial 3 months following transplantation. In these patients, abnormal mucosa on endoscopy has not been shown to correlate with biopsy results. There-fore, biopsies of normal and abnormal-appearing mucosa are indicated, especially of the distal colon, which has the highest diagnostic yield in patients undergoing endoscopy for gastroin-testinal symptoms [68]. Based on the location of highest diagnostic yield, a flexible sigmoido-scopy with distal colon biopsy is indicated in patients with diarrhea suspected of acute GVHD. However, some centers endorse combined upper GI endoscopy as well as colonoscopy in patients following hematopoietic stem cell transplantation to diagnose disease more quickly.

2.4. Therapeutic indications for colonoscopy

2.4.1. Excision and ablation of lesions

Endoscopic mucosal resection (EMR) is a method for treating early CRC. Most adenomas and intramucosal cancers can be removed by EMR. For tumors larger than 2 cm, EMR is less likely to achieve complete resection (histopathologically tumor-free lateral and vertical margins of the resected specimens) [69, 70]. Another method, known as endoscopic submucosal dissection (ESD) is also performed in several countries. The procedure is simpler than the laparoscopic colectomy but is time-consuming and carries a higher risk of perforation than EMR. ESD is indicated in lesions >2 cm, lesions that are suspected to be invasive submucosal cancer, and mucosal lesions with fibrosis or local residual early cancer after endoscopic resection. The rate of complete resection for large colorectal tumors by ESD has been reported to be 80-98.9% [71-74]. However, both procedures are operator-dependent and have limited data supporting their use.

2.4.2. Treatment of lower GI bleeding

Treatment of acute lower GI bleeding from any sources described earlier is indicated either urgently or as an elective procedure. In case of urgent colonoscopy, the colon is prepared using polyethylene glycol based solution administered orally or via nasogastric tube. Currently, metallic clip placement, thermal coagulation, and epinephrine injection are the available methods. Depending on the lesion and the severity of bleeding, colonoscopic intervention with any one of these methods is indicated as the first step in achieving hemostasis. In case of persistent diverticular bleeding, a bleeding vessel can be treated with metallic clip placement [75, 76]. Vascular ectasias can be treated with either thermal or epinephrine injection, though thermal cauterization has 87% of success rate [77]. Cases where a definite bleeding site cannot be located or cases where the visualization of the bleeding source is poor due to inadequate views due to bleeding need referral for angiographic or surgical treatment.

2.4.3. Colonic decompression

Acute colonic obstruction is a common presentation of colon cancer and, often, the presenting patient is in poor overall health making surgical intervention a suboptimal choice. Since 1990, the utility of colonoscopic interventions via either self-expanding metal stent (SEMS), place-ment of a decompression tube, or tumor debulking has become very popular and has been studied more frequently in recent years in various populations. Endoscopic interventions serve as a bridge to surgery or as a palliative measure in patients who are poor surgical candidates. A majority of the studies comparing SEMS placement with surgery has reported high clinical success rates (92%), better symptomatic relief, lower complication rates (<5%), cost-effectiveness, and higher patient acceptance and shorter hospital stay with endoscopic SEMS placement [78-83]. Argon plasma coagulation (APC) and snare polypectomy have been used to treat colonic obstruction and maintain luminal patency, and are good alternatives to endoscopic SEMS in treating colonic obstruction [84-86].

Endoscopic decompression of an acute colonic pseudo-obstruction or Ogilvie syndrome is another therapeutic indication for colonoscopy. The etiology of this condition is multifactorial (post-intraabdominal surgery, sepsis, hypothyroidism, neurological disorder, spinal cord injury, etc.) in the absence of a true mechanical obstruction. Bowel ischemia and perforation are dreaded complications and management is often conservative, involving the correction of the underlying disorder. However, in cases where the initial management fails, colonoscopic decompression is indicated [87, 88].

Colonoscopy is also used for decompression of sigmoid and cecal volvulus. Volvulus is a condition in which a part of colon twists upon itself. Due to venous congestion and obstruction to blood flow, tissue viability becomes a major issue. Patients presenting with signs of perforation, peritonitis, bowel necrosis or profound hemodynamic instability need immediate surgery. However, patients with less severe sigmoid and cecal volvulus can be managed endoscopically [89, 90]. Endoscopic correction of sigmoid volvulus achieves better success rates than the correction of cecal volvulus and is associated with a lesser need for surgical intervention [91]. A study by Oren and colleagues reported that sigmoidoscopic correction of sigmoid volvulus with a rectal tube was successful in 78% of patients [92]. Nevertheless, the rate of recurrence of sigmoid volvulus is high, ultimately requiring surgical treatment [93]. Cecal volvulus has been treated endoscopically but due to the high failure rate, often requires surgical intervention for most patients. Surgeons usually combine operative detorsion of cecal volvulus with right hemicolectomy (to prevent recurrence) and either a primary anastomosis or an ileostomy with mucus fistula. In medically unstable, high-risk patients who are poor surgical candidates or have poor vascular supplies to the cecum, cecal volvulus detorsion may be achieved with a cecostomy and cecopexy, which also are associated with significant morbidity and mortality [94]. Colonic volvuluses in other areas such as flexural territories are less common and the indication to perform colonoscopic interventions in these situations is not well studied.

2.4.4. Dilation of colonic stenosis

Colonoscopic intervention of stenotic lesions such as anastomotic strictures and strictures caused by IBD are among the common indications for performing colonoscopy. Several studies have reported high success rate with a low complications rate. However, recurrence is common. The methods commonly employed for the treatment of colonic stenosis are balloon dilation with or without steroid injection and electro-incision, all of which have been shown to have a variable amount of success [95-101].

2.4.5. Foreign body removal

The current management of the foreign bodies lying in the lower GI tract is based on the type of foreign body, the proximity to the anus, the injury to the adjacent structure, as well as the surgical and endoscopic expertise at the health care center. A foreign body in the GI tract presents after voluntary or involuntary insertion or ingestion of the foreign body. Very often, the patient tries to manipulate the object and attempts self-exploration to remove it before presenting to the hospital. Endoscopy provides an opportunity to avoid abdominal explora-tion. However if the radiological exam or clinical presentation indicates perforation or higher-lying object(s), colonoscopy may fail and may pose a delay in surgical management [102-106].

2.5. Miscellaneous indications

2.5.1. Abnormal radiological examination

Colonoscopy is commonly performed after an abnormal or suspicious radiological finding in the search for true pathological lesions such as cancers or ulcerative lesions. Filling defect or mucosal defect on barium enema or a luminal narrowing on barium enema or CT scan is routinely evaluated with a colonoscopy. Patients presenting with symptoms suggestive of acute diverticulitis with supportive CT scan findings also need to be evaluated with colono-scopy, but only after the acute inflammation has resolved. Air insufflation during colonoscopy in acute diverticulitis can lead to the bowel perforation and is considered a contraindication. A luminal defect or polyp(s) on CT scan or CT colonography is usually followed-up by a colonoscopy when feasible. However, controversy exists between the American College of Radiology, the American Gastroenterology Association, and American College of Gastroen-terology regarding the size and number of polyps on CT colonography that meet the require-ment for colonoscopy [107-109]. Patients with abnormal positron emission tomography (PET) scan showing a possible colorectal lesion should undergo colonoscopic evaluation. Neverthe-less, in the light of insufficient clinical data, the indications for colonoscopy after abnormal radiological exam are based on individual presentation, availability of the endoscopist, age, and other comorbidities of the patient.

2.5.2. Isolated unexplained abdominal pain

Patients presenting with symptoms of chronic (>3 months) abdominal pain and nonspecific abdominal discomfort might require colonoscopy. In the era of thorough radiologic studies, the need for colonoscopy emerges after noninvasive diagnostic modalities fail and symptoms persist. There is no clear indication for performing colonoscopy in patients presenting with unexplained abdominal pain or discomfort. A detailed history and physical examination provide diagnostic clues but a diagnostic workup often ends up requiring colonoscopy. The diagnostic yield of colonoscopy has been previously studied in retrospective studies. For example, in a study by Neugut et al., a total of 7% of patients who presented with abdominal pain (n=113) either had carcinoma or a polyp >1 cm in size on colonoscopy [110]. It is worth mentioning that detection of the pathological process does not offer symptomatic relief in these cases. In a more recent study by Kueh and colleagues, the diagnostic yield of colonoscopy was evaluated from 2005 to 2010 in a tertiary center in New Zealand among the patients who presented with isolated abdominal pain, which accounted for 1.2% of all colonoscopies (n=2633). The diagnostic yield of colonoscopy for a cancer, adenoma, diverticulosis, or hemorrhoid in the patients with abdominal pain was significantly lower in this cohort than the yield of colonoscopy performed for other symptoms such as rectal bleeding and/or iron deficiency anemia [111].

2.5.3. Chronic constipation

Chronic constipation, as defined by the Rome III criteria [112], is reported to be associated with an increased risk of colon cancer in retrospective studies from the United States [113, 114], Australia [115], and Japan [116]. In contrast, no such association was found in several other studies [117-119]. Interestingly, the yield of colon cancer in colonoscopy performed for constipation alone was lower than in colonoscopy performed for routine colorectal cancer screening [120]. Patients with chronic constipation who present with alarming symptoms such as rectal bleeding, melena, iron-deficiency anemia, unintentional weight loss, or are >50 years should be evaluated with a colonoscopy to identify the etiology of the obstruction, such as cancer, stricture, or extrinsic compression. Colonoscopy can be used to treat chronic constipation based on the etiology. In patients who have undergone prior abdominal surgery, have inflammatory bowel disease, or are prone to ischemia, colonoscopy is used to dilate fibrotic strictures that lead to constipation [121-123]. Patients suffering from chronic constipation due to neurogenic bowel or acute colonic pseudo-obstruction also benefit from a percutaneous endoscopic colostomy [124]. Importantly, chronic constipation as a procedural indication for colonoscopy is independently associated with poor colon preparation requiring a rigorous amount of laxative(s) or a longer duration of preparation [125, 126].

2.5.4. Preoperative and intraoperative localization of colonic lesions

Colonic lesions, depending on the size and consistency, may pose some difficulty in localization by surgeons during the surgical procedure, and this could be even more difficult for laparoscopic surgeries than for open procedures. In such cases, localization of a mass or polyp of interest is very important. Preoperative colonoscopy to localize the lesion using penetrating India ink, Spot, or indocyanine green is becoming a common practice [127, 128]. The dye migrates to the peritoneal surface and allows for accurate localization. An alternative colonoscopic method of applying clips around the area of interest has also been studied, which requires intraoperative ultrasound to precisely locate the site. Both methods have their own advantages and disadvantages, such as inflammatory reaction to the dye, micro-abscesses, broad spreading of the dye in the field in smaller lesions, migration of the metallic clips, false localization, or inadvertent injection of dye in the adjacent vital structures. A recent review reported that the accuracy of endoscopic tattooing is 70-100% and the incidence of intraoperative invisible lesions is 1.6-15% [129]. The complications reviewed were mostly related to transmural injection and the spillage rates varied from 2.4 to 13% and were asymptomatic. Intraoperative colonoscopy can also be performed to localize the site of a tumor or a polypectomy site. However, intraoperative colonoscopy is an understudied field and has reported problems with insufflated air in the colon which interferes with the surgical technique.

3. Contraindications for colonoscopy (table 2)

A patient who is either unwilling to give informed consent, or has given informed consent but is uncooperative and/or unable to achieve adequate sedation for colonoscopy, should not undergo colonoscopy. Colonoscopy is also contraindicated for known or suspected colonic perforation. Medical conditions associated with a high risk of perforation such as severe toxic megacolon and fulminant colitis are considered contraindications to colonoscopy. Although not strictly contraindicated, severe IBD with deep ulceration in the rectum/distal sigmoid colon and acute diverticulitis increase the risk of colonic perforation. The risk factors for colonic perforation during colonoscopy are age > 65, low body mass index, female gender, hypoalbuminemia, inpatient status, critically ill condition, multiple morbidities, IBD, and other forms of colitis such as ischemic colitis, colonic stricture dilation, polypectomy, foreign body removal, and hemostasis such as cautery [130-132].

Patients who are or are suspected of becoming hemodynamically unstable should be medically stabilized before colonoscopy. In patients who have had a myocardial infarction, a colonoscopy performed in the first 3 weeks following the infarction can provoke an arrhythmia although the only reported complications during colonoscopy in the 30 days following an myocardial infarction are hypotension and bradycardia [133]. Adequate bowel preparation is necessary because inadequate or poor bowel preparation increases colonoscopy duration with an increase in complications as well as an increase in the number of missed adenomas and high-risk lesions [134].

Contraindications for colonoscopy:
1. Patient refusal
2. Uncooperative patients
3. Inadequate sedation
4. Known or suspected colonic perforation
5. Severe toxic megacolon and fulminant colitis
6. Clinically unstable patients
7. Recent myocardial infarction
8. Inadequate bowel preparation
9. Peritonism

Table 2. Contraindications for colonoscopy

Patients with severe abdominal pain and peritoneal signs may be at risk for possible complete obstruction or gangrenous bowel and should be evaluated by other modalities first. These patients should not undergo colonoscopy due to the risk of bowel perforation from air insufflation of a distended bowel [135]. Colonoscopic decompression of cecal volvulus, though reported, has a high failure rate. Therefore, cecal volvulus should be managed surgically [94]. Failure of endoscopic bowel detorsion, or colonic volvulus with bowel perforation, bowel infarction, or peritonitis are indications for emergent surgery [135].

Author details

Jigar Bhagatwala, Arpit Singhal, Summer Aldrugh, Muhammed Sherid, Humberto Sifuentes and Subbaramiah Sridhar*

*Address all correspondence to: jbhagatwala@gru.edu

Georgia Regents University, Augusta, GA, USA

References

[1] Wolff WI. Colonoscopy: history and development. *Am J Gastroenterol.* 1989;84(9): 1017-25. PubMed PMID: 2672788.

[2] Telford JJ. Inappropriate uses of colonoscopy. *Gastroenterol Hepatol.* 2012;8(5):342-4. PubMed PMID: 22933868; PubMed Central PMCID: PMC3424432.

[3] Committee ASoP, Pasha SF, Shergill A, Acosta RD, Chandrasekhara V, Chathadi KV, et al. The role of endoscopy in the patient with lower GI bleeding. *Gastrointest Endosc.* 2014;79(6):875-85. doi: 10.1016/j.gie.2013.10.039. PubMed PMID: 24703084.

[4] Committee ASoP, Early DS, Ben-Menachem T, Decker GA, Evans JA, Fanelli RD, et al. Appropriate use of GI endoscopy. *Gastrointest Endosc.* 2012;75(6):1127-31. doi: 10.1016/j.gie.2012.01.011. PubMed PMID: 22624807.

[5] Peytremann-Bridevaux I, Arditi C, Froehlich F, O'Malley J, Fairclough P, Le Moine O, et al. Appropriateness of colonoscopy in Europe (EPAGE II). Iron-deficiency anemia and hematochezia. *Endoscopy.* 2009;41(3):227-33. doi: 10.1055/s-0028-1119644. PubMed PMID: 19280534.

[6] Talley NJ, Jones M. Self-reported rectal bleeding in a United States community: prevalence, risk factors, and health care seeking. *Am J Gastroenterol.* 1998;93(11):2179-83. doi: 10.1111/j.1572-0241.1998.00530.x. PubMed PMID: 9820393.

[7] Caos A, Benner KG, Manier J, McCarthy DM, Blessing LD, Katon RM, et al. Colonoscopy after Golytely preparation in acute rectal bleeding. *J Clin Gastroenterol*. 1986;8(1):46-9. PubMed PMID: 3486210.

[8] Tedesco FJ, Waye JD, Raskin JB, Morris SJ, Greenwald RA. Colonoscopic evaluation of rectal bleeding: a study of 304 patients. *Ann Intern Med*. 1978;89(6):907-9. PubMed PMID: 309745.

[9] Irvine EJ, O'Connor J, Frost RA, Shorvon P, Somers S, Stevenson GW, et al. Prospective comparison of double contrast barium enema plus flexible sigmoidoscopy v colonoscopy in rectal bleeding: barium enema v colonoscopy in rectal bleeding. *Gut*. 1988;29(9):1188-93. PubMed PMID: 3273756; PubMed Central PMCID: PMC1434375.

[10] Jensen DM, Machicado GA, Jutabha R, Kovacs TO. Urgent colonoscopy for the diagnosis and treatment of severe diverticular hemorrhage. *N Eng J Med*. 2000;342(2): 78-82. doi: 10.1056/NEJM200001133420202. PubMed PMID: 10631275.

[11] Bloomfeld RS, Rockey DC, Shetzline MA. Endoscopic therapy of acute diverticular hemorrhage. *Am J Gastroenterol*. 2001;96(8):2367-72. doi: 10.1111/j. 1572-0241.2001.04048.x. PubMed PMID: 11513176.

[12] Angtuaco TL, Reddy SK, Drapkin S, Harrell LE, Howden CW. The utility of urgent colonoscopy in the evaluation of acute lower gastrointestinal tract bleeding: a 2-year experience from a single center. *Am J Gastroenterol*. 2001;96(6):1782-5. doi: 10.1111/j. 1572-0241.2001.03871.x. PubMed PMID: 11419829.

[13] Whitlow CB. Endoscopic treatment for lower gastrointestinal bleeding. Clinic Colon Rect Surg. 2010;23(1):31-6. doi: 10.1055/s-0030-1247855. PubMed PMID: 21286288; PubMed Central PMCID: PMC2850164.

[14] Hwang JH, Fisher DA, Ben-Menachem T, Chandrasekhara V, Chathadi K, Decker GA, et al. The role of endoscopy in the management of acute non-variceal upper GI bleeding. *Gastrointest Endosc*. 2012;75(6):1132-8. doi: 10.1016/j.gie.2012.02.033. PubMed PMID: 22624808.

[15] Espey DK, Wu XC, Swan J, Wiggins C, Jim MA, Ward E, et al. Annual report to the nation on the status of cancer, 1975-2004, featuring cancer in American Indians and Alaska Natives. *Cancer*. 2007;110(10):2119-52. doi: 10.1002/cncr.23044. PubMed PMID: 17939129.

[16] Rex DK, Johnson DA, Anderson JC, Schoenfeld PS, Burke CA, Inadomi JM, et al. American College of Gastroenterology guidelines for colorectal cancer screening 2009 [corrected]. *Am J Gastroenterol*. 2009;104(3):739-50. doi: 10.1038/ajg.2009.104. PubMed PMID: 19240699.

[17] Sung JJ, Ng SC, Chan FK, Chiu HM, Kim HS, Matsuda T, et al. An updated Asia Pacific Consensus Recommendations on colorectal cancer screening. *Gut*. 2015;64(1): 121-32. doi: 10.1136/gutjnl-2013-306503. PubMed PMID: 24647008.

[18] Frazier AL, Colditz GA, Fuchs CS, Kuntz KM. Cost-effectiveness of screening for colorectal cancer in the general population. *Jama*. 2000;284(15):1954-61. PubMed PMID: 11035892.

[19] Vijan S, Hwang EW, Hofer TP, Hayward RA. Which colon cancer screening test? A comparison of costs, effectiveness, and compliance. *Am J Med*. 2001;111(8):593-601. PubMed PMID: 11755501.

[20] Thiis-Evensen E, Hoff GS, Sauar J, Majak BM, Vatn MH. Flexible sigmoidoscopy or colonoscopy as a screening modality for colorectal adenomas in older age groups? Findings in a cohort of the normal population aged 63-72 years. *Gut*. 1999;45(6):834-9. PubMed PMID: 10562581; PubMed Central PMCID: PMC1727750.

[21] Hewitson P, Glasziou P, Irwig L, Towler B, Watson E. Screening for colorectal cancer using the faecal occult blood test, Hemoccult. *The Cochrane Database of Systematic Reviews*. 2007(1):CD001216. doi: 10.1002/14651858.CD001216.pub2. PubMed PMID: 17253456.

[22] Foutch PG, Mai H, Pardy K, DiSario JA, Manne RK, Kerr D. Flexible sigmoidoscopy may be ineffective for secondary prevention of colorectal cancer in asymptomatic, average-risk men. *Dig Dis Sci*. 1991;36(7):924-8. PubMed PMID: 2070706.

[23] Lieberman DA, Smith FW. Screening for colon malignancy with colonoscopy. *Am J Gastroenterol*. 1991;86(8):946-51. PubMed PMID: 1858758.

[24] Johns LE, Kee F, Collins BJ, Patterson CC, Houlston RS. Colorectal cancer mortality in first-degree relatives of early-onset colorectal cancer cases. *Dis Colon Rectum*. 2002;45(5):681-6. PubMed PMID: 12004220.

[25] Johns LE, Houlston RS. A systematic review and meta-analysis of familial colorectal cancer risk. *Am J Gastroenterol*. 2001;96(10):2992-3003. doi: 10.1111/j.1572-0241.2001.04677.x. PubMed PMID: 11693338.

[26] Butterworth AS, Higgins JP, Pharoah P. Relative and absolute risk of colorectal cancer for individuals with a family history: a meta-analysis. *Eur J Can*. 2006;42(2):216-27. doi: 10.1016/j.ejca.2005.09.023. PubMed PMID: 16338133.

[27] McLeod RS, Canadian Task Force on Preventive Health C. Screening strategies for colorectal cancer: a systematic review of the evidence. *Canadian J Gastroenterol = J Canadien Gastroenterol*. 2001;15(10):647-60. PubMed PMID: 11694901.

[28] Rex DK, Johnson DA, Lieberman DA, Burt RW, Sonnenberg A. Colorectal cancer prevention 2000: screening recommendations of the American College of Gastroenterology. American College of Gastroenterology. *Am J Gastroenterol*. 2000;95(4):868-77. doi: 10.1111/j.1572-0241.2000.02059.x. PubMed PMID: 10763931.

[29] Smith RA, Cokkinides V, Eyre HJ. American Cancer Society guidelines for the early detection of cancer, 2006. *CA: A Cancer Journal for Clinicians*. 2006;56(1):11-25; quiz 49-50. PubMed PMID: 16449183.

[30] Force USPST. Screening for colorectal cancer: recommendation and rationale. *Am Fam Physician*. 2002;66(12):2287-90. PubMed PMID: 12507168.

[31] Lynch HT, Smyrk T, Lynch J, Fitzgibbons R, Jr., Lanspa S, McGinn T. Update on the differential diagnosis, surveillance and management of hereditary non-polyposis colorectal cancer. *Eur J Can*. 1995;31A(7-8):1039-46. PubMed PMID: 7576988.

[32] Lieberman DA, De Garmo PL, Fleischer DE, Eisen GM, Helfand M. Patterns of endoscopy use in the United States. *Gastroenterology*. 2000;118(3):619-24. PubMed PMID: 10702214.

[33] Ladabaum U, Song K. Projected national impact of colorectal cancer screening on clinical and economic outcomes and health services demand. *Gastroenterology*. 2005;129(4):1151-62. doi: 10.1053/j.gastro.2005.07.059. PubMed PMID: 16230069.

[34] Lieberman DA, Weiss DG, Harford WV, Ahnen DJ, Provenzale D, Sontag SJ, et al. Five-year colon surveillance after screening colonoscopy. *Gastroenterology*. 2007;133(4):1077-85. doi: 10.1053/j.gastro.2007.07.006. PubMed PMID: 17698067.

[35] Leung WK, Lau JY, Suen BY, Wong GL, Chow DK, Lai LH, et al. Repeat-screening colonoscopy 5 years after normal baseline-screening colonoscopy in average-risk Chinese: a prospective study. *Am J Gastroenterol*. 2009;104(8):2028-34. doi: 10.1038/ajg. 2009.202. PubMed PMID: 19455125.

[36] Brenner H, Chang-Claude J, Seiler CM, Hoffmeister M. Long-term risk of colorectal cancer after negative colonoscopy. *J Clin Oncol*: Official journal of the American Society of Clinical Oncology. 2011;29(28):3761-7. doi: 10.1200/JCO.2011.35.9307. PubMed PMID: 21876077.

[37] Brenner H, Haug U, Arndt V, Stegmaier C, Altenhofen L, Hoffmeister M. Low risk of colorectal cancer and advanced adenomas more than 10 years after negative colonoscopy. *Gastroenterology*. 2010;138(3):870-6. doi: 10.1053/j.gastro.2009.10.054. PubMed PMID: 19909750.

[38] Miller HL, Mukherjee R, Tian J, Nagar AB. Colonoscopy surveillance after polypectomy may be extended beyond five years. *J Clin Gastroenterol*. 2010;44(8):e162-6. doi: 10.1097/MCG.0b013e3181e5cd22. PubMed PMID: 20628313.

[39] Chung SJ, Kim YS, Yang SY, Song JH, Kim D, Park MJ, et al. Five-year risk for advanced colorectal neoplasia after initial colonoscopy according to the baseline risk stratification: a prospective study in 2452 asymptomatic Koreans. *Gut*. 2011;60(11): 1537-43. doi: 10.1136/gut.2010.232876. PubMed PMID: 21427200.

[40] Brenner H, Chang-Claude J, Seiler CM, Rickert A, Hoffmeister M. Protection from colorectal cancer after colonoscopy: a population-based, case-control study. *Ann Internal Med*. 2011;154(1):22-30. doi: 10.7326/0003-4819-154-1-201101040-00004. PubMed PMID: 21200035.

[41] Rex DK, Kahi CJ, Levin B, Smith RA, Bond JH, Brooks D, et al. Guidelines for colonoscopy surveillance after cancer resection: a consensus update by the American Can-

cer Society and US Multi-Society Task Force on Colorectal Cancer. *CA: A Cancer Journal for Clinicians.* 2006;56(3):160-7; quiz 85-6. PubMed PMID: 16737948.

[42] Meyerhardt JA, Mangu PB, Flynn PJ, Korde L, Loprinzi CL, Minsky BD, et al. Follow-up care, surveillance protocol, and secondary prevention measures for survivors of colorectal cancer: American Society of Clinical Oncology clinical practice guideline endorsement. *J Clin Oncol*: Official journal of the American Society of Clinical Oncology. 2013;31(35):4465-70. doi: 10.1200/JCO.2013.50.7442. PubMed PMID: 24220554.

[43] Labianca R, Nordlinger B, Beretta GD, Brouquet A, Cervantes A, Group EGW. Primary colon cancer: ESMO Clinical Practice Guidelines for diagnosis, adjuvant treatment and follow-up. *Ann Oncology*: Official journal of the European Society for Medical Oncology/ESMO. 2010;21 Suppl 5:v70-7. doi: 10.1093/annonc/mdq168. PubMed PMID: 20555107.

[44] Glimelius B, Pahlman L, Cervantes A, Group EGW. Rectal cancer: ESMO Clinical Practice Guidelines for diagnosis, treatment and follow-up. *Ann Oncol*: Official journal of the European Society for Medical Oncology/ESMO. 2010;21 Suppl 5:v82-6. doi: 10.1093/annonc/mdq170. PubMed PMID: 20555109.

[45] Dignass A, Eliakim R, Magro F, Maaser C, Chowers Y, Geboes K, et al. Second European evidence-based consensus on the diagnosis and management of ulcerative colitis part 1: definitions and diagnosis. *J Crohn's Colitis.* 2012;6(10):965-90. doi: 10.1016/j.crohns.2012.09.003. PubMed PMID: 23040452.

[46] Van Assche G, Dignass A, Reinisch W, van der Woude CJ, Sturm A, De Vos M, et al. The second European evidence-based Consensus on the diagnosis and management of Crohn's disease: special situations. *J Crohn's Colitis.* 2010;4(1):63-101. doi: 10.1016/j.crohns.2009.09.009. PubMed PMID: 21122490.

[47] Mowat C, Cole A, Windsor A, Ahmad T, Arnott I, Driscoll R, et al. Guidelines for the management of inflammatory bowel disease in adults. *Gut.* 2011;60(5):571-607. doi: 10.1136/gut.2010.224154. PubMed PMID: 21464096.

[48] Leighton JA, Shen B, Baron TH, Adler DG, Davila R, Egan JV, et al. ASGE guideline: endoscopy in the diagnosis and treatment of inflammatory bowel disease. *Gastrointest Endosc.* 2006;63(4):558-65. doi: 10.1016/j.gie.2006.02.005. PubMed PMID: 16564852.

[49] Horsthuis K, Stokkers PC, Stoker J. Detection of inflammatory bowel disease: diagnostic performance of cross-sectional imaging modalities. *Abdom Imaging.* 2008;33(4):407-16. doi: 10.1007/s00261-007-9276-3. PubMed PMID: 17619923; PubMed Central PMCID: PMC2386533.

[50] Marshall JK, Cawdron R, Zealley I, Riddell RH, Somers S, Irvine EJ. Prospective comparison of small bowel meal with pneumocolon versus ileo-colonoscopy for the diagnosis of ileal Crohn's disease. *Am J Gastroenterol.* 2004;99(7):1321-9. doi: 10.1111/j.1572-0241.2004.30499.x. PubMed PMID: 15233672.

[51]   Richards ME, Rickert RR, Nance FC. Crohn's disease-associated carcinoma. A poorly recognized complication of inflammatory bowel disease. *Ann Surg.* 1989;209(6): 764-73. PubMed PMID: 2543338; PubMed Central PMCID: PMC1494126.

[52]   Ekbom A, Helmick C, Zack M, Adami HO. Increased risk of large-bowel cancer in Crohn's disease with colonic involvement. *Lancet.* 1990;336(8711):357-9. PubMed PMID: 1975343.

[53]   Farraye FA, Odze RD, Eaden J, Itzkowitz SH. AGA technical review on the diagnosis and management of colorectal neoplasia in inflammatory bowel disease. *Gastroenterology.* 2010;138(2):746-74, 74 e1-4; quiz e12-3. doi: 10.1053/j.gastro.2009.12.035. PubMed PMID: 20141809.

[54]   Friedman S, Rubin PH, Bodian C, Goldstein E, Harpaz N, Present DH. Screening and surveillance colonoscopy in chronic Crohn's colitis. *Gastroenterology.* 2001;120(4): 820-6. PubMed PMID: 11231935.

[55]   Maykel JA, Hagerman G, Mellgren AF, Li SY, Alavi K, Baxter NN, et al. Crohn's colitis: the incidence of dysplasia and adenocarcinoma in surgical patients. *Dis Colon Rectum.* 2006;49(7):950-7. doi: 10.1007/s10350-006-0555-9. PubMed PMID: 16729218.

[56]   Jess T, Loftus EV, Jr., Velayos FS, Harmsen WS, Zinsmeister AR, Smyrk TC, et al. Risk of intestinal cancer in inflammatory bowel disease: a population-based study from olmsted county, Minnesota. *Gastroenterology.* 2006;130(4):1039-46. doi: 10.1053/ j.gastro.2005.12.037. PubMed PMID: 16618397.

[57]   Karlen P, Kornfeld D, Brostrom O, Lofberg R, Persson PG, Ekbom A. Is colonoscopic surveillance reducing colorectal cancer mortality in ulcerative colitis? A population based case control study. *Gut.* 1998;42(5):711-4. PubMed PMID: 9659169; PubMed Central PMCID: PMC1727094.

[58]   Lutgens MW, Oldenburg B, Siersema PD, van Bodegraven AA, Dijkstra G, Hommes DW, et al. Colonoscopic surveillance improves survival after colorectal cancer diagnosis in inflammatory bowel disease. *Brit J Can.* 2009;101(10):1671-5. doi: 10.1038/ sj.bjc.6605359. PubMed PMID: 19826420; PubMed Central PMCID: PMC2778537.

[59]   Ananthakrishnan AN, Cagan A, Cai T, Gainer VS, Shaw SY, Churchill S, et al. Colonoscopy is associated with a reduced risk for colon cancer and mortality in patients with inflammatory bowel diseases. *Clin Gastroenterol Hepatol*: Official clinical practice journal of the American Gastroenterological Association. 2014. doi: 10.1016/j.cgh. 2014.07.018. PubMed PMID: 25041865; PubMed Central PMCID: PMC4297589.

[60]   Cairns SR, Scholefield JH, Steele RJ, Dunlop MG, Thomas HJ, Evans GD, et al. Guidelines for colorectal cancer screening and surveillance in moderate and high risk groups (update from 2002). *Gut.* 2010;59(5):666-89. doi: 10.1136/gut.2009.179804. PubMed PMID: 20427401.

[61]   Van Assche G, Dignass A, Bokemeyer B, Danese S, Gionchetti P, Moser G, et al. Second European evidence-based consensus on the diagnosis and management of ulcer-

ative colitis part 3: special situations. *J Crohn's Colitis*. 2013;7(1):1-33. doi: 10.1016/j.crohns.2012.09.005. PubMed PMID: 23040453.

[62] Cancer Council Australia Colonoscopy Surveillance Working Party. Clinical practice guidelines for surveillance colonoscopy – in adenoma follow-up; following curative resection of colorectal cancer; and for cancer surveillance in inflammatory bowel disease. Sydney (Australia): Cancer Council Australia; 2011 Dec. 144 p. Available from: http://www.guideline.gov/content.aspx?id=47635.

[63] Lasson A, Kilander A, Stotzer PO. Diagnostic yield of colonoscopy based on symptoms. *Scand J Gastroenterol*. 2008;43(3):356-62. PubMed PMID: 18938663.

[64] Shah RJ, Fenoglio-Preiser C, Bleau BL, Giannella RA. Usefulness of colonoscopy with biopsy in the evaluation of patients with chronic diarrhea. *Am J Gastroenterol*. 2001;96(4):1091-5. doi: 10.1111/j.1572-0241.2001.03745.x. PubMed PMID: 11316152.

[65] Tanaka M, Mazzoleni G, Riddell RH. Distribution of collagenous colitis: utility of flexible sigmoidoscopy. *Gut*. 1992;33(1):65-70. PubMed PMID: 1740280; PubMed Central PMCID: PMC1373867.

[66] McHugh JB, Appelman HD, McKenna BJ. The diagnostic value of endoscopic terminal ileum biopsies. *Am J Gastroenterol*. 2007;102(5):1084-9. doi: 10.1111/j.1572-0241.2007.01194.x. PubMed PMID: 17391315.

[67] Kearney DJ, Steuerwald M, Koch J, Cello JP. A prospective study of endoscopy in HIV-associated diarrhea. *Am J Gastroenterol*. 1999;94(3):596-602. doi: 10.1111/j.1572-0241.1999.00920.x. PubMed PMID: 10086637.

[68] Khan K, Schwarzenberg SJ, Sharp H, Jessurun J, Gulbahce HE, Defor T, et al. Diagnostic endoscopy in children after hematopoietic stem cell transplantation. *Gastrointest Endosc*. 2006;64(3):379-85; quiz 89-92. doi: 10.1016/j.gie.2005.08.040. PubMed PMID: 16923486.

[69] Saito Y, Fukuzawa M, Matsuda T, Fukunaga S, Sakamoto T, Uraoka T, et al. Clinical outcome of endoscopic submucosal dissection versus endoscopic mucosal resection of large colorectal tumors as determined by curative resection. *Surg Endosc*. 2010;24(2):343-52. doi: 10.1007/s00464-009-0562-8. PubMed PMID: 19517168.

[70] Tajika M, Niwa Y, Bhatia V, Kondo S, Tanaka T, Mizuno N, et al. Comparison of endoscopic submucosal dissection and endoscopic mucosal resection for large colorectal tumors. *Eur J Gastroenterol Hepatol*. 2011;23(11):1042-9. doi: 10.1097/MEG.0b013e32834aa47b. PubMed PMID: 21869682.

[71] Isomoto H, Nishiyama H, Yamaguchi N, Fukuda E, Ishii H, Ikeda K, et al. Clinicopathological factors associated with clinical outcomes of endoscopic submucosal dissection for colorectal epithelial neoplasms. *Endoscopy*. 2009;41(8):679-83. doi: 10.1055/s-0029-1214979. PubMed PMID: 19670135.

[72] Yoshida N, Naito Y, Sakai K, Sumida Y, Kanemasa K, Inoue K, et al. Outcome of en-doscopic submucosal dissection for colorectal tumors in elderly people. *Int J Colorectal Dis.* 2010;25(4):455-61. doi: 10.1007/s00384-009-0841-9. PubMed PMID: 19921221.

[73] Yoshida N, Wakabayashi N, Kanemasa K, Sumida Y, Hasegawa D, Inoue K, et al. En-doscopic submucosal dissection for colorectal tumors: technical difficulties and rate of perforation. *Endoscopy.* 2009;41(9):758-61. doi: 10.1055/s-0029-1215028. PubMed PMID: 19746316.

[74] oshida N, Yagi N, Naito Y, Yoshikawa T. Safe procedure in endoscopic submucosal dissection for colorectal tumors focused on preventing complications. *World J Gastro-enterol: WJG.* 2010;16(14):1688-95. PubMed PMID: 20379999; PubMed Central PMCID: PMC2852815.

[75] Savides TJ, Jensen DM. Colonoscopic hemostasis for recurrent diverticular hemor-rhage associated with a visible vessel: a report of three cases. *Gastrointest Endosc.* 1994;40(1):70-3. PubMed PMID: 8163141.

[76] Binmoeller KF, Thonke F, Soehendra N. Endoscopic hemoclip treatment for gastroin-testinal bleeding. *Endoscopy.* 1993;25(2):167-70. doi: 10.1055/s-2007-1010277. PubMed PMID: 8491134.

[77] Santos JC, Jr., Aprilli F, Guimaraes AS, Rocha JJ. Angiodysplasia of the colon: endo-scopic diagnosis and treatment. *Brit J Surg.* 1988;75(3):256-8. PubMed PMID: 3258173.

[78] Sagar J. Colorectal stents for the management of malignant colonic obstructions. *The Cochrane Database of Systematic Reviews.* 2011(11):CD007378. doi: 10.1002/14651858.CD007378.pub2. PubMed PMID: 22071835.

[79] Frago R, Ramirez E, Millan M, Kreisler E, del Valle E, Biondo S. Current management of acute malignant large bowel obstruction: a systematic review. *Am J Surg.* 2014;207(1):127-38. doi: 10.1016/j.amjsurg.2013.07.027. PubMed PMID: 24124659.

[80] Cheung DY, Kim JY, Hong SP, Jung MK, Ye BD, Kim SG, et al. Outcome and safety of self-expandable metallic stents for malignant colon obstruction: a Korean multi-center randomized prospective study. *Surg Endosc.* 2012;26(11):3106-13. doi: 10.1007/s00464-012-2300-x. PubMed PMID: 22609981.

[81] Varadarajulu S, Roy A, Lopes T, Drelichman ER, Kim M. Endoscopic stenting versus surgical colostomy for the management of malignant colonic obstruction: compari-son of hospital costs and clinical outcomes. *Surg Endosc.* 2011;25(7):2203-9. doi: 10.1007/s00464-010-1523-y. PubMed PMID: 21293882; PubMed Central PMCID: PMC3116133.

[82] Kavanagh DO, Nolan B, Judge C, Hyland JM, Mulcahy HE, O'Connell PR, et al. A comparative study of short- and medium-term outcomes comparing emergent sur-gery and stenting as a bridge to surgery in patients with acute malignant colonic ob-

struction. *Dis Colon Rectum*. 2013;56(4):433-40. doi: 10.1097/DCR.0b013e3182760506. PubMed PMID: 23478610.

[83] van Hooft JE, Bemelman WA, Oldenburg B, Marinelli AW, Lutke Holzik MF, Grubben MJ, et al. Colonic stenting versus emergency surgery for acute left-sided malignant colonic obstruction: a multicentre randomised trial. *Lancet Oncol*. 2011;12(4): 344-52. doi: 10.1016/S1470-2045(11)70035-3. PubMed PMID: 21398178.

[84] Gevers AM, Macken E, Hiele M, Rutgeerts P. Endoscopic laser therapy for palliation of patients with distal colorectal carcinoma: analysis of factors influencing long-term outcome. *Gastrointest Endosc*. 2000;51(5):580-5. PubMed PMID: 10805846.

[85] Solecki R, Zajac A, Richter P, Szura M. Bifocal esophageal and rectal cancer palliatively treated with argon plasma coagulation. *Surgical Endosc*. 2004;18(2):346. doi: 10.1007/s00464-003-4232-y. PubMed PMID: 15106621.

[86] Baumhoer D, Armbrust T, Ramadori G. Nonsurgical treatment of the primary tumor in four consecutive cases of metastasized colorectal carcinoma. *Endoscopy*. 2005;37(12):1232-6. doi: 10.1055/s-2005-870225. PubMed PMID: 16329023.

[87] Saunders MD. Acute colonic pseudo-obstruction. *Best Pract Res Clin Gastroenterol*. 2007;21(4):671-87. doi: 10.1016/j.bpg.2007.03.001. PubMed PMID: 17643908.

[88] Tsirline VB, Zemlyak AY, Avery MJ, Colavita PD, Christmas AB, Heniford BT, et al. Colonoscopy is superior to neostigmine in the treatment of Ogilvie's syndrome. *Am J Surg*. 2012;204(6):849-55; discussion 55. doi: 10.1016/j.amjsurg.2012.05.006. PubMed PMID: 23021196.

[89] Renzulli P, Maurer CA, Netzer P, Buchler MW. Preoperative colonoscopic derotation is beneficial in acute colonic volvulus. *Dig Surg*. 2002;19(3):223-9. PubMed PMID: 12119526.

[90] Swenson BR, Kwaan MR, Burkart NE, Wang Y, Madoff RD, Rothenberger DA, et al. Colonic volvulus: presentation and management in metropolitan Minnesota, United States. *Dis Colon Rectum*. 2012;55(4):444-9. doi: 10.1097/DCR.0b013e3182404b3d. PubMed PMID: 22426269.

[91] Halabi WJ, Jafari MD, Kang CY, Nguyen VQ, Carmichael JC, Mills S, et al. Colonic volvulus in the United States: trends, outcomes, and predictors of mortality. *Ann Surg*. 2014;259(2):293-301. doi: 10.1097/SLA.0b013e31828c88ac. PubMed PMID: 23511842.

[92] Oren D, Atamanalp SS, Aydinli B, Yildirgan MI, Basoglu M, Polat KY, et al. An algorithm for the management of sigmoid colon volvulus and the safety of primary resection: experience with 827 cases. *Dis Colon Rectum*. 2007;50(4):489-97. doi: 10.1007/s10350-006-0821-x. PubMed PMID: 17205203.

[93] Ballantyne GH. Review of sigmoid volvulus: history and results of treatment. *Dis Colon Rectum*. 1982;25(5):494-501. PubMed PMID: 7047106.

[94]   Madiba TE, Thomson SR. The management of cecal volvulus. *Dis Colon Rectum.* 2002;45(2):264-7. PubMed PMID: 11852342.

[95]   Hassan C, Zullo A, De Francesco V, Ierardi E, Giustini M, Pitidis A, et al. Systematic review: Endoscopic dilatation in Crohn's disease. *Alim Pharmacol Therapeut.* 2007;26(11-12):1457-64. doi: 10.1111/j.1365-2036.2007.03532.x. PubMed PMID: 17903236.

[96]   Ramboer C, Verhamme M, Dhondt E, Huys S, Van Eygen K, Vermeire L. Endoscopic treatment of stenosis in recurrent Crohn's disease with balloon dilation combined with local corticosteroid injection. *Gastrointest Endosc.* 1995;42(3):252-5. PubMed PMID: 7498692.

[97]   Lucha PA, Jr., Fticsar JE, Francis MJ. The strictured anastomosis: successful treatment by corticosteroid injections – report of three cases and review of the literature. *Dis Colon Rectum.* 2005;48(4):862-5. doi: 10.1007/s10350-004-0838-y. PubMed PMID: 15747075.

[98]   East JE, Brooker JC, Rutter MD, Saunders BP. A pilot study of intrastricture steroid versus placebo injection after balloon dilatation of Crohn's strictures. *Clin Gastroenterol Hepatol*: The official clinical practice journal of the American Gastroenterological Association. 2007;5(9):1065-9. doi: 10.1016/j.cgh.2007.04.013. PubMed PMID: 17627903.

[99]   Brooker JC, Beckett CG, Saunders BP, Benson MJ. Long-acting steroid injection after endoscopic dilation of anastomotic Crohn's strictures may improve the outcome: a retrospective case series. *Endoscopy.* 2003;35(4):333-7. doi: 10.1055/s-2003-38145. PubMed PMID: 12664391.

[100] Brandimarte G, Tursi A, Gasbarrini G. Endoscopic treatment of benign anastomotic colorectal stenosis with electrocautery. *Endoscopy.* 2000;32(6):461-3. doi: 10.1055/s-2000-651. PubMed PMID: 10863912.

[101] Hagiwara A, Togawa T, Yamasaki J, Shirasu M, Sakakura C, Yamagishi H. Endoscopic incision and balloon dilatation for cicatricial anastomotic strictures. *Hepatogastroenterology.* 1999;46(26):997-9. PubMed PMID: 10370654.

[102] Koornstra JJ, Weersma RK. Management of rectal foreign bodies: description of a new technique and clinical practice guidelines. World journal of gastroenterology : WJG. 2008;14(27):4403-6. PubMed PMID: 18666334; PubMed Central PMCID: PMC2731197.

[103] Goldberg JE, Steele SR. Rectal foreign bodies. *Surg Clin N Am.* 2010;90(1):173-84, Table of Contents. doi: 10.1016/j.suc.2009.10.004. PubMed PMID: 20109641.

[104] Singaporewalla RM, Tan DE, Tan TK. Use of endoscopic snare to extract a large rectosigmoid foreign body with review of literature. *Surgical Laparosc, Endosc Percut Tech.* 2007;17(2):145-8. doi: 10.1097/SLE.0b013e318045bf1a. PubMed PMID: 17450100.

[105] Humes D, Lobo DN. Removal of a rectal foreign body by using a Foley catheter passed through a rigid sigmoidoscope. *Gastrointestinal Endosc.* 2005;62(4):610. PubMed PMID: 16185979.

[106] Billi P, Bassi M, Ferrara F, Biscardi A, Villani S, Baldoni F, et al. Endoscopic removal of a large rectal foreign body using a large balloon dilator: report of a case and description of the technique. *Endoscopy.* 2010;42 Suppl 2:E238. doi: 10.1055/s-0030-1255573. PubMed PMID: 20931459.

[107] Rex DK, Lieberman D, Acg. ACG colorectal cancer prevention action plan: update on CT-colonography. *Am Journal of Gastroenterol.* 2006;101(7):1410-3. doi: 10.1111/j.1572-0241.2006.00585.x. PubMed PMID: 16863539.

[108] Rockey DC, Barish M, Brill JV, Cash BD, Fletcher JG, Sharma P, et al. Standards for gastroenterologists for performing and interpreting diagnostic computed tomographic colonography. *Gastroenterology.* 2007;133(3):1005-24. doi: 10.1053/j.gastro.2007.06.001. PubMed PMID: 17678924.

[109] Zalis ME, Barish MA, Choi JR, Dachman AH, Fenlon HM, Ferrucci JT, et al. CT colonography reporting and data system: a consensus proposal. *Radiology.* 2005;236(1):3-9. doi: 10.1148/radiol.2361041926. PubMed PMID: 15987959.

[110] Neugut AI, Garbowski GC, Waye JD, Forde KA, Treat MR, Tsai JL, et al. Diagnostic yield of colorectal neoplasia with colonoscopy for abdominal pain, change in bowel habits, and rectal bleeding. *Am J Gastroenterol.* 1993;88(8):1179-83. PubMed PMID: 8338084.

[111] Kueh SH, Zhou L, Walmsley RS. The diagnostic yield of colonoscopy in patients with isolated abdominal pain. *N Zea Med J.* 2013;126(1382):36-44. PubMed PMID: 24154768.

[112] Longstreth GF, Thompson WG, Chey WD, Houghton LA, Mearin F, Spiller RC. Functional bowel disorders. *Gastroenterology.* 2006;130(5):1480-91. doi: 10.1053/j.gastro.2005.11.061. PubMed PMID: 16678561.

[113] Roberts MC, Millikan RC, Galanko JA, Martin C, Sandler RS. Constipation, laxative use, and colon cancer in a North Carolina population. *Am J Gastroenterol.* 2003;98(4):857-64. doi: 10.1111/j.1572-0241.2003.07386.x. PubMed PMID: 12738468.

[114] Jacobs EJ, White E. Constipation, laxative use, and colon cancer among middle-aged adults. *Epidemiology.* 1998;9(4):385-91. PubMed PMID: 9647901.

[115] Kune GA, Kune S, Field B, Watson LF. The role of chronic constipation, diarrhea, and laxative use in the etiology of large-bowel cancer. Data from the Melbourne colorectal cancer study. *Dis Colon Rectum.* 1988;31(7):507-12. PubMed PMID: 3391059.

[116] Watanabe T, Nakaya N, Kurashima K, Kuriyama S, Tsubono Y, Tsuji I. Constipation, laxative use and risk of colorectal cancer: The Miyagi Cohort Study. *Eur J Can.* 2004;40(14):2109-15. doi: 10.1016/j.ejca.2004.06.014. PubMed PMID: 15341986.

[117] Dukas L, Willett WC, Colditz GA, Fuchs CS, Rosner B, Giovannucci EL. Prospective study of bowel movement, laxative use, and risk of colorectal cancer among women. *Am J Epidemiol*. 2000;151(10):958-64. PubMed PMID: 10853634.

[118] Anderson JC, Lacy BE. Editorial: Constipation and colorectal cancer risk: a continuing conundrum. *Am J Gastroenterol*. 2014;109(10):1650-2. doi: 10.1038/ajg.2014.292. PubMed PMID: 25287089.

[119] Power AM, Talley NJ, Ford AC. Association between constipation and colorectal cancer: systematic review and meta-analysis of observational studies. *Am J Gastroenterol*. 2013;108(6):894-903; quiz 4. doi: 10.1038/ajg.2013.52. PubMed PMID: 23481143.

[120] Obusez EC, Lian L, Kariv R, Burke CA, Shen B. Diagnostic yield of colonoscopy for constipation as the sole indication. *Colorect Dis*: The official journal of the Association of Coloproctology of Great Britain and Ireland. 2012;14(5):585-91. doi: 10.1111/j.1463-1318.2011.02664.x. PubMed PMID: 21689337.

[121] Virgilio C, Cosentino S, Favara C, Russo V, Russo A. Endoscopic treatment of postoperative colonic strictures using an achalasia dilator: short-term and long-term results. *Endoscopy*. 1995;27(3):219-22. doi: 10.1055/s-2007-1005674. PubMed PMID: 7664698.

[122] Sabate JM, Villarejo J, Bouhnik Y, Allez M, Gornet JM, Vahedi K, et al. Hydrostatic balloon dilatation of Crohn's strictures. *Alim Pharmacol Therapeut*. 2003;18(4):409-13. PubMed PMID: 12940926.

[123] Morini S, Hassan C, Lorenzetti R, Zullo A, Cerro P, Winn S, et al. Long-term outcome of endoscopic pneumatic dilatation in Crohn's disease. *Dig Liver Dis*: Official journal of the Italian Society of Gastroenterology and the Italian Association for the Study of the Liver. 2003;35(12):893-7. PubMed PMID: 14703886.

[124] Ramage JI, Jr., Baron TH. Percutaneous endoscopic cecostomy: a case series. *Gastrointest Endosc*. 2003;57(6):752-5. doi: 10.1067/mge.2003.197. PubMed PMID: 12709715.

[125] Ness RM, Manam R, Hoen H, Chalasani N. Predictors of inadequate bowel preparation for colonoscopy. Am J Gastroenterol. 2001;96(6):1797-802. doi: 10.1111/j.1572-0241.2001.03874.x. PubMed PMID: 11419832.

[126] Van Dongen M. Enhancing bowel preparation for colonoscopy: an integrative review. *Gastroenterol Nurs*: The official journal of the Society of Gastroenterology Nurses and Associates. 2012;35(1):36-44. doi: 10.1097/SGA.0b013e3182403413. PubMed PMID: 22306728.

[127] Committee AT, Kethu SR, Banerjee S, Desilets D, Diehl DL, Farraye FA, et al. Endoscopic tattooing. *Gastrointest Endosc*. 2010;72(4):681-5. doi: 10.1016/j.gie.2010.06.020. PubMed PMID: 20883844.

[128] Park JW, Sohn DK, Hong CW, Han KS, Choi DH, Chang HJ, et al. The usefulness of preoperative colonoscopic tattooing using a saline test injection method with pre-

packaged sterile India ink for localization in laparoscopic colorectal surgery. *Surg Endosc*. 2008;22(2):501-5. doi: 10.1007/s00464-007-9495-2. PubMed PMID: 17704874.

[129] Trakarnsanga A, Akaraviputh T. Endoscopic tattooing of colorectal lesions: Is it a risk-free procedure? *World J Gastrointest Endosc*. 2011;3(12):256-60. doi: 10.4253/wjge.v3.i12.256. PubMed PMID: 22195235; PubMed Central PMCID: PMC3244942.

[130] Hamdani U, Naeem R, Haider F, Bansal P, Komar M, Diehl DL, et al. Risk factors for colonoscopic perforation: a population-based study of 80118 cases. *World J Gastroenterol: WJG*. 2013;19(23):3596-601. doi: 10.3748/wjg.v19.i23.3596. PubMed PMID: 23801860; PubMed Central PMCID: PMC3691036.

[131] Polter DE. Risk of colon perforation during colonoscopy at Baylor University Medical Center. *Proceedings*. 2015;28(1):3-6. PubMed PMID: 25552784; PubMed Central PMCID: PMC4264696.

[132] Rex DK, Petrini JL, Baron TH, Chak A, Cohen J, Deal SE, et al. Quality indicators for colonoscopy. *Am J Gastroenterol*. 2006;101(4):873-85. doi: 10.1111/j.1572-0241.2006.00673.x. PubMed PMID: 16635231.

[133] Cappell MS. Safety and efficacy of colonoscopy after myocardial infarction: an analysis of 100 study patients and 100 control patients at two tertiary cardiac referral hospitals. *Gastrointest Endosc*. 2004;60(6):901-9. PubMed PMID: 15605004.

[134] Chokshi RV, Hovis CE, Hollander T, Early DS, Wang JS. Prevalence of missed adenomas in patients with inadequate bowel preparation on screening colonoscopy. *Gastrointest Endosc*. 2012;75(6):1197-203. doi: 10.1016/j.gie.2012.01.005. PubMed PMID: 22381531.

[135] Committee ASoP, Harrison ME, Anderson MA, Appalaneni V, Banerjee S, Ben-Menachem T, et al. The role of endoscopy in the management of patients with known and suspected colonic obstruction and pseudo-obstruction. Gastrointest Endosc. 2010;71(4):669-79. doi: 10.1016/j.gie.2009.11.027. PubMed PMID: 20363408.

2

Acquired and Intrinsic Resistance to Colorectal Cancer Treatment

Romina Briffa, Simon P. Langdon,
Godfrey Grech and David J. Harrison

Abstract

First line therapy for colorectal cancer (CRC) is usually fluoropyrimidine monotherapy and oxaliplatin, or irinotecan-based therapy. Additionally, targeted therapies such as bevacizumab, aflibercept, ramucirumab, regorafenib, cetuximab and panitumumab are indicated in combination with chemotherapy in metastatic CRC. Resistance of CRC to treatment is the principal rationale for treatment failure. Resistance can be intrinsic (primary resistance) or acquired (secondary resistance). Here, we discuss the classical model of resistance, which focuses primarily on mechanisms involving alterations in drug metabolism, increased drug efflux, secondary mutations in drug targets, inactivation of apoptotic pathways, p53 and DNA damage repair. Other resistance mechanisms, including the Warburg effect, cancer stem cells, intra-tumor heterogeneity and pharmacoepigenomic mechanisms will also be discussed. We conclude the chapter with a systems medicine approach to predict response to treatment for the discovery and validation of predictive biomarkers that are urgently needed.

Keywords: colorectal cancer, chemotherapy, targeted therapy, intrinsic resistance, acquired resistance, predictive biomarkers

1. Introduction

The mainstay of colorectal cancer (CRC) treatment is curative surgery, although in some cases patients are administered neo-adjuvant therapy. Surgery is usually followed by adjuvant therapy in patients presenting with Stage III and Stage IV disease. Additionally, adjuvant therapy is sometimes administered to high risk stratified Stage II patients. Adjuvant treatment for stage III CRC patients consists of chemotherapy including 5-fluorouracil (5-FU), oxaliplatin and capecitabine—usually administered combination therapy [1]. Patients having advanced CRC are frequently treated with targeted therapy in combination with chemotherapy, or as a single agent, and more recently with immunotherapy (**Table 1**). The rationale for using combination therapy is to avoid treatment resistance, promote a synergistic effect and reduce potential toxicity (refer to **Table 2**).

Therapeutic agent	Class	Colorectal cancer indications	Date of first launch worldwide [1–6]
5-Fluorouracil (5-FU)	Antimetabolite, pyrimidine analogue	Used as a single agent or in combination	1962
Epirubicin	Cytotoxic antibiotics	Used as a single agent or in combination	1984
Irinotecan	Topoisomerase I inhibitor	1. Indicated for the treatment of mCRC: • in combination with 5-FU and folinic acid in chemotherapy naïve patients • as a single agent in patients who have failed a 5-FU-based regimen 2. In combination with cetuximab is indicated for the treatment of patients with EGFR-expressing KRAS wild-type mCRC, who had not received prior treatment for metastatic disease or after failure of irinotecan-including cytotoxic therapy 3. In combination with 5-FU, folinic acid and bevacizumab is indicated for first-line treatment of patients with mCRC 4. In combination with capecitabine with or without bevacizumab is indicated for first-line treatment of patients with mCRC	1994
Oxaliplatin	Platinum derivative, alkylating agent	Oxaliplatin in combination with 5-FU and folinic acid is indicated for: 1. adjuvant treatment of stage III colon cancer after complete resection of primary tumor 2. treatment of mCRC	1996
Raltitrexed	Antimetabolite	Palliative treatment of advanced colorectal cancer where 5-FU and folinic acid-based regimens are either not tolerated or inappropriate	1996
Capecitabine	Antimetabolite	1. Used as a single agent or in combination 2. Used for the adjuvant treatment of stage III colon cancer patients 3. Used in mCRC	1998
Cetuximab	Monoclonal antibody, EGFR inhibitor	Indicated for the treatment of patients with EGFR-expressing, RAS wt mCRC: • in combination with irinotecan-based chemotherapy • in first-line in combination with FOLFOX • as a single agent in patients who have failed oxaliplatin- and irinotecan-based therapy and who are intolerant to irinotecan	2003

Therapeutic agent	Class	Colorectal cancer indications	Date of first launch worldwide [1–6]
Bevacizumab	Monoclonal antibody, VEGF inhibitor	In combination with fluoropyrimidine-based chemotherapy is indicated for treatment of mCRC	2004
Panitumumab	Monoclonal antibody, EGFR inhibitor	Indicated for the treatment of wt *RAS* mCRC: 1. first-line in combination with FOLFOX or FOLFIRI 2. second-line in combination with FOLFIRI for patients who have received first-line fluoropyrimidine-based chemotherapy (excluding irinotecan) 3. monotherapy after failure of fluoropyrimidine-, oxaliplatin-, and irinotecan-containing chemotherapy regimens	2006
Regorafenib	Angiogenesis inhibitor, tyrosine kinase inhibitor	mCRC patients who have been previously treated with, or are not considered candidates for available therapies	2013
Aflibercept	Angiogenesis inhibitor, tyrosine kinase inhibitor	In combination with FOLFIRI is indicated in mCRC that is resistant to or has progressed after an oxaliplatin-containing regimen	2013
Trifluridine/ tipiracil hydrochloride	Antimetabolite	Treatment of mCRC patients who have been previously treated with, or are not considered candidates for available therapies	2015
Pembrolizumab	Anti-PD1 immunotherapy	Unresectable or metastatic, MSI-H or dMMR CRC that has progressed following treatment with a fluoropyrimidine, oxaliplatin, and irinotecan	2017

Table 1. Colorectal cancer drugs currently on the market.

Combination regimens	Therapeutic agents
deGramont/modified de Gramont	5-Fluorouracil, folinic acid
FOLFIRINOX	Folinic acid, 5-fluorouracil, irinotecan, oxaliplatin
FOLFIRI	Folinic acid, 5-fluorouracil, irinotecan
FOLFOX	Folinic acid, 5-fluorouracil, oxaliplatin
XELOX	Oxaliplatin, capecitabine
FOLFIRI + cetuximab	Folinic acid, 5-fluorouracil, irinotecan, cetuximab
FOLFOX + cetuximab	Folinic acid, 5-fluorouracil, oxaliplatin, cetuximab
FOLFIRI + panitumumab	Folinic acid, 5-fluorouracil, irinotecan, panitumumab
FOLFOX + panitumumab	Folinic acid, 5-fluorouracil, oxaliplatin, panitumumab
FOLFIRI + aflibercept	Folinic acid, 5-fluorouracil, irinotecan, aflibercept
FOLFIRI + bevacizumab	Folinic acid, 5-fluorouracil, irinotecan, bevacizumab

Table 2. Drug combinations to treat colorectal cancer.

Patients' responses to treatment are limited, and in fact less than one-third of patients respond to 5-fluorouracil as a single agent [2, 3]. However, when used in combination, for instance, with oxaliplatin-based therapy, 50% response rate is obtained [4]. Resistance to 5-fluorouracil can be due to loss of SMAD4 [5], thymidylate synthase (TYMS) amplification [6], defective mismatch repair (MMR) genes [7], high level expression of thymidylate synthase (TS) [8], increased DPD activity [9], microsatellite instability [9], modulation of the Bcl2 family members [10], cell cycle perturbation [11], decreased ATP synthase [12] and adaptation to oxidative stress [13]. General mechanisms attributed to oxaliplatin resistance include cellular transport, detoxification, DNA repair, cell death, epigenetic alteration and NF-κβ signaling pathway [14].

Although, the use of cetuximab and panitumumab in combination with other agents is very effective, they are not sufficiently potent as single agents and are reported to work in only around 10% of cases [15]. Over the last decade, a number of papers on anti-epidermal growth factor receptor (EGFR) resistance mechanisms have been published [16–18]. Resistance mechanisms attributed to EGFR resistance include, but are not limited to, low EGFR gene copy number, low expression of AREG and EREG, EGFR S492R mutation, RAS mutation, BRAF V600E mutation, PIK3CA exon 20 mutation, PTEN loss, STAT3 phosphorylation, activated IGF1R, MET amplification, HER2 amplification, altered VEGF/VEGFR and EMT [16, 19].

Unfortunately, the lack of predictive markers would allow clinicians to select patients who are most likely to benefit from a specific therapy remains a challenge. A recent review by Wu et al. reported that in the context of metastatic cancer, approximately 90% of treatment failure is due to multi-drug resistance [20]. Currently, the only markers that predict potential toxicity to 5-FU treatment are DPD deficiency, DPYD mutation, UGT1A1 and high TS expression [21]. Moreover, the only marker that predicts lack of response to 5-FU is mismatch repair deficiency (dMMR), while pembrolizumab, dMMR predicts increase in response [7]. With respect to anti-EGFR treatment, KRAS, NRAS and BRAF mutations are the only biological markers that predict lack of response and hence pose a contraindication to treatment administration [21].

Both intrinsic resistance, which is characterized by cancer cells having only a slight or no response to treatment from the beginning, and acquired resistance that is described as, initially, having a clinical response, ensued by development of resistance will be discussed [22]. Several studies that discuss resistance to specific chemotherapeutic agents have been published and therefore we will be solely referring to salient resistance mechanisms to CRC therapies.

2. The classical model of resistance

2.1. Drug metabolism

Chemotherapeutic agents are extensively metabolized by Phase I, Phase II and Phase III enzymes. Phase I enzymes, which are mostly involved in chemical modification, include the heme protein cytochrome superfamily CYP450, which is sub-divided into 74 gene families and is involved in oxidation reactions. CYP3A is involved in irinotecan metabolism while CYP2A6, CYP2C8 and CYP1A2 are involved in tegafur activation [23].

Increased expression of dihydropyrimidine dehydrogenase (DYPD) or thymidine phosphorylase (TP) is correlated with resistance to 5-FU chemotherapy [24]. On the other hand, in a cohort of 177 CRC patients, there was a correlation between high TP expression and a better survival rate in the doxifluridine arm (p = 0.025) [25]. TP has also been reported to increase in both hypoxic and hypoglycemic environments, which will be discussed later [26]. Furthermore, polymorphic changes in DYPD account for life-threatening adverse effects in patients treated with 5-FU or its derivatives [27]. On the other hand, patients having a low expression of DYPD cannot metabolize 5-FU efficiently [28]. Decreased orotate phosphoribosyl transferase (OPRT) expression in gastric cancer is associated with resistance to 5-FU [29].

Phase II enzymes are involved in conjugation and include glutathione (GSH), glutathione-S-transferase (GSTs), uridine diphosphate glucuronosyltransferases (UGT) and NADH quinone oxidases (NQO). One of the oxaliplatin resistance mechanisms entails elevation of glutathione mediated by γ-glutamyl transpeptidase [30]. Additionally, GSTπ1 is associated with oxaliplatin and cisplatin resistance mechanisms [31]. SN-38, the active metabolite of irinotecan, is inactivated by way of glucuronidation by UGT [32]. UGT1A1 is one of the main genes involved in glucuronidation and is reported as being highly polymorphic; subsequently patients having UGT1A1*28 polymorphisms tend to suffer from increased risks of toxicity as reported in a cohort of colorectal cancer patients [33]. Both CYP450 and GSTs have been implicated in the metabolism of chemotherapeutic agents, but their predictive value is still uncertain [32].

Members of the ATP-binding cassette (ABC) superfamily are involved in Phase III drug metabolism [34] and to date 49 ABC transporters have been documented in humans [35]. The role of ABC transporters is to use energy from ATP hydrolysis to move their substrates across biological membranes and against concentration gradients, thereby limiting cellular accumulation of their substrates [36]. ABC members include P-glycoprotein (MDR1/ABCB1), breast cancer resistance protein (BCRP/ABCG2) and transporters of the multidrug resistance-associated protein (MRP/ABCC) family like the multi-drug resistance protein 5 (ABCC5), which bestows resistance to 5 FU via transporting the monophosphate metabolites in colorectal and breast cancers [37]. MDR1 is found to be highly expressed in the epithelial cells of the colon, overexpressed in a number of tumors, and has been associated with treatment failure [38]. At least 12 ABC transporters from 4 ABC sub-families have been shown to have a role in *in vitro* drug resistance (reviewed in Ref. [39]). MRP5 has been reported to confer cross-resistance to a number of anti-cancer agents including 5-FU, oxaliplatin and a number of antifolates [37]. The authors postulated that resistance might be instigated via drug efflux mechanisms which interfere with 5-FU's ability to impede both DNA and RNA synthesis. P-glycoprotein is a drug efflux pump and exerts its mode of action by lowering the intracellular concentration of a number of drugs, which subsequently leads to increased drug resistance [40]. BCRP is also involved in irinotecan efflux and is reported to be overexpressed in colon cancer, subsequently increasing chemoresistance.

2.2. Drug targets

5-FU naive CRC patients exhibiting high expression of TS and disturbed folate pools are intrinsically resistant to 5-FU [9]. A meta-analysis of over 3000 pooled CRC cases by Popat and colleagues concluded that the variation of TS expression in CRC patients could explain inter-individual variation in clinical outcome, and patients with low TS expression treated with 5-FU had better overall survival [41]. CRC patients who are chemoresponsive to 5-FU have lower TS enzymatic activity compared to those patients who fail to respond [42]. Furthermore, the low availability of 5,10-methylenetetrahydrofolate and its polyglutamates also contrib-uted to intrinsic resistance [43]. An indirect resistance mechanism reported in hepatocellular carcinoma cells is the induction of the expression of the transcription factor Late SV40 Factor (LSF) that regulates TS expression, by way of the astrocyte elevated gene-1 (AEG-1) [44].

Additionally, TS mRNA increases in a number of patients treated with 5-FU, resulting in acquired resistance [45]. In a review by Holohan et al., the authors explained further that 5-FU can post-transcriptionally upregulate the TS expression as a result of the inhibition of a negative feedback loop where the substrate free TS binds to and inhibits the translation of thymidylate synthase mRNA [38].

Watson and colleagues reported that patients with TYMS amplification treated with adjuvant chemotherapy had a median overall survival of 18 months shorter when compared to patients with low or normal TYMS copy number [46]. A total of 113 mCRC patients were enrolled in this study (62 exposed and 51 unexposed to 5-FU prior to resection) and the investigators con-cluded that TYMS copy number gain was associated with patients treated with 5-FU-based neoadjuvant treatment [46].

Guo and colleagues have demonstrated that a possible mechanism of acquired 5-FU resis-tance can be due to disruption in cell cycle. Using two 5-FU resistant and two sensitive cell lines, Guo and colleagues showed that the protein expression of CDK2 (total and phosphory-lated threonine 160), Cyclin D3, and Cyclin A was significantly decreased in the 5-FU resistant cell lines. On the other hand, p21^{WAF1} expression was modestly increased in both resistant cell lines [11]. The authors postulated that the G1 and S phase delay in the 5-FU resistant cell lines occurs because of Cyclin E−CDK2 complex deficiency. Additionally, the Cyclin A−CDK2 complex is also deficient and may assist in bringing about a delay in the S phase of 5-FU resis-tance cell lines [11]. Guo and colleagues speculated that the slowing down of the cell cycle might interfere with the active 5-FU metabolites being incorporated into DNA and also allows the cells to repair the DNA damage [11].

Montagut and colleagues confirmed one mechanism of acquired resistance to cetuximab, where they showed that an acquired EGFR ectodomain mutation (S492R) prevented the effec-tive binding of cetuximab to the receptor [47]. On the other hand, overexpression of EGFR in CRC has been poorly correlated with response to anti-EGFR therapy [48]. One of the determi-nants of poor response is because KRAS mutant patients have a constantly activated KRAS, irrelevant to the phosphorylation status of EGFR. Fluorescence in situ hybridisation (FISH) analysis was carried out on a cohort of 58 mCRC patients treated with panitumumab and it was observed that patients that did not exhibit an EGFR copy number gain or chromosome 7 polysomy or amplification were associated with treatment failure ($p = 0.0009$, $p = 0.0007$) [49]. Another possible mechanism of resistance using an in vitro model postulated that increased Src family kinases activity leads to lengthened EGFR activity, increased EGFR-modulated HER3 activity, and activation of the PI3K/AKT pathway [50].

A study by Lievre and colleagues on a cohort of 30 mCRC patients reported a highly significant association between non-response to cetuximab and mutant KRAS (n = 19, p = 0.0003) [51]. This association was further confirmed by other larger studies [52, 53]. A study by Misale and colleagues unprecedentedly described that a significant number of wild-type KRAS CRC patients, who are initially responsive to anti-EGFR therapies, acquire resistance due to *de novo* KRAS mutations resulting from continuing mutagenesis [54]. Another somatic mutation, associated with treatment resistance in CRC is PIK3CA [55], is mutated in 25–32% of CRC patients [56].

2.3. DNA damage repair

Mismatch repair deficiency (dMMR) can occur because of both sporadic and hereditary CRC. In the autosomal dominant hereditary non-polyposis colon cancer (HNPCC), which is also referred to as Lynch Syndrome, dMMR arises primarily due to inactivating germline mutations in either MLH1, MSH2, PMS2, or MSH6 [57]. Furthermore, loss of function of the remaining allele can occur via various mechanisms, namely loss of heterozygosity, mutations, gene conversion, and also promoter methylation [58]. On the other hand, epigenetic hypermethylation of MLH1 accounts for the majority of sporadic dMMR in CRC [59]. A recent study by Ye and colleagues concluded that miR-1290 promotes 5-FU resistance by directly targeting hMSH2 [60].

An *in vitro* study on CRC cell lines showed that MMR-proficient cell lines were more sensitive to the therapeutic doses of 5-FU (5–10 μM) compared to MMR-deficient cell lines [61]. Furthermore, patients who are high microsatellite instable (MSI-H) do not show any survival advantage when administered 5-FU-based chemotherapies [62]. The scientific literature not only alludes to the fact that dMMR tumor cells have a distinct response to standard chemotherapies, but also to many emerging therapies for CRC [58]. In an *in vitro* study, Tajima and colleagues showed that resistance of dMMR cancer cells to 5-FU can arise due to the incorporation of 5-FU metabolites in DNA [63].

Mechanisms attributed to resistance to oxaliplatin include increased DNA repair, impaired DNA adduct formation, over-expression of copper transporters (increased levels of ATP7B correlated with poor outcome in CRC patients) [64], enhanced drug detoxification, and increased tolerance to DNA damage. While NER and recombination repair mechanisms do not distinguish between cisplatin and oxaliplatin adducts, mismatch repair, damage-recognition proteins, and translesion DNA polymerases do distinguish between the two [65].

Increased excision repair cross complementation group 1 (ERCC1) mRNA expression correlates with resistance to oxaliplatin [66]. A polymorphism (Gln mutant allele) in X-ray repair cross complementation group 1 (XRCC1), which is involved in single strand break, adduct formation, and base excision repair, was associated with treatment resistance in a cohort of 61 patients treated with 5-FU and oxaliplatin [67].

2.4. p53

An *in vitro* study on the NCI-60 panel investigated the relationship between a group of p53 mutant and p53 wild-type cell lines and chemosensitivity to 123 drugs used in cancer treatment.

One of the findings was that the median GI50 for p53 mutant cell lines treated with 5-FU was sixfold higher than the GI50 of p53 wild-type cell lines [68].

The TP53 Colorectal Cancer International Collaborative Study published a study consisting of a patient cohort of 3583 samples from 25 different research groups in 17 countries. One of the aims of this study was to investigate whether there was a prognostic impact of TP53 mutations and treatment subgroups. In 1334 Dukes' C patients (792 wild-type TP53 and 542 mutant TP53), the wild-type TP53 patients treated with chemotherapy showed significantly better survival in the proximal and rectal tumor groups ($p = 0.006$ and $p = <0.001$, respectively) and a trend towards statistical significance ($p = 0.022$) was observed for the distal tumor group [69]. In the mutant TP53 group, patients receiving chemotherapy had better survival only in the proximal colon group ($p = <0.001$), with the authors concluding that TP53 mutation had no predictive value within Dukes' C patients treated by surgery alone or surgery and chemotherapy [69]. The authors advised caution in interpreting these observations, since the chemotherapy treatment was not always 5-FU based. When the 5-FU-based regimens were grouped together, the authors reported that chemotherapy can have an impact on survival based on TP53 mutational status and tumor sites [69]. Furthermore, this study showed that wild-type TP53 rectal patients received a significant survival benefit from 5-FU-based chemotherapy, irrespective of whether or not radiotherapy was received [69].

In 2008, Ahmed and colleagues carried out a study on 41 Dukes' C CRC patients that had a curative resection of the primary tumor and were administered 5-FU adjuvant treatment. The p53 mutation status was confirmed by gene sequencing and the study concluded that there was significant advantage for the wild type p53 patients in the time to develop metastasis and overall survival within the two groups receiving 5-FU adjuvant treatment [70].

2.5. Apoptosis

Failure of cells to undergo apoptosis may affect treatment efficacy [71]. Apoptosis can occur via two main signaling pathways: extrinsic (receptor-mediated pathway) and/or intrinsic (mitochondrial-mediated pathway [72]. Although a number of studies have reported the involvement of extrinsic pathway in treatment resistance, namely CD95 (Fas), it has been shown that under certain situations most chemotherapy-treated cells undergo intrinsic apoptosis [71, 73].

By way of an *in vitro* model, Gourdier and colleagues demonstrated that acquired resistance to oxaliplatin can occur via a defect in the intrinsic apoptosis pathway [74]. Furthermore, expression of cleaved caspase-3 and Bax was lost in the 68-fold oxaliplatin-trained resistant cell line, while the expression of Bcl-2, Bak, and Bcl-X$_L$ remained unaltered, suggesting that they are not involved in the acquired resistance mechanism to oxaliplatin [74]. Transcription factor NFκβ is known to be constitutively activated in colorectal cancers and although it has been associated with pro-apoptotic function, it is not always the case [75]. 5-FU has been shown to induce NFκβ expression via IKKβ and consequently chemoresistance in colorectal cell lines [76]. Apart from the fact that oxaliplatin, like 5-FU, can cause NFκβ constitutive activation, this activation imparts chemoresistance via c-FLIP and Mcl-1 [77].

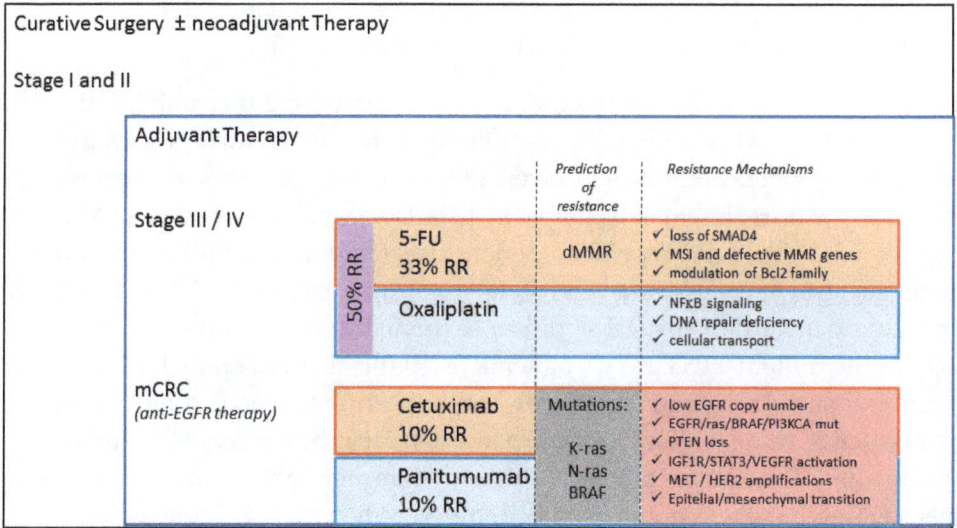

RR: Response Rate
MMR: Mismatch Repair Genes
MSI: microsatellite instability
mCRC: metastatic colorectal cancer

Figure 1. Treatment for colorectal cancer patients according to the stage at diagnosis.

A study identified double stranded RNA dependent protein kinase (PKR), as a key molecule in inducing apoptosis in colon cancer cells—irrelevant of the p53 status [78]. The authors proceeded by demonstrating that PKR knockdown cells responded poorly to treatment with 5-FU. The importance of integrins and apoptosis in chemoresistance is being investigated by a number of groups. A study by Liu and colleagues focussed on the involvement of the β6-integrin-ERK-MAP kinase pathway in conferring chemoresistance to 5-FU in colon cancer lines (**Figure 1**) [79].

3. Novel resistance mechanisms

3.1. Warburg effect

Over the past decade, the significance of the Warburg effect in the field of oncology has gained momentum and a number of original research papers [80, 81] and reviews have been published on this topic [82]. The Warburg effect, also referred to as the glycolytic phenotype, is singularized by an increased rate of aerobic glycolysis together with irreversible injury to mitochondrial oxidative phosphorylation [83] and is favored by the majority of tumors [84]. Subsequently, Tong and colleagues showed that aerobic glycolysis is involved in cancer cell proliferation and tumorigenesis in a model of HCT116 colorectal cell lines [85]. A number of mechanisms that affect increased glycolysis, and therefore contribute to the Warburg effect, include mitochondrial defects, adaptation to hypoxic conditions, oncogenic signals, and altered metabolic enzymes [86]. A number of these mechanisms occur via hypoxia inducible factor-1 (HIF-1) [87].

A putative major player in the Warburg effect and cancer is the uncoupling protein coding-2 (UCP2) [88]. UCP2 is located in the mitochondrial inner membrane and its main function is that of a mitochondrial transporter protein, that creates proton leaks across the inner mitochondrial membrane, ergo uncoupling oxidative phosphorylation from ATP synthesis [89]. Furthermore, UCP2 might act as a negative regulator of ROS production [90].

Horimoto et al. postulated that UCP2 is involved in colon tumor adaptation and is correlated with neoplastic changes [91]. UCP2 gene expression and protein expression was assessed on a small cohort of 10 patients, where a paired normal and tumor sample for each patient was processed. Gene expression results demonstrated an average of 3.88 ± 0.85-fold difference in UCP2 mRNA expression between the tumor (T) and peritumoral (P) paired samples. The same ratio was found for UCP2 protein expression and furthermore a strong linear correlation between T/P ratio of UCP mRNA and protein expression ($r = 0.91$, $p = 0.0015$) was confirmed. Additionally, immunohistochemistry (IHC) for UCP2 was carried out on a cohort of 9 hyperplastic polyps, 17 adenomas, and 107 adenocarcinoma and positive scores were 11.1, 58.8, and 86%, respectively.

A comparable study was undertaken on a larger cohort of colon cancer patients and it yielded the same results and correlations in addition to association of UCP2 expression and metastasis [88]. Altered colon cancer metabolism, as confirmed through measurement of UCP2 expression in these studies, can also contribute to resistance to cancer therapies. An *in vitro* study investigated the rate of cell death caused by 5-FU, with respect to different metabolic rates, as quantified by the bioenergetic signature [92]. This study demonstrated the bioenergetic signature directly correlates with the apoptotic response to treatment with 5-FU [92].

Tumor adaptation to hypoxic and acidic microenvironments strongly selects for tumor cells that are resistant to chemo- and radiotherapy [93]. The slowing down of cell cycling induces a decreased rate of cell division, thereby decreasing chemotherapy activity [93]. Furthermore, hypoxia dysregulates several DNA damage response pathways and prevents effective functioning of proteins involved in homologous recombination (HR), non-homologous end joining (NHEJ), and the mismatch repair (MMR) pathways, thereby driving genetic instability [94]. The cascade of events triggered by chronic hypoxia may also bring about amplification of multidrug resistant gene ABCB1 via induction of chromosomal fragile sites [94].

An *in vitro* study on colon carcinoma cell lines demonstrated that low oxygen concentration resulted in decreased protein expression of Bid, Bad, and Bax [87]. A further series of experiments illustrated that all three CRC cell lines studied expressed a functional HIF-1 pathway and the authors showed that in a hypoxic environment Bid down-regulation occurs via HIF-1, while down-regulation of Bax and Bad occurs independently of HIF-1 function [87]. Additionally, under anoxic conditions, SW480, HCT116, and HT29 were resistant to etoposide treatment and SW480 was also resistant to oxaliplatin. Further investigation by Erler and colleagues demonstrated that down regulation of Bid and/or Bax contributed to etoposide resistance in this model [87]. An important observation from this study was that Bak was least responsive to hypoxia and thereby it might be crucial for drug-induced apoptosis [87].

The PI3K/Akt signaling pathway enhances aerobic glycolysis, and dual PI3K/mTOR inhibitors can influence the cancer cell metabolic programme [95]. Oncogenic mutations involving this pathway, MAPK, and Src pathways have been shown to increase HIF-1 expression in both hypoxic and normoxic conditions [96]. Inhibiting HIF1 decreases proliferation, influences anaerobic glycolysis, encourages apoptosis, and reduces resistance to chemo- and radiotherapy [93].

Moderate evidence in the literature demonstrates that 18q LOH/SMAD4 loss has potential for it being used as a marker to predict response to 5-FU-based therapies [97]. Papageorgis and colleagues demonstrated that a SMAD4 defect suppresses hypoxia-induced cell death, induces aerobic glycolysis, and promotes 5-FU resistance in the HCT116 cell line model [98]. Furthermore, the authors observed a physical interaction between SMAD4 and HIF1α and postulated that the acquired chemoresistance in 18q-deficient CRC may be explained by Smad4 negatively regulating HIF1α-induced GLUT1 expression and the rate of aerobic glycolysis [98]. Other oncogenes/tumor suppressor genes known to be involved in the stimulation of glycolytic energy include Ras, c-myc, Src, and p53 [99].

Downregulation of pyruvate kinase M2 (PKM2) is also known to promote the Warburg effect metabolic phenotype and tumorigenesis [80]. Additionally, PKM2 is a HIF-1 target gene and concurrently a co-activator of HIF-1 [93]. A study by Tamada and colleagues on a number of cancer cell lines, which also comprised of CRC cell lines HCT116 p53 wild-type and HCT116 p53 null, demonstrated CD44-regulated glycolysis in p53 deficient cells via interaction with PKM2 [100]. Furthermore, the authors speculated that CD44 functions as a scaffold between a tyrosine kinase and PKM2 near the cell membrane, ergo down-regulating the activity of PKM2 [100]. By means of a set of elegant experiments, the authors showed evidence that CD44 silencing in p53 deficient cell lines sensitized the cells to cisplatin, 5-FU, and adriamycin in normoxia, and that CD44 silencing of p53 wild-type cells under hypoxic conditions increased sensitivity to these three chemotherapeutic agents [100].

The relationship of hypoxia and resistance to both radio- and chemotherapy has been explored for the last decade and several mechanisms have been postulated. As evidenced by a number of studies referred above, the Warburg effect is an adaptive mechanism used by solid tumors to overcome stress caused by hypoxia and also contributes to resistance to both chemotherapy and targeted inhibitors.

3.2. Clonal evolution

Another contributor to therapy failure is the innate Darwinian aspect of cancer [101]. In a review of clonal evolution, Greaves and Maley describe the complexity of cancer and the selective pressure for resistant cells to thrive when treated with chemotherapeutic agents. Similarly, adaptive microenvironmental mechanisms such as hypoxia and acidosis lead to both phenotypic and genotypic heterogeneity [102]. This evolution not only affects the genomic instability of the tumor but also contributes towards resistance to therapy, including targeted therapies [102].

A retrospective study analyzing circulating tumor DNA from a cohort of 28 mCRC patients suggested that development of resistance to panitumumab can occur in metastatic lesions, having a sub-clone encompassing just 1 of 42 mutations associated with resistance to panitumumab. Subsequently, the time for recurrence is basically the time taken for that sub-clone to repopulate the lesion [103]. Furthermore, the authors concluded that resistance mutation in KRAS and other genes were likely to be present prior to starting panitumumab therapy [103].

A number of mechanisms contributing to acquired resistance to 5-FU-based therapies include alteration of the drug's specific target, drug inactivation, influx and efflux of drugs in the cells, drug-induced damage, and evasion of apoptosis [104]. In an attempt to comprehend these complex mechanisms, Tentes et al. investigated 5-FU acquired resistance in the SW620 cell line model [105]. A significant finding reported in this study consisted of the maintenance of a 5-FU resistant phenotype, albeit by culturing the trained cell line in drug-free media for 15 weeks. The authors concluded that the resistant clones may have acquired an altered genetic background and unique gene expression patterns due to long-term exposure to 5-FU, and that this scenario might explain relapses caused by residual disease of chemo-resistant cells. Besides, overlapping mechanisms of resistance to 5-FU could be observed in the trained resistant cell line [105].

3.3. Intra-tumor heterogeneity

A published study evidenced that intra-tumor heterogeneity is a considerable hurdle to both predictive and prognostic biomarker development [106]. One of the principal results in this study highlighted that 63–69% of all somatic mutations are not detectable across every tumor area, hence confirming that one biopsy is not representative of the whole tumor [106]. Intra-tumor heterogeneity is one of the main challenges to patients being successfully treated and can also contribute to patients having relapses [107].

Chromosomal instability (CIN) is associated with both intrinsic- and acquired-drug resistance and also involved in intra-tumor heterogeneity [108]. A number of hypotheses surrounding CIN, Darwinian selection, and intra-tumoural heterogeneity are currently being investigated. Evidence has been obtained to indicate that cells having a high degree of chromosomal instability are more predisposed to exhibit intrinsic resistance [108].

Lee and colleagues conducted a study on a panel of 27 CRC cell lines (18 of which were CIN$^+$) and demonstrated that CIN$^+$ cell lines were significantly more intrinsically resistant to the inhibitors used (Kolmogorov-Smirnov test p < 0.0001) and, even at similar proliferation rates, CIN$^+$ cell lines were more resistant to treatment when compared to CIN$^-$ (one sided Wilcoxon-Mann-Whitney test, p = 0.049) [55]. Furthermore, according to previous reports, patients treated with 5-FU-based therapy who exhibited CIN$^+$ did not obtain as much benefit from the treatments, when compared to patients having diploid CRC [109]. This acquired multidrug resistance has been attributed to cell heterogeneity due to multiple chromosomal re-assortments in these aneuploid cells [55]. One of the hypotheses that Lee and colleagues discussed is that there is a distinct CIN$^+$ survival phenotype that triggers an endurance to ongoing chromosomal rearrangements which is also related to drug resistance [55].

Phenotypic heterogeneity arises from both genetic and non-genetic influences [110]. Non-genetic influences can emerge from phenotypic plasticity and differentiation of cancer stem cells [107]. The cellular phenotype is affected by several factors namely, stochastic fluctuations (noise), genotypes, microenvironment, and the gene regulatory network [110]. In their review, Marusyk and colleagues remark that even though genetic heterogeneity is not likely to contribute considerably to phenotypic heterogeneity, it still supports tumor evolution during tumorigenesis and treatment resistance [110]. Phenotypic heterogeneity manifests as phenotypic diverse subpopulations of subpopulation of tumor cells, histologic alterations, different patterns of disease progression, prognosis, diagnosis, and also responses to therapy [111]. This necessitates further investigations on therapeutic resistance of CRC with respect to phenotypic heterogeneity.

3.4. Pharmacoepigenomics

Epigenetic modifications are implicated in the progression of chemoresistance [112]. They bring about changes in gene expression that are autonomous of changes in DNA sequence and persevere over numerous cell divisions. In contrast to genetic modifications, epigenetic transformations are reversible [113]. As a result, the field of pharmacoepigenomics is now gaining more popularity. One of the main mechanisms of action of chemotherapeutic agents is by inducing DNA damage which subsequently leads to either DNA repair, apoptosis, or cell-cycle arrest [114]. A number of genes implicated in these biological processes in cancer cells are epigenetically regulated [115]. Drug resistance has been associated with hypermethyl-ation of promoter regions of pro-apoptotic genes, hypomethylation of drug efflux promoters, and also modified promoter methylation patterns of DNA repair genes [116]. Furthermore, global histone modification patterns may also be involved in drug resistance [117].

Sugita and colleagues conducted a study on a cohort of 80 gastric cancer patients and inves-tigated the relationship between methylation of BNIP3 and DAPK with respect to response to 5-FU-based therapy. This study confirmed a relationship between poor response rate and methylation of one or both genes when compared to patients that did not have methyla-tion (p = 0.003) [118]. Furthermore, a study on 112 primary colorectal patients substantiated that BNIP3 is methylated in CRC patients, with approximately 58% of the cohort exhibiting methylation [119]. Additionally, 30 patients having BNIP3 methylation were non-responsive to irinotecan therapy [119]. An *in vitro* study demonstrated that cells having a methylated p16[Ink4A] were more resistant to irinotecan-induced cell cycle arrest [120] . Cheetham and col-leagues presented support that hypermethylation of the SPARC promoter is frequently found in both CRC tumor and cell lines when compared to normal colon (p = 0.03) [121]. A previous *in vitro* study by the same group showed that mRNA and protein expression of SPARC were low in chemoresistant tumors and thereby the authors concluded that hypermethylation of the SPARC promoter might be a potential mechanism of low SPARC expression, leading to resistance to therapy [121, 122].

Dynamic chromatin modification can also influence resistance to treatment and a publication by Sharma and colleagues illustrated this resistance mechanism. "Drug-tolerant persisters" were detected while studying the acute response of human cell lines with respect to different treatments. These cells remained viable in conditions where other cells failed to thrive, and since they were encountered at a higher frequency than expected, the authors associated this observation to epigenetic regulation [123]. Following several elegant experiments, the authors concluded that this transiently acquired drug resistant phenotype is capable of arising *de novo* and requires the histone demethylase KDM5A/RBP2/Jarid1A. This particular histone demethylase secures a metastable chromatin state which contributes towards the ability of cells to tolerate drug exposure. Additionally, this chromatin state is dependent on IGF-1R signaling, which has also been associated with drug resistance in a number of other studies [124, 125].

3.5. Additional mechanisms

Resistance to the newest drug, trifluridine was attributed to decreased changes in expression of mRNA and miRNA located on chromosome 9. This could have been due to either genome deletion or LOH of let-7d-5p, a miRNA inversely associated to trifluridine-induced proliferative effects; hence low expression would lead to decreased effectiveness [126] .

Resistance-promoting adaptive responses include the (1) epithelial-mesenchymal transition (EMT) which is associated with invasive capacity, increased motility and related to chemotherapy, and targeted therapy resistance [38]; (2) Oncogenic bypass and pathway redundancy, also referred to as compensatory signaling pathway via crosstalk mechanisms is involved in acquired resistance to cetuximab. With EGFR deregulated, HER2, HER3, cMET, MAPK, and Akt are subsequently switched on and as a result, acquired resistance can ensue since some RTKs share signaling pathways involved in proliferation and survival [127]. (3) Activation of pro-survival signaling: ADAM17, known to be deregulated in CRC, is also known to be activated with chemotherapy and has been implicated with growth factor shedding, growth factor receptor activation, and drug resistance [128].

Another downstream resistance mechanism is autophagy. In CRC, BRAF V600E induces autophagic properties. Recently, Goulielmaki and colleagues reported that PI3K/AKT/MTOR inhibitors induce autophagic tumor properties, whereas RAF/MEK/ERK signaling inhibitors reduce expression of autophagic markers. They showed that pre-treatment of autophagy inhibitor 3-MA followed by its combination with BRAFV600E targeting drug PLX4720 can synergistically sensitize resistant colorectal tumors [129].

Another recent review highlighted the involvement of telomerase in drug resistance in cancer [130]. The main telomerase-related mechanism highlighted in this review included hTERT translocation, hTERT and cell resistance to stress, G-quadruplex inhibitors specific, telomerase inhibition and the mechanism by which telomerase helps cancer cells resistance to DNA damage/apoptosis. Recent literature also implicates the mammalian vault complexes in drug resistance [130].

4. Conclusion

During the last decade, a number of groups have started taking a systems medicine approach to better understand treatment resistance in colorectal cancer. As described by the Coordinating Action Systems Medicine, this approach comprises the iterative and reciprocal feedback between clinical investigations and practice with computational, statistical and mathematical multi-scale analysis and modeling of pathogenic mechanisms, disease progression and remission, disease spread and cure, treatment responses and adverse events, as well as disease prevention both at the epidemiological and individual patient level [131].

We are already witnessing a number of success stories and by integrating data, especially with respect to understanding mechanisms of resistance, we are now moving away from clinical trials directed to specific tumors towards umbrella trials (multiple molecular targets in a single tumor) and basket trials (single molecular abnormality across multiple cancer types). This evolution can be clearly seen in CRC, where we started with one gene, one drug approach, and moved towards a multi-gene, multi-drug approach and currently we are at a multi-molecular, multi-drug approach [132].

This systems medicine approach is helping to accelerate bench to bedside developments and an example is the EXACT trial, where treatment-refractory cancer patients are administered an individualized treatment concept based on prospective biomarkers assessed in a real-time biopsy [133].

All of the above has had a major impact on the clinic and as we can now witness, we have achieved a better patient stratification, earlier and more sensitive diagnostics and drug repurposing. Nonetheless, it is important that we continue working to overcome the major challenges we are still facing. These include, but are not limited to morphologic and molecular heterogeneity of cancer, treatment resistance, drug addiction, and other challenges such as standardization of methods, infrastructure, and cost and big data. Hence, it will be important to have appropriate biomarkers to inform clinicians on administering the most effective treatment to the individual patient at the right time.

Acknowledgements

RB is supported by a REACH HIGH Scholars Programme – Post-Doctoral Grants. The grant is part-financed by the European Union, Operational Programme II — Cohesion Policy 2014–2020 investing in human capital to create more opportunities and promote the wellbeing of society – European Social Fund.

Author details

Romina Briffa[1,2]*, Simon P. Langdon[3], Godfrey Grech[2] and David J. Harrison[1]

*Address all correspondence to: rb228@st-andrews.ac.uk

1 School of Medicine, University of St Andrews, Fife, United Kingdom

2 Department of Pathology, Faculty of Medicine and Surgery, University of Malta, Msida, Malta

3 Cancer Research UK Edinburgh Centre and Division of Pathology Laboratory, Institute of Genetics and Molecular Medicine, University of Edinburgh, Edinburgh, United Kingdom

References

[1] Bastos DA, Ribeiro SC, de Freitas D, Hoff PM. Combination therapy in high-risk stage II or stage III colon cancer: Current practice and future prospects. Therapeutic Advances in Medical Oncology 2010 Jul;**2**(4):261-272

[2] Weidlich S, Walsh K, Crowther D, Burczynski ME, Feuerstein G, Carey FA, et al. Pyrosequencing-based methods reveal marked inter-individual differences in onco-gene mutation burden in human colorectal tumours. British Journal of Cancer. 2011 Jul 12;**105**(2):246-254

[3] Rô Me Viguier J, Rie Boige V, Miquel C, Pocard M, Giraudeau B, Sabourin J-C, et al. ERCC1 codon 118 polymorphism is a predictive factor for the tumor response to oxaliplatin/5-flu-orouracil combination chemotherapy in patients with advanced colorectal cancer. Clinical Cancer Research. 2005;**11**(17):6212-6217

[4] Virag P, Fischer-Fodor E, Perde-Schrepler M, Brie I, Tatomir C, Balacescu L, et al. Oxaliplatin induces different cellular and molecular chemoresistance patterns in colorec-tal cancer cell lines of identical origins. BMC Genomics. 2013;**14**(1):480

[5] Zhang B, Zhang B, Chen X, Bae S, Singh K, Washington MK, et al. Loss of Smad4 in colorectal cancer induces resistance to 5-fluorouracil through activating Akt pathway. British Journal of Cancer. 2014 Feb 18;**110**(4):946-957

[6] Watson RG, Muhale F, Thorne LB, Yu J, O'Neil BH, Hoskins JM, et al. Amplification of thymidylate synthetase in metastatic colorectal cancer patients pretreated with 5-fluoro-uracil-based chemotherapy. European Journal of Cancer. 2017 Jun 15;**46**(18):3358-3364

[7] Sargent DJ, Marsoni S, Monges G, Thibodeau SN, Labianca R, Hamilton SR, et al. Defective mismatch repair as a predictive marker for lack of efficacy of fluorouracil-based adju-vant therapy in colon cancer. Journal of Clinical Oncology. 2010 Jul 10;**28**(20):3219-3226

[8] van Triest B, Pinedo HM, van Hensbergen Y, Smid K, Telleman F, Schoenmakers PS, et al. Thymidylate synthase level as the main predictive parameter for sensitivity to 5-fluoro-uracil, but not for folate-based thymidylate synthase inhibitors, in 13 nonselected colon cancer cell lines. Clinical Cancer Research. 1999 Mar;**5**(3):643-654

[9] Zhang N, Yin Y, S-J X, Chen W-S. 5-Fluorouracil: Mechanisms of resistance and reversal strategies. Molecules. 2008 Aug 5;**13**(8):1551-1569

[10] Sasaki S, Watanabe T, Kobunai T, Konishi T, Nagase H, Sugimoto Y, et al. hRFI overex-pressed in HCT116 cells modulates Bcl-2 family proteins when treated with 5-fluoroura-cil. Oncology Reports. 2006 May;**15**(5):1293-1298

[11] Guo X, Goessl E, Jin G, Collie-Duguid ESR, Cassidy J, Wang W, et al. Cell cycle perturba-tion and acquired 5-fluorouracil chemoresistance. Anticancer Research. 2008;**28**(1A):9-14

[12] Shin Y-K, Yoo BC, Chang HJ, Jeon E, Hong S-H, Jung M-S, et al. Down-regulation of mitochondrial F1F0-ATP synthase in human colon cancer cells with induced 5-fluoro-uracil resistance. Cancer Research. 2005 Apr 15;**65**(8):3162-3170

[13] Hwang IT, Chung YM, Kim JJ, Chung JS, Kim BS, Kim HJ, et al. Drug resistance to 5-FU linked to reactive oxygen species modulator 1. Biochemical and Biophysical Research Communications. 2007 Jul 27;359(2):304-310

[14] Martinez-Balibrea E, Martínez-Cardús A, Ginés A, Ruiz de Porras V, Moutinho C, Layos L, et al. Tumor-related molecular mechanisms of oxaliplatin resistance. Molecular Cancer Therapeutics. 2015;14(8):1767-1776

[15] Van Emburgh BO, Sartore-Bianchi A, Di Nicolantonio F, Siena S, Bardelli A. Acquired resistance to EGFR-targeted therapies in colorectal cancer. Molecular Oncology. 2014 Sep;8(6):1084-1094

[16] Zhao B, Wang L, Qiu H, Zhang M, Sun L, Peng P, et al. Mechanisms of resistance to anti-EGFR therapy in colorectal cancer. Oncotarget. 2017 Jan 17;8(3):3980-4000

[17] Misale S, Di Nicolantonio F, Sartore-Bianchi A, Siena S, Bardelli A. Resistance to anti-EGFR therapy in colorectal cancer: From heterogeneity to convergent evolution. Cancer Discovery. 2014;4(11):1269-1280

[18] Dienstmann R, Salazar R, Tabernero J. Overcoming resistance to anti-EGFR therapy in colorectal cancer. American Society of Clinical Oncology Educational Book. 2015;35: e149-e156

[19] Sartore-Bianchi A, Loupakis F, Argilés G, Prager GW. Challenging chemoresistant metastatic colorectal cancer: Therapeutic strategies from the clinic and from the laboratory. Annals of Oncology. 2016 Aug;27(8):1456-1466

[20] Wu G, Wilson G, George J, Liddle C, Hebbard L. Overcoming treatment resistance in cancer: Current understanding and tactics. Cancer Letters. 2017;387:69-76

[21] Al-Hajeili M, Shields AF, Hwang JJ, Wadlow RC, Marshall JL. Molecular testing to optimize and personalize decision making in the management of colorectal cancer. Oncology (Williston Park, N.Y.). 2017;31(4):301-312

[22] Martinez-Rivera M, Siddik ZH. Resistance and gain-of-resistance phenotypes in cancers harboring wild-type p53. Biochemical Pharmacology. 2012 Apr 15;83(8):1049-1062

[23] Purnapatre K, Khattar SK, Saini KS. Cytochrome P450s in the development of target-based anticancer drugs. Cancer Letters. 2008 Jan 18;259(1):1-15

[24] Muhale FA, Wetmore BA, Thomas RS, McLeod HL. Systems pharmacology assessment of the 5-fluorouracil pathway. Pharmacogenomics. 2011 Mar;12(3):341-350

[25] Hasegawa S, Seike K, Koda K, Takiguchi N, Oda K, Hasegawa R, et al. Thymidine phosphorylase expression and efficacy of adjuvant doxifluridine in advanced colorectal cancer patients. Oncology Reports. 2005 Apr;13(4):621-626

[26] Griffiths L, Dachs GU, Bicknell R, Harris AL, Stratford IJ. The influence of oxygen tension and pH on the expression of platelet-derived endothelial cell growth factor/thymidine phosphorylase in human breast tumor cells grown in vitro and in vivo. Cancer Research. 1997 Feb 15;57(4):570-572

[27] Diasio RB, Beavers TL, Carpenter JT. Familial deficiency of dihydropyrimidine dehydro-
      genase. Biochemical basis for familial pyrimidinemia and severe 5-fluorouracil-induced
      toxicity. The Journal of Clinical Investigation. 1988 Jan;**81**(1, 1):47-51

[28] Dervieux T, Meshkin B, Neri B. Pharmacogenetic testing: Proofs of principle and pharma-
      coeconomic implications. Mutation Research-Fundamental and Molecular Mechanisms
      of Mutagenesis. 2005 Jun;**573**(1-2):180-194

[29] Tsutani Y, Yoshida K, Sanada Y, Wada Y, Konishi K, Fukushima M, et al. Decreased oro-
      tate phosphoribosyltransferase activity produces 5-fluorouracil resistance in a human
      gastric cancer cell line. Oncology Reports. 2008 Dec;**20**(6):1545-1551

[30] Hector S, Bolanowska-Higdon W, Zdanowicz J, Hitt S, Pendyala L. In vitro studies on
      the mechanisms of oxaliplatin resistance. Cancer Chemotherapy and Pharmacology.
      2001 Nov 21;**48**(5):398-406

[31] Stoehlmacher J, Park DJ, Zhang W, Groshen S, Tsao-Wei DD, MC Y, et al. Association
      between glutathione S-transferase P1, T1, and M1 genetic polymorphism and survival of
      patients with metastatic colorectal cancer. Journal of the National Cancer Institute. 2002
      Jun 19;**94**(12):936-942

[32] Imyanitov EN, Moiseyenko VM. Molecular-based choice of cancer therapy: Realities and
      expectations. Clinica Chimica Acta. 2007 Apr;**379**(1-2):1-13

[33] Marcuello E, Altés A, Menoyo A, Del Rio E, Gómez-Pardo M, Baiget M. UGT1A1 gene
      variations and irinotecan treatment in patients with metastatic colorectal cancer. British
      Journal of Cancer. 2004 Aug 16;**91**(4):678-682

[34] Lee C, Raffaghello L, Longo VD. Starvation, detoxification, and multidrug resistance in
      cancer therapy. Drug Resistance Updates. 2012;**15**(1-2):114-122

[35] Vasiliou V, Vasiliou K, Nebert DW. Human ATP-binding cassette (ABC) transporter fam-
      ily. Human Genomics. 2009 Apr;**3**(3):281-290

[36] DeGorter MK, Xia CQ, Yang JJ, Kim RB. Drug transporters in drug efficacy and toxicity.
      Annual Review of Pharmacology and Toxicology. 2012 Feb 10;**52**(1):249-273

[37] Pratt S, Shepard RL, Kandasamy RA, Johnston PA, Perry Iii W, Dantzig AH. The mul-
      tidrug resistance protein 5 (ABCC5) confers resistance to 5-fluorouracil and transports
      its monophosphorylated metabolites. Molecular Cancer Therapeutics. May 1 2005;**4**(5):
      855-863

[38] Holohan C, Van Schaeybroeck S, Longley DB, Johnston PG. Cancer drug resistance: An
      evolving paradigm. Nature Reviews. Cancer. 2013 Oct;**13**(10):714-726

[39] Szakacs G, Paterson JK, Ludwig JA, Booth-Genthe C, Gottesman MM. Targeting mul-
      tidrug resistance in cancer. Nature Reviews. Drug Discovery. 2006 Mar 1;**5**(3):219-234

[40] Abraham J, Earl HM, Pharoah PD, Caldas C. Pharmacogenetics of cancer chemotherapy.
      Biochimica et Biophysica Acta. 2006 Dec;**1766**(2):168-183

[41] Popat S, Matakidou A, Houlston RS. Thymidylate synthase expression and prognosis in colorectal cancer: A systematic review and meta-analysis. Journal of Clinical Oncology. 2004 Feb 1;**22**(3):529-536

[42] Etienne M-C, Chazal M, Laurent-Puig P, Magné N, Rosty C, Formento J-L, et al. Prognostic value of tumoral thymidylate synthase and p53 in metastatic colorectal cancer patients receiving fluorouracil-based chemotherapy: Phenotypic and genotypic analyses. Journal of Clinical Oncology. 2002 Jun 15;**20**(12):2832-2843

[43] Aschele C, Sobrero A, Faderan MA, Bertino JR. Novel mechanism(s) of resistance to 5-fluorouracil in human colon cancer (HCT-8) sublines following exposure to two different clinically relevant dose schedules. Cancer Research. 1992 Apr 1;**52**(7):1855-1864

[44] Yoo BK, Gredler R, Vozhilla N, Su Z-Z, Chen D, Forcier T, et al. Identification of genes conferring resistance to 5-fluorouracil. Proceedings of the National Academy of Sciences. 2009 Aug 4;**106**(31):12938-12943

[45] Libra M, Navolanic PM, Talamini R, Cecchin E, Sartor F, Tumolo S, et al. Thymidylate synthetase mRNA levels are increased in liver metastases of colorectal cancer patients resistant to fluoropyrimidine-based chemotherapy. BMC Cancer. 2004 Mar 25;**4**:11

[46] Watson RG, Muhale F, Thorne LB, Yu J, O?Neil BH, Hoskins JM, et al. Amplification of thymidylate synthetase in metastatic colorectal cancer patients pretreated with 5-fluorouracil-based chemotherapy. European Journal of Cancer. 2010 Dec;**46**(18):3358-3364

[47] Montagut C, Dalmases A, Bellosillo B, Crespo M, Pairet S, Iglesias M, et al. Identification of a mutation in the extracellular domain of the epidermal growth factor receptor conferring cetuximab resistance in colorectal cancer. Nature Medicine. 2012 Jan 22;**18**(2): 221-223

[48] Ibrahim AEK, Arends MJ. Molecular typing of colorectal cancer: Applications in diagnosis and treatment. Diagnostic Histopathology. 2012 Feb;**18**(2):70-80

[49] Sartore-Bianchi A, Moroni M, Veronese S, Carnaghi C, Bajetta E, Luppi G, et al. Epidermal growth factor receptor gene copy number and clinical outcome of metastatic colorectal cancer treated with panitumumab. Journal of Clinical Oncology. 2007 Aug 1;**25**(22):3238-3245

[50] Wheeler DL, Iida M, Kruser TJ, Nechrebecki MM, Dunn EF, Armstrong EA, et al. Epidermal growth factor receptor cooperates with Src family kinases in acquired resistance to cetuximab. Cancer Biology & Therapy. 2009 Apr;**8**(8):696-703

[51] Lievre A, Bachet J-B, Le Corre D, Boige V, Landi B, Emile J-F, et al. KRAS mutation status is predictive of response to cetuximab therapy in colorectal cancer. Cancer Research. 2006 Apr 15;**66**(8):3992-3995

[52] Di Fiore F, Blanchard F, Charbonnier F, Le Pessot F, Lamy A, Galais MP, et al. Clinical relevance of KRAS mutation detection in metastatic colorectal cancer treated by cetuximab plus chemotherapy. British Journal of Cancer. 2007 Apr 23;**96**(8):1166-1169

[53] De Roock W, Piessevaux H, De Schutter J, Janssens M, De Hertogh G, Personeni N, et al. KRAS wild-type state predicts survival and is associated to early radiological response in metastatic colorectal cancer treated with cetuximab. Annals of Oncology. 2008 Mar;**19**(3):508-515

[54] Misale S, Yaeger R, Hobor S, Scala E, Janakiraman M, Liska D, et al. Emergence of KRAS mutations and acquired resistance to anti-EGFR therapy in colorectal cancer. Nature. 2012 Jun 13;**486**(7404):532-536

[55] Lee AJX, Endesfelder D, Rowan AJ, Walther A, Birkbak NJ, Futreal PA, et al. Chromosomal instability confers intrinsic multidrug resistance. Cancer Research. 2011 Mar 1; **71**(5):1858-1870

[56] Samuels Y, Velculescu VE. Oncogenic mutations of PIK3CA in human cancers. Cell Cycle. 2004 Oct 12;**3**(10):1221-1224

[57] Arnold CN, Goel A, Boland CR. Role of hMLH1 promoter hypermethylation in drug resistance to 5-fluorouracil in colorectal cancer cell lines. International Journal of Cancer. 2003 Aug 10;**106**(1):66-73

[58] Hewish M, Lord CJ, Martin SA, Cunningham D, Ashworth A. Mismatch repair deficient colorectal cancer in the era of personalized treatment. Nature Reviews. Clinical Oncology. 2010 Apr 23;**7**(4):197-208

[59] Veigl ML, Kasturi L, Olechnowicz J, Ma AH, Lutterbaugh JD, Periyasamy S, et al. Biallelic inactivation of hMLH1 by epigenetic gene silencing, a novel mechanism causing human MSI cancers. Proceedings of the National Academy of Sciences of the United States of America. 1998 Jul 21;**95**(15):8698-8702

[60] Ye L, Jiang T, Shao H, Zhong L, Wang Z, Liu Y, et al. miR-1290 Is a biomarker in DNA-mismatch-repair-deficient colon cancer and promotes resistance to 5-fluorouracil by directly targeting hMSH2. Molecular Therapy. Nucleic Acids. 2017;**7**:453-464

[61] Carethers JM, Chauhan DP, Fink D, Nebel S, Bresalier RS, Howell SB, et al. Mismatch repair proficiency and in vitro response to 5-fluorouracil. Gastroenterology. 1999 Jul;**117**(1):123-131

[62] Carethers JM, Smith EJ, Behling CA, Nguyen L, Tajima A, Doctolero RT, et al. Use of 5-fluorouracil and survival in patients with microsatellite-unstable colorectal cancer. Gastroenterology. 2004 Feb;**126**(2):394-401

[63] Tajima A, Hess MT, Cabrera BL, Kolodner RD, Carethers JM. The mismatch repair complex hMutS alpha recognizes 5-fluorouracil-modified DNA: Implications for chemosensitivity and resistance. Gastroenterology. 2004 Dec;**127**(6):1678-1684

[64] Martinez-Cardús A, Martinez-Balibrea E, Bandrés E, Malumbres R, Ginés A, Manzano JL, et al. Pharmacogenomic approach for the identification of novel determinants of acquired resistance to oxaliplatin in colorectal cancer. Molecular Cancer Therapeutics. 2009;**8**(1):194-202

[65] Chaney SG, Campbell SL, Bassett E, Wu Y. Recognition and processing of cisplatin- and oxaliplatin-DNA adducts. Critical Reviews in Oncology/Hematology. 2005 Jan;**53**(1):3-11

[66] Shirota Y, Stoehlmacher J, Brabender J, Xiong Y-P, Uetake H, Danenberg KD, et al. ERCC1 and thymidylate synthase mRNA levels predict survival for colorectal cancer patients receiving combination oxaliplatin and fluorouracil chemotherapy. Journal of Clinical Oncology. 2001 Dec 1;**19**(23):4298-4304

[67] Stoehlmacher J, Ghaderi V, Iobal S, Groshen S, Tsao-Wei D, Park D, et al. A polymorphism of the XRCC1 gene predicts for response to platinum based treatment in advanced colorectal cancer. Anticancer Research. 2001;**21**(4B):3075-3079

[68] O'Connor PM, Jackman J, Bae I, Myers TG, Fan S, Mutoh M, et al. Characterization of the p53 tumor suppressor pathway in cell lines of the National Cancer Institute anticancer drug screen and correlations with the growth-inhibitory potency of 123 anticancer agents. Cancer Research. 1997 Oct 1;**57**(19):4285-4300

[69] Russo A, Bazan V, Iacopetta B, Kerr D, Soussi T, Gebbia N, et al. The TP53 colorectal cancer international collaborative study on the prognostic and predictive significance of *p53* mutation: Influence of tumor site, type of mutation, and adjuvant treatment. Journal of Clinical Oncology. 2005 Oct 20;**23**(30):7518-7528

[70] Ahmed IAM, Kelly SB, Anderson JJ, Angus B, Challen C, Lunec J. The predictive value of p53 and p33 (ING1b) in patients with Dukes'C colorectal cancer. Colorectal Disease. 2008 May;**10**(4):344-351

[71] Fulda S, Debatin K-M. Extrinsic versus intrinsic apoptosis pathways in anticancer chemotherapy. Oncogene. 2006 Aug 7;**25**(34):4798-4811

[72] Indran IR, Tufo G, Pervaiz S, Brenner C. Recent advances in apoptosis, mitochondria and drug resistance in cancer cells. Biochimica et Biophysica Acta (BBA) – Bioenergetics. 2011 Jun;**1807**(6):735-745

[73] Yang SY, Sales KM, Fuller B, Seifalian AM, Winslet MC. Apoptosis and colorectal cancer: Implications for therapy. Trends in Molecular Medicine. 2009 May;**15**(5):225-233

[74] Gourdier I, Del Rio M, Crabbé L, Candeil L, Copois V, Ychou M, et al. Drug specific resistance to oxaliplatin is associated with apoptosis defect in a cellular model of colon carcinoma. FEBS Letters. 2002 Oct 9;**529**(2-3):232-236

[75] Li F, Sethi G. Targeting transcription factor NF-κB to overcome chemoresistance and radioresistance in cancer therapy. Biochimica et Biophysica Acta (BBA) – Reviews on Cancer. 2010 Apr;**1805**(2):167-180

[76] Fukuyama R, Ng KP, Cicek M, Kelleher C, Niculaita R, Casey G, et al. Role of IKK and oscillatory NFκB kinetics in MMP-9 gene expression and chemoresistance to 5-fluorouracil in RKO colorectal cancer cells. Molecular Carcinogenesis. 2007 May;**46**(5):402-413

[77] Jani TS, DeVecchio J, Mazumdar T, Agyeman A, Houghton JA. Inhibition of NF-κB signaling by quinacrine is cytotoxic to human colon carcinoma cell lines and is synergistic

in combination with tumor necrosis factor-related apoptosis-inducing ligand (TRAIL) or oxaliplatin. The Journal of Biological Chemistry. 2010 Jun 18;**285**(25):19162-19172

[78] Garcia MA, Carrasco E, Aguilera M, Alvarez P, Rivas C, Campos JM, et al. The chemotherapeutic drug 5-fluorouracil promotes PKR-mediated apoptosis in a p53- independent manner in colon and breast cancer cells. Ulasov I, editor. PLoS One 2011 Aug 24;**6**(8):e23887

[79] Liu S, Wang J, Niu W, Liu E, Wang J, Peng C, et al. The β6-integrin-ERK/MAP kinase pathway contributes to chemo resistance in colon cancer. Cancer Letters. 2013 Jan 28;**328**(2): 325-334

[80] Christofk HR, Vander Heiden MG, Harris MH, Ramanathan A, Gerszten RE, Wei R, et al. The M2 splice isoform of pyruvate kinase is important for cancer metabolism and tumour growth. Nature. 2008 Mar 13;**452**(7184):230-233

[81] Derdak Z, Mark NM, Beldi G, Robson SC, Wands JR, Baffy G. The mitochondrial uncoupling protein-2 promotes chemoresistance in cancer cells. Cancer Research. 2008 Apr 15;**68**(8):2813-2819

[82] Bensinger SJ, Christofk HR. New aspects of the Warburg effect in cancer cell biology. Seminars in Cell & Developmental Biology. 2012 Jun;**23**(4):352-361

[83] Ayyasamy V, Owens KM, Desouki MM, Liang P, Bakin A, Thangaraj K, et al. Cellular model of Warburg effect identifies tumor promoting function of UCP2 in breast cancer and its suppression by genipin. Lewin A, editor. PLoS One 2011 Sep 15;**6**(9):e24792

[84] Warburg O, Wind F, Negelein E. The metabolism of tumors in the body. The Journal of General Physiology. 1927 Mar 7;**8**(6):519-530

[85] Tong X, Zhao F, Mancuso A, Gruber JJ, Thompson CB. The glucose-responsive transcription factor ChREBP contributes to glucose-dependent anabolic synthesis and cell proliferation. Proceedings of the National Academy of Sciences. 2009 Dec 22;**106**(51): 21660-21665

[86] Pelicano H, Martin DS, R-H X, Huang P. Glycolysis inhibition for anticancer treatment. Oncogene. 2006 Aug 7;**25**(34):4633-4646

[87] Erler JT, Cawthorne CJ, Williams KJ, Koritzinsky M, Wouters BG, Wilson C, et al. Hypoxia-mediated down-regulation of Bid and Bax in tumors occurs via hypoxia-inducible factor 1-dependent and -independent mechanisms and contributes to drug resistance. Molecular and Cellular Biology. 2004 Apr;**24**(7):2875-2889

[88] Kuai X-Y, Ji Z-Y, Zhang H-J. Mitochondrial uncoupling protein 2 expression in colon cancer and its clinical significance. World Journal of Gastroenterology. 2010 Dec 7;**16**(45): 5773-5778

[89] Rousset S, Mozo J, Dujardin G, Emre Y, Masscheleyn S, Ricquier D, et al. UCP2 is a mitochondrial transporter with an unusual very short half-life. FEBS Letters. 2007 Feb 6;**581**(3):479-482

[90] Arsenijevic D, Onuma H, Pecqueur C, Raimbault S, Manning BS, Miroux B, et al. Disruption of the uncoupling protein-2 gene in mice reveals a role in immunity and reactive oxygen species production. Nature Genetics. 2000 Dec 1;**26**(4):435-439

[91]   Horimoto M, Resnick MB, Konkin TA, Routhier J, Wands JR, Baffy G. Expression of uncou-
       pling protein-2 in human colon cancer. Clinical Cancer Research. 2004 Sep 15;**10**(18):
       6203-6207

[92]   Sánchez-Aragó M, Cuezva JM. The bioenergetic signature of isogenic colon cancer cells
       predicts the cell death response to treatment with 3-bromopyruvate, iodoacetate or
       5-fluorouracil. Journal of Translational Medicine. 2011 Feb 8;**9**:19

[93]   Ward C, Langdon SP, Mullen P, Harris AL, Harrison DJ, Supuran CT, et al. New strat-
       egies for targeting the hypoxic tumour microenvironment in breast cancer. Cancer
       Treatment Reviews. 2013 Apr;**39**(2):171-179

[94]   Bristow RG, Hill RP. Hypoxia and metabolism: Hypoxia, DNA repair and genetic insta-
       bility. Nature Reviews. Cancer. 2008 Mar;**8**(3):180-192

[95]   Zhang J, Roberts TM, Shivdasani RA. Targeting PI3K signaling as a therapeutic
       approach for colorectal cancer. Gastroenterology. 2011 Jul;**141**(1):50-61

[96]   Semenza GL. Targeting HIF-1 for cancer therapy. Nature Reviews. Cancer. 2003 Oct;
       3(10):721-732

[97]   Pritchard CC, Grady WM. Colorectal cancer molecular biology moves into clinical
       practice. Gut. 2011 Jan 1;**60**(1):116-129

[98]   Papageorgis P, Cheng K, Ozturk S, Gong Y, Lambert AW, Abdolmaleky HM, et al.
       Smad4 inactivation promotes malignancy and drug resistance of colon cancer. Cancer
       Research. 2011 Feb 1;**71**(3):998-1008

[99]   Sosa V, Moliné T, Somoza R, Paciucci R, Kondoh H, LLeonart ME. Oxidative stress and
       cancer: An overview. Ageing Research Reviews. 2013 Jan;**12**(1):376-390

[100] Tamada M, Nagano O, Tateyama S, Ohmura M, Yae T, Ishimoto T, et al. Modulation of
       glucose metabolism by CD44 contributes to antioxidant status and drug resistance in
       cancer cells. Cancer Research. 2012 Mar 15;**72**(6):1438-1448

[101] Greaves M, Maley CC. Clonal evolution in cancer. Nature. 2012 Jan 18;**481**(7381):306-313

[102] Gillies RJ, Verduzco D, Gatenby RA. Evolutionary dynamics of carcinogenesis and why
       targeted therapy does not work. Nature Reviews. Cancer. 2012 Jun 14;**12**(7):487-493

[103] Diaz Jr LA, Williams RT, Wu J, Kinde I, Hecht JR, Berlin J, et al. The molecular evolution
       of acquired resistance to targeted EGFR blockade in colorectal cancers. Nature 2012 Jun
       13;**486**(7404):537-540

[104] Longley DB, Allen WL, Johnston PG. Drug resistance, predictive markers and phar-
       macogenomics in colorectal cancer. Biochimica et Biophysica Acta (BBA) – Reviews on
       Cancer. 2006 Dec;**1766**(2):184-196

[105] Tentes IK, Schmidt WM, Krupitza G, Steger GG, Mikulits W, Kortsaris A, et al. Long-
       term persistence of acquired resistance to 5-fluorouracil in the colon cancer cell line
       SW620. Experimental Cell Research. 2010 Nov;**316**(19):3172-3181

[106] Gerlinger M, Rowan AJ, Horswell S, Larkin J, Endesfelder D, Gronroos E, et al. Intratumor Heterogeneity and Branched Evolution Revealed by Multiregion Sequencing. The New England Journal of Medicine. 2012 Mar 8;**366**(10):883-892

[107] Marusyk A, Polyak K. Tumor heterogeneity: Causes and consequences. Biochimica et Biophysica Acta (BBA) – Reviews on Cancer. 2010 Jan;**1805**(1):105-117

[108] McGranahan N, Burrell RA, Endesfelder D, Novelli MR, Swanton C. Cancer chromosomal instability: Therapeutic and diagnostic challenges. EMBO Reports. 2012 May 18;**13**(6):528-538

[109] Barratt PL, Seymour MT, Stenning SP, Georgiades I, Walker C, Birbeck K, et al. DNA markers predicting benefit from adjuvant fluorouracil in patients with colon cancer: A molecular study. Lancet (London, England). 2002 Nov 2;**360**(9343):1381-1391

[110] Marusyk A, Almendro V, Polyak K. Intra-tumour heterogeneity: A looking glass for cancer? Nature Reviews. Cancer. 2012 Apr 19;**12**(5):323-334

[111] Urbach D, Lupien M, Karagas MR, Moore JH. Cancer heterogeneity: Origins and implications for genetic association studies. Trends in Genetics. 2012 Nov;**28**(11):538-543

[112] Crea F, Nobili S, Paolicchi E, Perrone G, Napoli C, Landini I, et al. Epigenetics and chemoresistance in colorectal cancer: An opportunity for treatment tailoring and novel therapeutic strategies. Drug Resistance Updates. 2011 Dec;**14**(6):280-296

[113] Kelly TK, De Carvalho DD, Jones PA. Epigenetic modifications as therapeutic targets. Nature Biotechnology. 2010 Oct 13;**28**(10):1069-1078

[114] Jeggo PA, L?brich M. Contribution of DNA repair and cell cycle checkpoint arrest to the maintenance of genomic stability. DNA Repair (Amst). 2006 Sep 8;**5**(9-10):1192-1198

[115] Lahtz C, Pfeifer GP. Epigenetic changes of DNA repair genes in cancer. Journal of Molecular Cell Biology. 2011 Feb;**3**(1):51-58

[116] Wilting RH, Dannenberg J-H. Epigenetic mechanisms in tumorigenesis, tumor cell heterogeneity and drug resistance. Drug Resistance Updates. 2012 Feb;**15**(1-2):21-38

[117] Feinberg AP, Ohlsson R, Henikoff S. The epigenetic progenitor origin of human cancer. Nature Reviews. Genetics. 2006 Jan 1;**7**(1):21-33

[118] Sugita H, Iida S, Inokuchi M, Kato K, Ishiguro M, Ishikawa T, et al. Methylation of BNIP3 and DAPK indicates lower response to chemotherapy and poor prognosis in gastric cancer. Oncology Reports. 2011 Feb 1;**25**(2):513-518

[119] Shimizu S, Iida S, Ishiguro M, Uetake H, Ishikawa T, Takagi Y, et al. Methylated BNIP3 gene in colorectal cancer prognosis. Oncology Letters. 2010 Sep 1;**1**(5):865-872

[120] Crea F, Giovannetti E, Cortesi F, Mey V, Nannizzi S, Gallegos Ruiz MI, et al. Epigenetic mechanisms of irinotecan sensitivity in colorectal cancer cell lines. Molecular Cancer Therapeutics. 2009 Jul 1;**8**(7):1964-1973

[121] Cheetham S, Tang MJ, Mesak F, Kennecke H, Owen D, Tai IT. SPARC promoter hypermethylation in colorectal cancers can be reversed by 5-Aza-2′deoxycytidine to increase

SPARC expression and improve therapy response. British Journal of Cancer. 2008 Jun 3;**98**(11):1810-1819

[122] Tai IT, Dai M, Owen DA, Chen LB. Genome-wide expression analysis of therapy-resistant tumors reveals SPARC as a novel target for cancer therapy. The Journal of Clinical Investigation. 2005 Jun;**115**(6):1492-1502

[123] Sharma SV, Lee DY, Li B, Quinlan MP, Takahashi F, Maheswaran S, et al. A chromatin-mediated reversible drug-tolerant state in cancer cell subpopulations. Cell. 2010 Apr 2;**141**(1):69-80

[124] Spitzner M, Emons G, Kramer F, Gaedcke J, Rave-Frank M, Scharf J-G, et al. A gene expression signature for chemoradiosensitivity of colorectal cancer cells. International Journal of Radiation Oncology. 2010 Nov 15;**78**(4):1184-1192

[125] Dallas NA, Xia L, Fan F, Gray MJ, Gaur P, van Buren G, et al. Chemoresistant colorectal cancer cells, the cancer stem cell phenotype, and increased sensitivity to insulin-like growth factor-I receptor inhibition. Cancer Research. March 1 2009;**69**(5):1951-1957

[126] Tsunekuni K, Konno M, Asai A, Koseki J, Kobunai T, Takechi T, et al. MicroRNA profiles involved in trifluridine resistance. Oncotarget. 2017;**8**:53017-53027

[127] Wheeler DL, Huang S, Kruser TJ, Nechrebecki MM, Armstrong EA, Benavente S, et al. Mechanisms of acquired resistance to cetuximab: Role of HER (ErbB) family members. Oncogene. 2008 Jun 26;**27**(28):3944-3956

[128] Kyula JN, Van Schaeybroeck S, Doherty J, Fenning CS, Longley DB, Johnston PG. Chemotherapy-induced activation of ADAM-17: A novel mechanism of drug resistance in colorectal cancer. Clinical Cancer Research. 2010 Jul 1;**16**(13):3378-3389

[129] Goulielmaki M, Koustas E, Moysidou E, Vlassi M, Sasazuki T, Shirasawa S, et al. BRAF associated autophagy exploitation: BRAF and autophagy inhibitors synergise to efficiently overcome resistance of BRAF mutant colorectal cancer cells. Oncotarget. 2016 Feb 22;**7**(8):9188-9221

[130] Lipinska N, Romaniuk A, Paszel-Jaworska A, Toton E, Kopczynski P, Rubis B. Telomerase and drug resistance in cancer. Cellular and Molecular Life Sciences. 2017 Jun;**16**:1-12

[131] CASYM Europe. CASyM and the Road to Systems Medicine [Internet]. Available from: https://www.casym.eu/casym-systems-medicine [Accessed Jul 21, 2017]

[132] Dienstmann R, Vermeulen L, Guinney J, Kopetz S, Tejpar S, Tabernero J. Consensus molecular subtypes and the evolution of precision medicine in colorectal cancer. Nature Reviews. Cancer. 2017 Jan 4;**17**(2):79-92

[133] Prager G, Mader RM, Wrba F, Zielinski C. The EXACT trial: An individualized treatment protocol for solid tumors. Journal of Clinical Oncology. 2014 May 20;**32**(15 Suppl):e14002-e14002

3

Building up the Future of Colonoscopy – A Synergy between Clinicians and Computer Scientists

Jorge Bernal, F. Javier Sánchez, Cristina Rodríguez de Miguel and Gloria Fernández-Esparrach

Abstract

Recent advances in endoscopic technology have generated an increasing interest in strengthening the collaboration between clinicians and computers scientist to develop intelligent systems that can provide additional information to clinicians in the different stages of an intervention. The objective of this chapter is to identify clinical drawbacks of colonoscopy in order to define potential areas of collaboration. Once areas are defined, we present the challenges that colonoscopy images present in order computational methods to provide with meaningful output, including those related to image formation and acquisition, as they are proven to have an impact in the performance of an intelligent system. Finally, we also propose how to define validation frameworks in order to assess the performance of a given method, making an special emphasis on how databases should be created and annotated and which metrics should be used to evaluate systems correctly.

Keywords: Intelligent systems, Image properties, Validation, Clinical drawbacks, Endoluminal scene description

1. Introduction

1.1. Motivation

During the last few years there has been an increasing effort in exploring the use of intelligent systems to assist and provide additional information to clinicians in the different stages of an intervention. In this context, we can find in the literature systems aiming at assisting the clinician in in-vivo diagnosis such as KARDIO proposed in [1], which can automatically analyze electrocardiograms, or methods that provide with data to help in the detection and diagnosis of breast [2] or prostate cancer [3]. The spread use of Computed Tomography has elicited a new set of methods that help clinicians in intervention planning as exposed in [4]. For instance, we can find systems which allow clinicians to follow the fastest and safest way to target a pulmonary lesion [5], perform laparoscopic surgery [6] or systems such as [7] in the domain of transcatheter aortic valve implantations. However, there is scarce experience with intelligent systems applied to endoscopy where there are only a few methods such as the works presented in [8] in the context of colonoscopy quality assessment which analyzes how clinical procedures have been performed to provide quality scores.

Endoscopic technology has rapidly evolved in the last decade and current equipment allows clinicians to observe the whole endoluminal scene in high definition and, moreover, makes it possible to get different views of the same scene for further analysis by applying automatic techniques of chromoendoscopy [9] as narrow band imaging (NBI) –proposed in [10]-, the Fujinon Intelligent Chromo-Endoscopy (FICE) presented in [11] or Pentax I-scan, which was published in [12]. These advances in endoscopy imaging have generated an increasing interest in strengthening partnerships between clinicians and computer scientists to build applications that can solve some of the challenges that colonoscopy procedures still present nowadays.

It is clear that this potential collaboration between these two domains of knowledge needs from each part to acknowledge the challenges that the analysis of colonoscopy images present related to their area of expertise. Related to this, clinicians need to identify which of the existing drawbacks could be mitigated with the aid of image processing tools and computer scientists must define clearly what can be achieved by means of image processing to provide clinicians with feasible and clinically applicable solutions. Endoscopy imaging analysis present some challenges that are not limited to the ones that the characterization of anatomical structures for detection or diagnosis purposes present; aspects that are rarely covered by existing methods such as image acquisition and formation should be considered as they are proven to have an impact on the output of a given method [13].

Considering this, the focus of this chapter is to present new advances on computer vision methods for colonoscopy and to identify potential clinical issues that may be solved with the aid of computer vision. As it can be observed, this chapter is not written from either a pure clinical or technical point of view but as a way to couple the necessities and challenges of each of the domains in order to build up feasible and clinically applicable systems.

2. Introduction to colonoscopy challenges

2.1. A brief history of endoscopy

The history of endoscopy, as stated in [14], starts in 1805 with P. Bozzini and his attempts to construct a cystoscope (See Table 1). Although this first endoscope was considered as having failed, the principles incorporated in its design - a light source, a reflective surface (lens) and a series of specula (mirrors)- are the basis of current endoscopes. The technical challenges posed since then have been overcome with the collaboration of physicians, engineers, scientists and optical experts among others. The progress has been slow but constant and initially rigid instruments have been changed by flexible endoscopes; candles and lamps have been replaced by electric filaments and, for vision, single lenses have been supplanted by optic fibers.

Year	Authorship	Development
1805	Philipp Bozzini (Physician)	Design of the first endoscope (Lichtleiter). Illumination is provided by candles.
1825	Pierre Solomon Ségalas (Urologist)	Design of an urethro-cystic speculum that incorporates mirrors for projecting light along the tube.
1827	John D. Fisher (Physician)	Development of a cystoscope. His principal innovation is the inclusion of a double convex lens to amplify the image.
1853	Antonin Jean Desormeaux (Urologist)	Demonstration of the first functional endoscope (cystoscope). Candles are replaced by mixture of alcohol and turpentine for illumination.
1865	Francis Richard Cruise (Urologist)	Improvement of the illumination using camphor and petrol and redesigns the lens and lamp system.
1867	Julius Brück (Dentist)	Design of an unusual instrument that uses a lamp lit by electric current.
1868	Adolf Kussmaul (Surgeon)	Attempt at the creation of the first gastroscopy using a rigid instrument based upon sword swallowers.
1870	Gustav Trouvé (Engineer)	Construction of the first electrical endoscopic instrument with optical system: the polyscope (mostly for laryngeal observations).
1877	Max Nitze (Urologist) Fritz Leiter (Manufacturer)	Development the first effective rigid endoscope that incorporates an optical system and an incandescent platinum wire lamp at the end of the cystoscope.
1880	David Newman (Surgeon)	Incorporation of the Edison incandescent lamp into a cystoscope.
1881	Johann Von Mikulicz (Surgeon) Fritz Leiter (Manufacturer)	Development the first practical and functional esophagoscope.
1894	Howard A. Kelly (Gynecologist)	Introduction the first long (30 cm) rigid rectosigmodoscope.
1911	Michael Hoffmann (Physician)	Proposal of a solution to the problem of bending light using multiple prisms and lenses and applies this concept to gastroscopy. This is the first attempt to construct a flexible gastroscope.
1911	Hans Elsner (Physician)	Construction of the first rigid gastroscope.
1922	Rudolf Schindler (Gastroenterologist)	Building of the second rigid gastroscope
1930	Heinrich Lamm (Medical student)	Images are successfully transmitted through glass fibers.

Year	Authorship	Development
1932	Rudolf Schindler (Gastroenterologist) Georg Wolf (Manufacturer)	Development of the first semiflexible gastroscope. Schindler is considered the founder of modern endoscopy.
1940	Cameron Surgical Co.	The first flexible gastroscope is made in the USA: the *Cameron Schindler Endoscope*.
1948	Edward B. Benedict (Surgeon)	Development of the operating gastroscope by incorporating both a biopsy forceps and a suction tube within the gastroscope itself.
1948	Harry Segal (Physician) James Watson (Physician)	Production of a viable endoscopic photographic system.
1952	Tatsuno Uji (Engineer)	Design of a miniature gastrocamera that can be introduced into the stomach.
1957	Basil Hirschowitz (Gastroenterologist) Larry Curtiss (Physicist)	Introduction of the first fiber optic gastroscope.
1960	Machida Endoscope Co. Olympus Optical Co.	Development of the first prototypes of flexible colonoscopes.
1971	William I. Wolff (Surgeon) Hiromi Shinya (Surgeon)	Performance of the first polypectomy with a wire loop snare.
1975	Masahiro Tada (Gastroenterologist)	Description of the first magnifying colonoscope.
1983	Welch Allyn Inc.	Development of an electronic sensor or charge coupled device that is inserted at the tip of the endoscope.
2002	Olympus Co.	HD endoscopes

Table 1. Evolution of endoscopy as a result of collaboration of different disciplines

Shortly after having successfully traversed the esophagus and reached the stomach, the assessment of the duodenum, small intestine and colon were the next steps that were progressively addressed and achieved. Other needs were also identified and solved: first, the evolution from diagnostic to operating endoscopes that allowed obtaining biopsies; second, the need of preserving the image of the lesion which was observed. The latter not only reflected clinical needs but also documentation and educational requirements. At that point, several corporations became involved in the development of endoscopic instrumentation and they also designed cameras specifically for endoscopic usage.

Once the fiber optic endoscope was established as a reality by late 1960s, numerous design modifications were performed with the collaboration of physicians in order to augment the utility of the device and increase its resolution. The decade of 1970 witnessed a series of rapid technological advances where a number of instrumental manufactures including ACMI, Olympus Optical Company and Machida Endoscope Company included a variety of innovations (length, flexibility, channel size...) that improved the performance of the instrument. In 1983 video endoscopy was introduced as the logical consequence of technical advances in microelectronics and all current endoscopes are based on this technology. Video endoscopy allows an easy exploration, instant image acquisition and further storage confirming its utility not only for clinical practice but also for educational purposes.

2.2. High definition endoscopy (The quality of image matters)

In the last years, most of the developments in endoscopy have been focused on improving the quality of images, as it is the case of high definition (HD) endoscopes that use a 1080-line television and a high resolution charge coupled device with up to 1.3 million pixels. This allows the acquisition and storage of images with double the resolution of normal television. Other capabilities available in some endoscopes are the following:

- Wide angle: the endoscope has a field of vision of 170º (30% more than the conventional model) that is supposed to improve the detection of lesions hidden behind the folds;

- Electronic zoom: that achieves a ×80–100 maximum effect;

- Narrow band imaging (NBI): a modification in the light beam enhances visualization of the network of the mucosa providing contrast and acting as a substitute of chromoendoscopy. This system offers the possibility to switch from conventional white light to blue NBI light alternatively (see Fig.1).

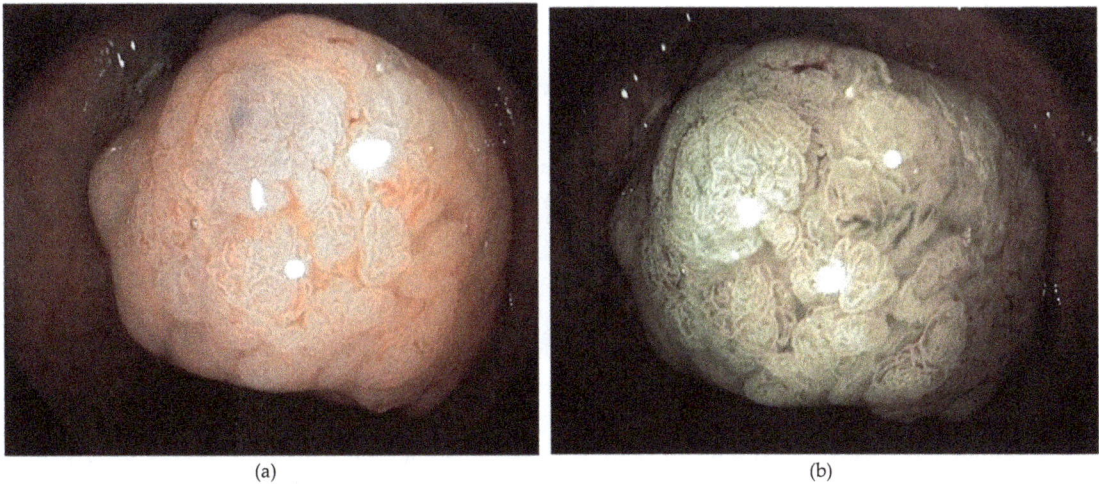

(a)　　　　　　　　　　　　　　　　　　　　(b)

Figure 1. Example of a same polyp observed with white light (a) and NBI (b).

HD endoscopes (particularly those with magnification function) facilitate the demonstration of the mucosal architectural and vascular patterns that are altered in dysplastic lesions as it can be observed in Fig.2. With regards to the detection rate of lesions, although it is logical to assume that a higher resolution endoscope could provide better results, the results of several studies [15, 16] do not support this hypothesis.

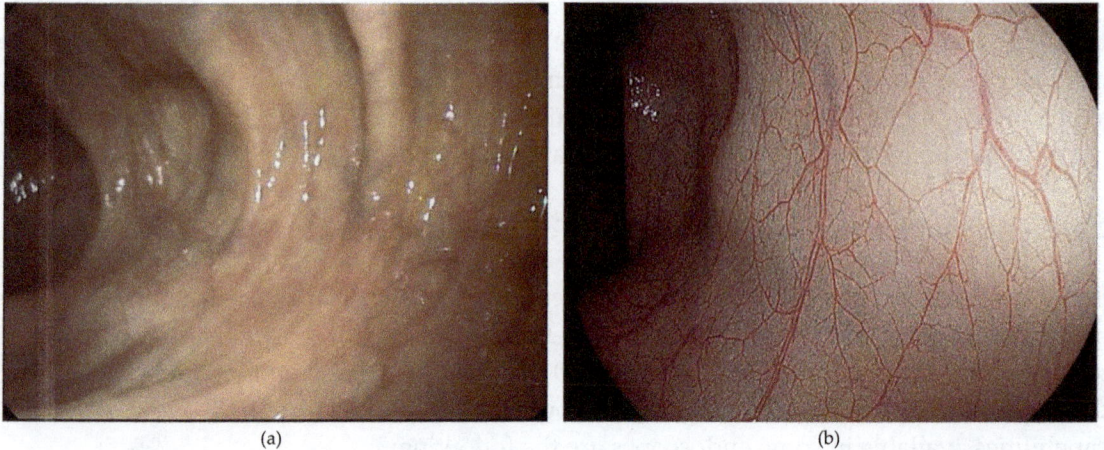

(a)   (b)

Figure 2. Example of a colonoscopy frame observed with conventional endoscope (a) and with high definition endoscope (b).

2.3. The problem of colonic polyps

Colorectal cancer (CRC) is a serious health problem in the general population and it is considered that at least two thirds of CRC develop through the adenoma–carcinoma pathway. Consequently, screening with colonoscopy for CRC and its precursor lesion has become an increasingly practice, as shown in [17]. Several actions have been proposed to optimize colonoscopy such as ensuring colon perfect preparation and carrying out a thorough examination of the mucosa which would imply a longer withdrawal inspection time, as indicated in [18].

However, colonoscopy still presents some drawbacks being the most relevant the polyp miss-rate -reported to be as high as 22%- resulting in a lack of total effectiveness [19]. The rate of polyps missed increases significantly in smaller sized polyps (2% for adenomas ≥ 10 mm versus 26% for adenomas < 5 mm) and this has a clinical impact, not only because the prevalence of high-grade dysplasia increases with the size as exposed in [20] but because of the risk of having an interval cancer. Interval colorectal cancers are described as cancers occurring after a negative screening test or examination and they are an important indicator of the quality and effectiveness of CRC screening and surveillance, as stated in [21].

The diagnosis of dysplasia has practical consequences on the management of polyps. There is general consensus on removing all polyps detected during colonoscopy but size is a limiting factor for endoscopic polypectomy. Therefore, having a histological diagnostic of presumption is very useful in order to make the decision of performing or not a polypectomy. In this regard, there are several classifications (NICE, Kudo…) that predict the histology of the lesion based on the characteristics of the image. Kudo [22] proposes a gross classification of pit patterns into 7 types: type I and II pit patterns are characteristic of non-neoplastic lesions such as normal mucosa or hyperplastic polyps whereas pattern types IIIS, IIIL, IV, and a subset of VI are intramucosal neoplastic lesions such as adenoma or intramucosal carcinoma and lesions with a type VN pattern and a subset of type VI suggest deep invasive carcinoma (see Fig. 3).

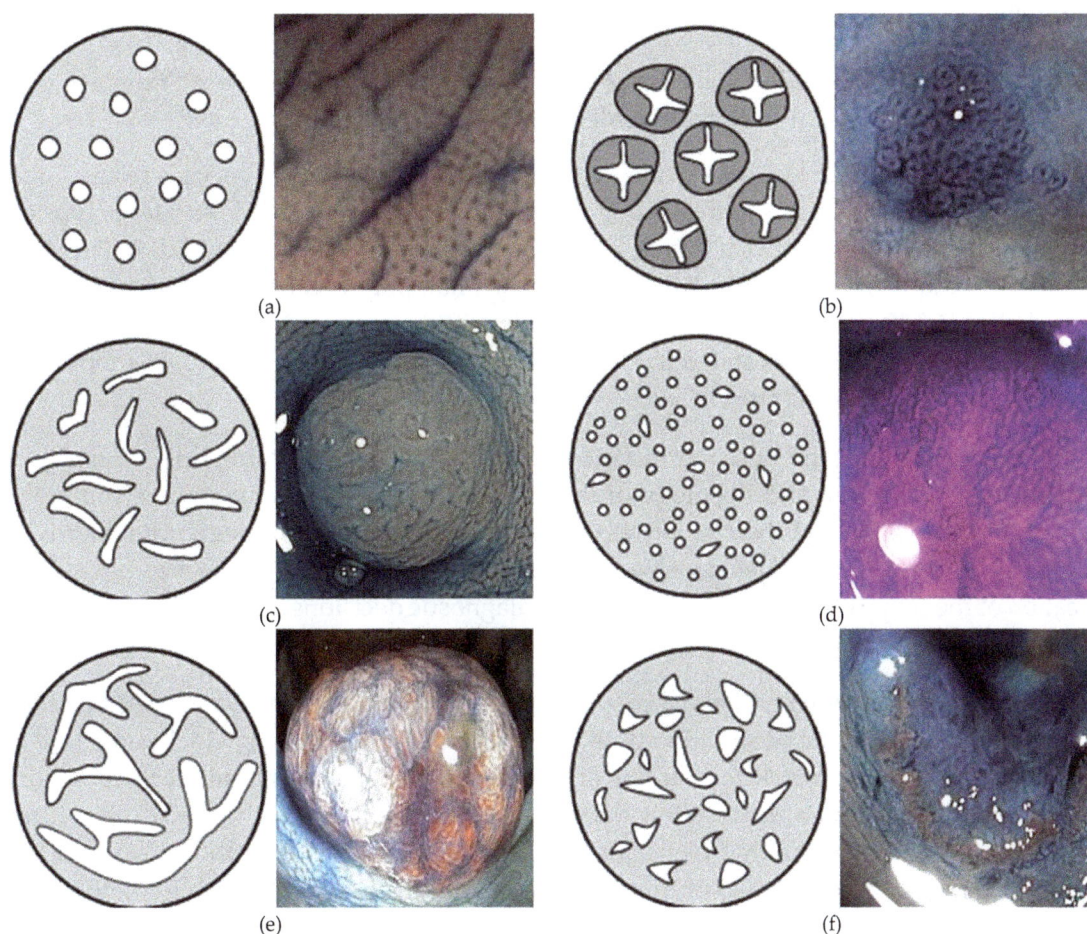

Figure 3. Examples of Kudo neoplastic lesion classification: (a) Type I; (b) Type II; (c) Type IIIL; (d) Type IIIS; (e) Type IV and (f) Type V.

As this classification applies for magnification endoscopy, when it is used with conventional endoscopy the results are worse. Contrarily, NICE is an international classification of colorectal tumors on the basis of NBI observation either with or without use of a magnifying endoscope [23]. NICE is a simple categorical classification defining three different types based on three characteristics: (i) lesion color; (ii) micro vascular architecture; and (iii) surface pattern. Type 1 is considered an index for hyperplastic lesions, type 2 an index for adenoma or mucosal/submucosal scanty invasive carcinoma, and type 3 an index for deeply submucosal-invasive carcinoma The problem with these classifications is that diagnostic derives from a subjective visual analysis and requires specific training and a high degree of experience.

Finally, the precise location of the polyps is another meaningful drawback of colonoscopy, not only when planning a surgery but also during successive colonoscopies. This limitation is especially remarkable in the presence of several polyps. In this case, an exhaustive analysis of the surface and boundaries of the polyp could be very helpful.

2.4. Identification of potential collaborative research areas between clinicians and computer scientists

Considering the mentioned drawbacks of colonoscopy, three potential areas in which computer science may play a role have been identified:

- Automatic polyp detection and localization: one of the exposed drawbacks is related to the difficulty on detecting certain types of polyps such as small or flat lesions. Flat polyps can be detected with the support of CT [24, 25] although its detection supposes additional patient radiation and is limited by the size. Detection of small polyps cannot be undertaken with the help of CT as the current available resolution makes it impossible to detect polyps with size smaller than 10 mm as stated in [26], therefore the diagnosis in these cases should only rely on endoscopic exploration.

- Polyp classification: the decision of performing polypectomy is commonly taken by an estimation of the size and histology of the detected lesion. This estimation is commonly made by means of visual observation and therefore incorporates some degree of subjectivity. In this context, a system that can objectively provide an estimation of the size and classification of the polyp could allow taking in-vivo diagnostic decisions and this would optimize the treatment timing.

- Patients lesion follow-up and endoscopy navigation: there is a necessity expressed by some clinicians regarding the recognition of the area that a lesion occupies, which can be useful for two different reasons: 1) for the case of polyps that have not been removed, an univocal recognition of the lesion would allow the study of the evolution of the lesion; 2) an accurate recognition of the marks that clinicians leave to identify the area of the polyp once it is removed would allow the exploration of areas nearby the lesion to search for new pathologies.

3. Image processing challenges for the analysis of colonoscopy videos

In order to provide clinicians with meaningful applications, the content of colonoscopy videos and frames must be thoroughly analyzed by computer scientists to search for lesions or indicators defined by clinicians. In this context, the majority of the literature has been focused on developing methods to characterize accurately the different elements of the endoluminal scene, paying special attention to polyps. Although it is clear that anatomical landmarks recognition is essential for application development, the acquisition and generation of high quality images is also crucial for computer vision methods in order to work as they are intended. For instance, the presence of image artifacts has been proven to have an impact in the performance of polyp localization methods, as shown in [13].

Considering this we present in this section a summary of the most important challenges that a given computer vision method must face in order to provide with efficient support to clinicians. We have divided the challenges in two groups: those related to image acquisition and formation and those related to the characterization of anatomical structures needed to build up the clinicians' support system.

3.1. Identification of endoscopy image particularities with impact in image processing analysis

Videos that endoscopes generate are created following common television standards in a way such they can provide with sufficiently moving image quality while allowing for efficient resource management in case endoscopy images and videos are stored for later inspection. It is important to mention that quality in this case is understood under human's observer point of view but not under computer visions; for instance there are some image processing techniques automatically performed – i.e. sharpening - that may improve how images are observed but, as they modify the original image, they create new elements that affect an automatic analysis by means of computer vision methods. Some of the features that can affect the performance of a computer vision method are listed below and in table 2:

- *Illumination effects:* The way colonoscope illuminates the scene produces an axial illumination which tends to generate *specular highlights* on shiny surfaces such as the mucosa. Mucosa is covered by a thin watery film which generates many specular highlights when it is illuminated in a perpendicular direction to its surface. Specular highlights position will vary with little movements of the colonoscope which will change the angle at which mucosa is illuminated therefore areas of the mucosa affected by specularities will change rapidly. The presence of specular highlights difficult strongly image processing [13] as they appear as very prominent structures which also hinder color and texture information about the surfaces in which they appear. Moreover, axial illumination introduces also an additional side-effect regarding its *lack of uniformity* in the way structures are illuminated: structures closer to the endoscope will appear brighter than others far from the endoscope (see Fig. 4).

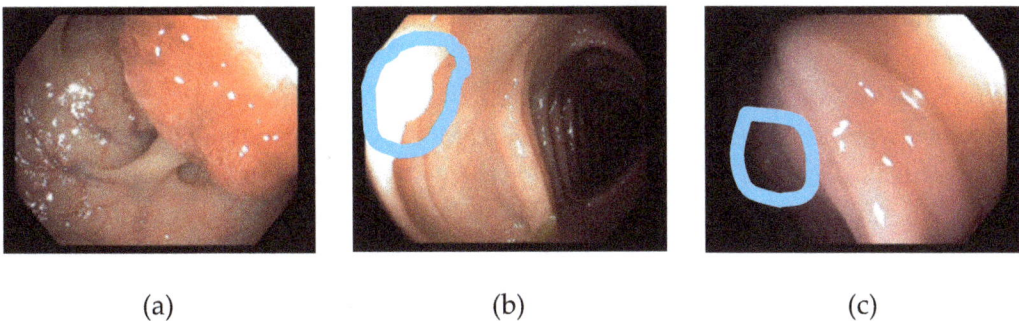

| (a) | (b) | (c) |

Figure 4. Examples of illumination effects: (a) specular highlights (b) overexposed polyp and (c) underexposed polyp. Polyps in images b and c are delimited with a blue mask to ease visualization.

- *Sensor acquisition effects: Color phantoms* appear due to temporal misalignment of color channels related to some endoscopes that still use monochrome sensors. In this case, color information is generated by illuminating the scene with the three primary colors (red, green and blue) successively. Consequently, three different images are needed to generate a color image. This process introduces some undesired side-effects associated to camera movement: as we acquire the images in different time instants, specular highlights generated by the light source in each of the three moments will be located in slightly different positions, causing instability in the final color image –Fig. 5(a).

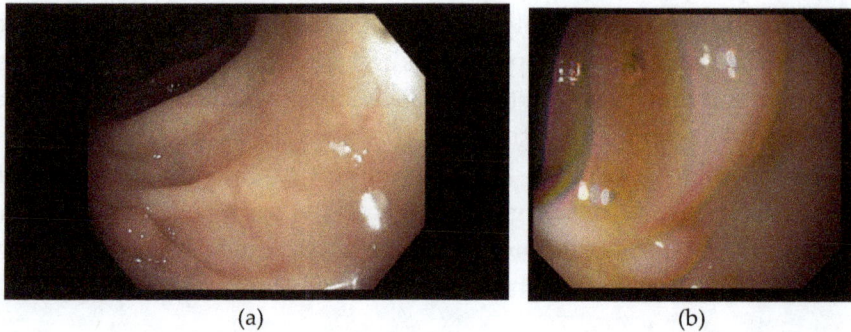

(a)   (b)

Figure 5. Effect of channel misalignment due to monochrome sensors: instability in specular highlights position (a) and apparition of color phantoms (b).

Moreover, as each color channel is acquired in different times, the three components (red, green and blue) will not be exactly aligned if the endoscope moves when the image is acquired. This lack of color channel alignment generates artificial color bands in the contours of the structures –Fig. 5(b) - that appear in the image which limits the performance of any color information-based structure characterization method.

- *Image resolution:* Commercial endoscopes generate videos in formats following television standards (PAL for Europe, NTSC for America and Japan). These formats are meant to generate motion images with enough quality to be observed by the general public but also minimizing the size of the information to be transmitted. By acting this way, videos generated by commercial endoscopes can be played in any standard system (TV, personal computers) without needing format conversion. Moreover, the minimization of the amount of transmitted information allows a reduction of the storage needs which is crucial in clinical settings where the amount of resources dedicated to information storage must be efficiently distributed.

Although the use of standard formats presents clear advantages for visualization and storage purposes, it does not benefit image processing by means of computer vision. Video standards offer images with lower resolution than the one that can be achieved by means of commercial cameras. For instance, NTSC standard provides as output 0.3 Megapixels images, HD standard offers images up to 2 Megapixels and a commercial camera easily exceeds 10 Megapixels [27]. Low resolution images lead to a loss of texture information associated to anatomical structures in the endoluminal scene, which can have an impact on the output of structure classification methods -Fig. 6-.

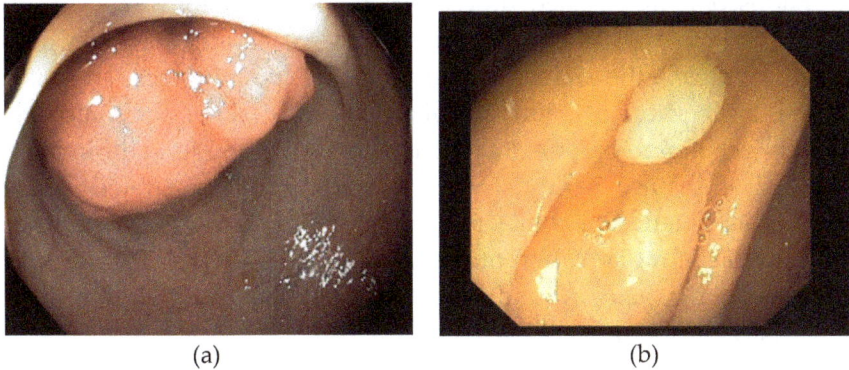

Figure 6. Different colonoscopy images acquired at different resolutions: (a) high resolution image and (b) low resolution image. We can observe greater texture details in the polyp from the highest resolution image.

- *Image interlacing:* As it has been mentioned before, from all available video standards those with lowest bandwidth –amount of information that needs to be transmitted-requirements are chosen for use in endoscopy. This reduction in bandwidth is achieved by interlacing image lines, which is performed by acquiring odd and even image lines in different time instants. By this we can double the image refresh rate without increasing the size of the information. This also makes video movement appear smoother and more continuous to the human eye but it has a counterpart that affects posterior image processing. The final image provided by the processor will be a mixture of two different images captured in different time instants: even lines will be from the first capture whereas odd lines will come from the second. As with color channel misalignment, interlacing impact will depend on the amount of endoscope movement between the two acquisitions. For instance, if camera moves horizontally we can observe sawtooth profiles in vertical contours, apart from change of position of specular highlights. We show in Fig. 7 a clear example on how interlacing can affect the quality of the image to be processed by, for instance, the apparition of double and shadowy contours surrounding the elements of the image.

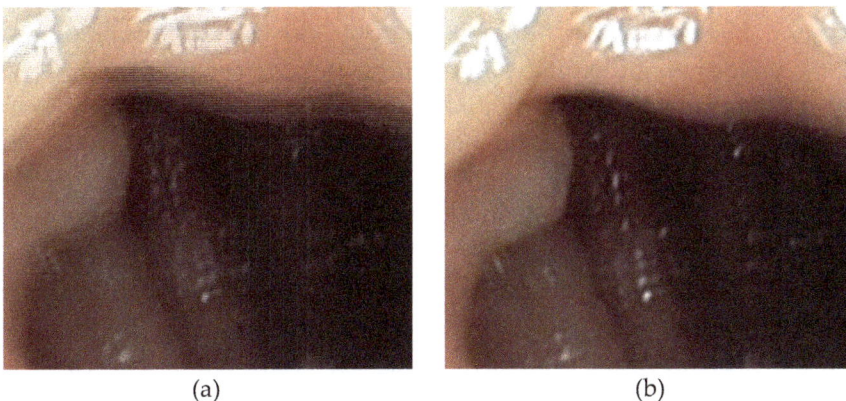

Figure 7. Impact of interlacing in image quality: (a) Interlaced image and (b) Separate field of an interlaced image.

- *Sharpening:* Endoscopes and video processors include functionalities that improve the quality of the image to be visualized by human observers, aiming to simplify the observation of particular structures in the images. One of the most common techniques is sharpening, which describes a subjective perception of sharpness related to edge contrast in an image. By applying this technique, contours that separate different objects in the image can be more clearly identified and consequently structures can be easily separated –Fig. 8 (b)-. This visualization enhancement [28] comes at a cost in terms of image processing as contour enhancement implies a modification of the original image which increases image noise. Sharpening also generate halos around structures that appear in the image such as specular highlights, as observed in Fig. 8 (b).

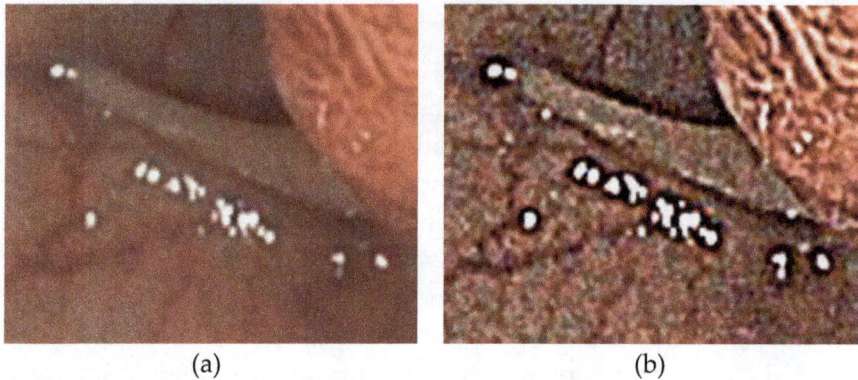

(a)   (b)

Figure 8. Examples of sharpening applied on colonoscopy images: (a) Original image and (b) image with sharpening applied.

- *Information overlay:* Video processors associated to endoscope do not present a specific output dedicated to its connection to a personal computer. Considering this, the image that the clinician is observing will be the same that will be stored for later processing. It is common that some information regarding the procedure such as patient information or procedure date is superimposed to the image provided by the colonoscope, as it can be observed in Fig. 9. The presence of this information precludes its use for research purposes, as this data should be anonymzed. Moreover the presence of this information superimposed to the original image may difficult the observation and characterization of structures in the images apart from introducing additional noise and elements (letters, numbers) to the image.

- *Black mask:* Endoscopes automatically add an octagonal or circular black mask surrounding the image acquired by the sensor. This mask covers those regions of the image that are strongly affected by geometric distortions introduced by wide angle optic used in endoscopes. These distortions, similar to fisheye effects present in some cameras, makes structures below the mask appear different to what they are in reality and consequently they should not be analyzed by clinicians. Unfortunately the presence of this black mask affects the performance of image processing methods, as the mask creates strong contours in the separation between the mask and the endoluminal scene, as it can be observed in Fig. 10.

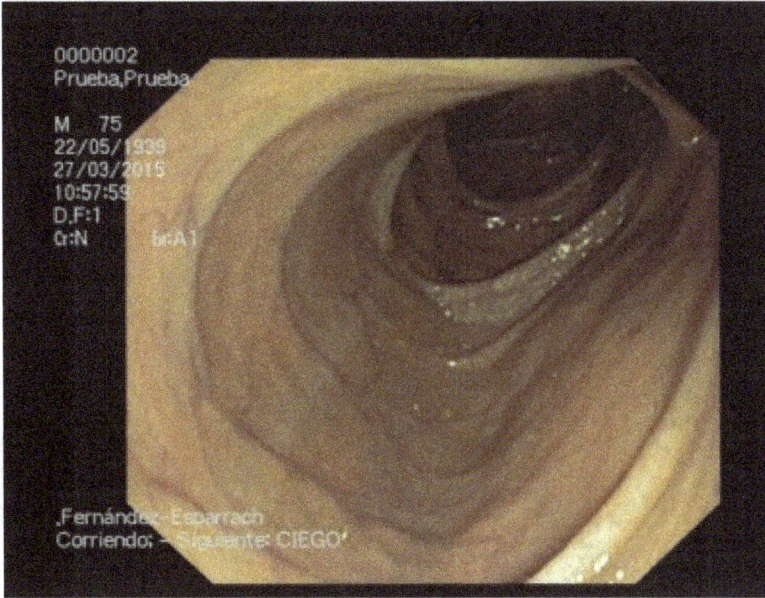

Figure 9. Examples of information overlay in colonoscopy images.

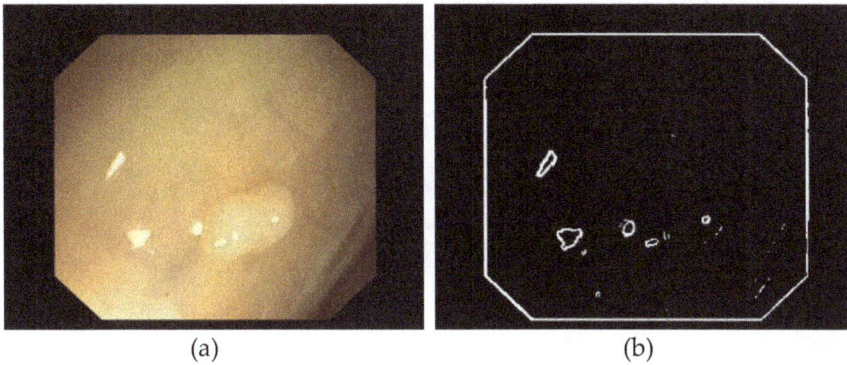

(a)   (b)

Figure 10. Impact of black mask in image processing algorithms. (a) shows the original image whereas (b) shows the output of an edge detection algorithm. Note that mask contours appear as strong as structural elements.

- *Data compression:* Image and video data are commonly compressed in order to save storage space but commonly used formats such as MPEG and JPEG lead to information loss along with the introduction of some artifacts they may difficult fine detail processing in images. In this case the lower the compression, the least impact it will have in further image processing.

3.2. Endoluminal scene description challenges

In order to provide with systems that can help clinicians to overcome some of the clinical challenges identified earlier, a description of the elements of the endoluminal scene is needed. We show in Fig.11 an example on how endoluminal scene looks like.

We can make a division of the elements that appear on a given scene into pure anatomical structures (polyps, luminal region, folds, blood vessels or intestinal content) and structures appearing as result of image acquisition and formation processes (specular highlights and black mask). It is clear that a potential intelligent system should focus on the characterization of anatomical structures in order to be clinically useful –being polyps the usual target structure– but, as recent studies demonstrate [29], the consideration of all the elements of the endoluminal scene may result in an improvement of the performance of a given system. Endoluminal structure characterization is not a straightforward task due to three main reasons:

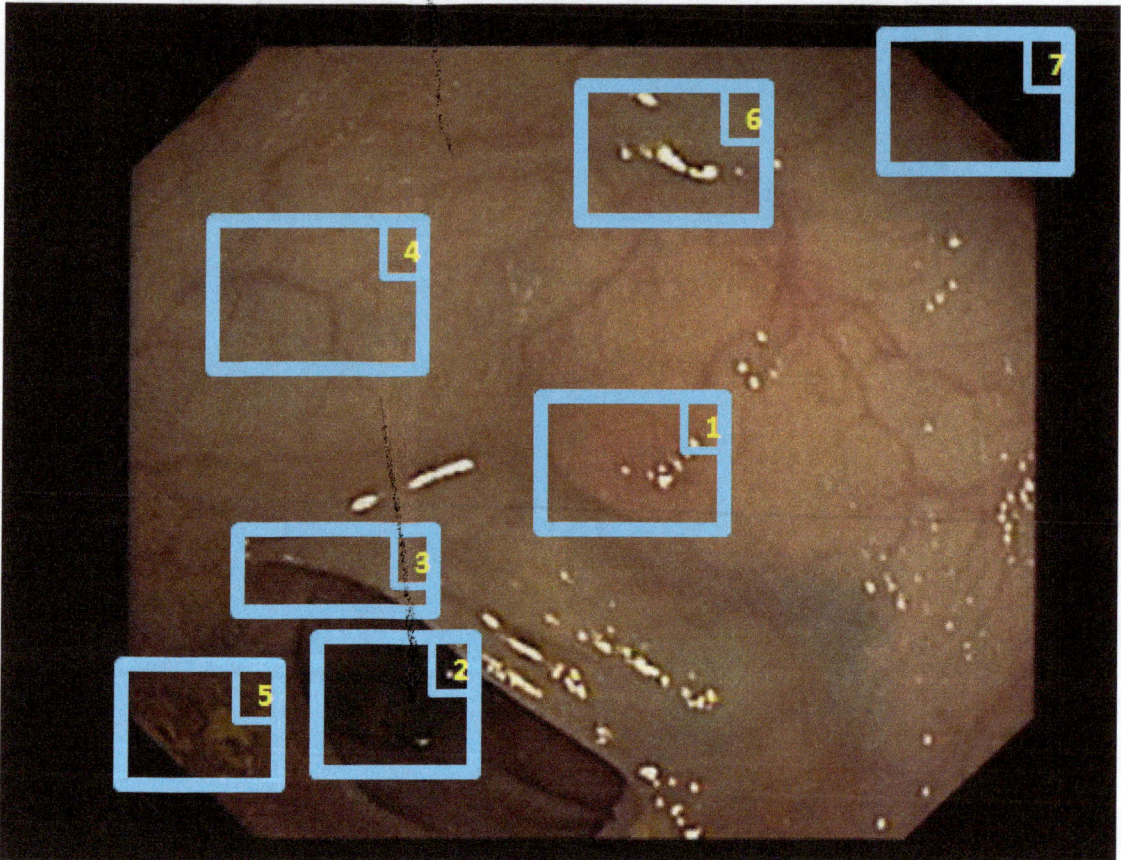

Figure 11. Elements of the endoluminal scene: (1) Polyp; (2) Luminal region; (3) Folds; (4) Blood vessels; (5) Intestinal content; (6) Specular highlights and (7) Black mask.

- *Lack of uniform structure appearance:* Anatomical structures appearance differs greatly in different interventions, which may difficult the development of characterization methods that can be widely applicable. For instance, polyp characterization is challenging because there is not an uniform and unique polyp appearance; in fact, polyp appearance depends greatly on the point of view in which it is observed and we can observe different particularities whether we are observing polyps in zenithal or lateral views –see Fig. 12-.

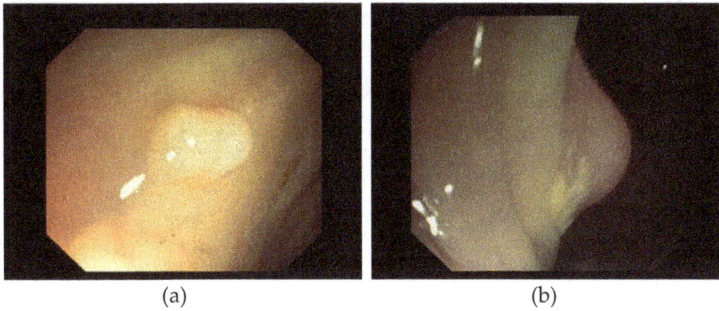

(a)   (b)

Figure 12. Variability in polyp appearance: (1) Zenithal view and (2) Lateral view.

Consequently a definition of a model of appearance for a given structure should consider this great variability in order to be widely applicable and, therefore, search for general features that can be attainable for the majority of the cases.

• *Impact of other elements of the scene on a particular element characterization:* Following with the polyp example, the majority of available works rely on polyp characterization from the identification of polyp boundaries but, in terms of image processing, there is not a big difference in terms of contour appearance between polyps, blood vessels and folds, as the three of them provide with similar response to contour detection operators, as it can be observed in Fig. 13. Considering this, a given intelligent system must consider the impact of all present structures when providing a characterization of a particular one and it will need to find additional cues to differentiate between these structures.

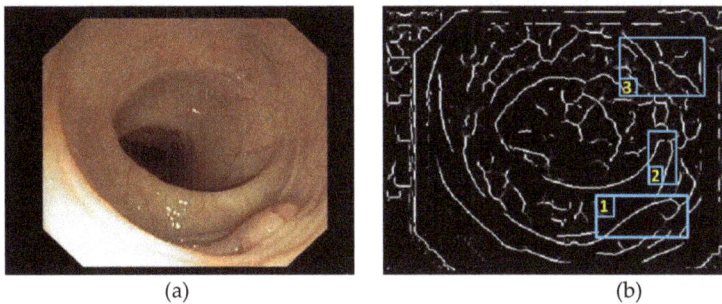

(a)   (b)

Figure 13. Example of similarity of response of different structures to a given operator. Number 1 represents a polyp, number 2 a fold and 3 represents blood vessels.

• *Difficulties on the definition of the structural element:* Another challenge is related to the visual definition of the structure itself, that is, sometimes the definition of the element itself is not clear, which makes it difficult to delimit the structure. For instance, recent studies show a great variability between observers when defining the luminal region –demonstrated in [30], which may have an impact on ground truth creation for assessing the performance of a given intelligent system. This difficult on the definition on the structure can also be applied for other elements such as fecal or intestinal content.

4. Equipment setting to favor optimal image processing analysis

We present in this section the optimal settings of clinical equipment to ensure the best possible quality of the images which will be analyzed by the intelligent system.

4.1. Endoscopic equipment settings

Chronologically, the first element to be considered is the configuration of both endoscope and video processor in order to obtain the best possible images for further analysis. In this case we propose the following configuration:

- Disable sharpening options, so we can avoid the apparition of artificial information (halos) surrounding image structure contours along with reducing image noise.

- Disable the superimposition of overlay information such as patient or procedure data to obtain a clean view of the endoluminal scene. This also allows a complete anonymization of the information easing its use for research purposes.

- If possible, allow the endoluminal view to occupy the largest portion of the scene without applying any kind of digital zooming operation.

- Configure storage options to obtain data with the minimum possible compression.

4.2. Image storage and anonymization

We have to consider that image or/and video data will be used in research projects from which several research publications will be generated. Access to this image or video data should be granted to other researchers in order to allow an easier comparison of the performance of different methods. Considering this, no information that can allow an identification of either the patient or the clinician should be provided in neither the images or in the metadata associated to them –such as time and date of image capture or endoscopy used-, preventing the association of a given image to a patient, clinician or hospital.

Considering the amount of endoscopic interventions performed in a hospital in a year, images or videos that are stored tend to be compressed. This compression has already been mentioned to have implications for image processing methods so; if possible, the configuration with less possible compression should be chosen.

4.3. Endoscopic naviagation guidelines

Endoscope movement when images are acquired impacts the quality of the images that are obtained. If there is no scope movement, effects such as interlacing or color phantoms can be almost inexistent -Fig. 14 (a)-. Considering this, we propose still images acquisition to be made being both the scope and the elements of the endoluminal scene static. For the case of video acquisition we suggest slow and smooth endoscope progression through the patient in order to maximize the reduction of movement-related artifacts generation.

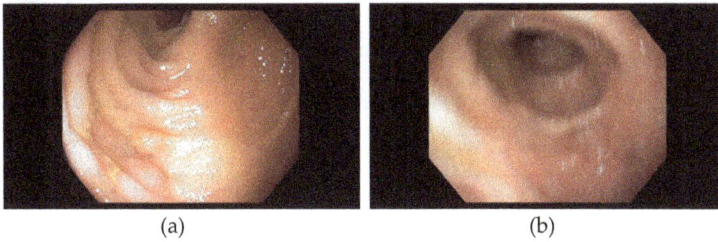

Figure 14. Difference in image quality related to endoscope movement when acquiring images: (a) still endoscope vs. (b) moving endoscope.

It is clear that even by considering all the suggestions expressed, there will still be a minor movement of the scope between the two time instants in which odd and even lines of the final image are acquired. In order to mitigate the impact of interlacing and to avoid loss of image resolution we propose to make a real-time analysis of the images when they are acquired in order to store only the one which less interlacing impact. This analysis will be made by comparing consecutive frames, where the difference in content between them is so minimal that there is no point on storing them all, considering the small changes that will appear in images extracted from a 30 frames per second video. In case interlacing can still be perceived, its impact can be completely removed by working with one of the two channels of the image [29], although this implies a decrease in final image resolution.

To close this section, we show in Table 2 a summary of the challenges related to image formation and acquisition depicted in Section 3 and our proposal on how to solve/mitigate them. As it can be seen from the table, there are some challenges that cannot be solved by applying specific settings to the devices involved. For instance, those related to image formation are highly device-dependent. In this sense, newer equipment has dedicated sensors for each color channel avoiding the apparition of color phantoms. There are other challenges that must be solved by means of image processing techniques, such as specular highlights. In this sense, the most accepted solution [29] consists of a specular highlight detection followed by a substitution of the pixels in the image belonging to specular highlights by a combination of valid values of neighbor pixels, as it can be observed in Fig. 15. The same operation is applied to mitigate the impact of strong contours created by the black mask.

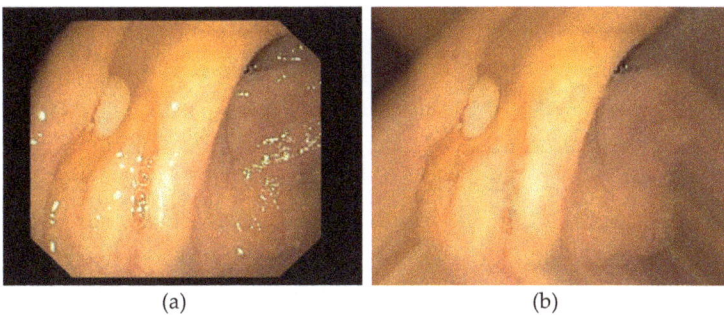

Figure 15. Application of image processing methods to mitigate impact of specular highlights and black mask. (a) Original image and (b) Processed image.

Source	Challenge		Proposed solution
Image formation	Illumination	Specular highlights	Specular highlights correction
		Lack of uniform illumination	Device-dependent
	Sensor acquisition	Color phantoms	Device-dependent
Image acquisition and visualization	Image acquisition and storage	Image resolution	Stabilization of endoscope, interlacing suppression and use of HD endoscopes
		Image interlacing	Interlacing suppression, neighbor frame frames, endoscope stabilization
	Image visualization capabilities enhancement	Sharpening	Disable sharpening
		Presence of patient and procedure information	Disable overlays
		Black mask	Black mask substitution
		Data compression	Use of lossless compression standards.

Table 2. Summary of image acquisition and formation challenges along with proposal of solutions

5. Current endoluminal scene description methods

We present in this section a review on the most recent works published on the topic of anatomical endoluminal scene elements description.

5.1. Polyps

As they are the main focus of colonoscopy explorations, the majority of already existing intelligent systems for colonoscopy deals with polyp characterization. We divide existing systems according to the application they are built for:

• *Polyp detection:* This group of methods aim to decide whether there is a polyp or not in the image. The majority of the works on polyp detection are built on the principle of applying a given feature detector/descriptor to the image in order to guide detection methods. In this sense, we can divide existing approaches in two groups: (a) shape and (b) texture and color-based. The first group aims to detect polyps by observing specific cues on the contours of the polyp –examples of this can be found in works presented in [31-33], or by fitting candidate objects in the image to the most common shapes that polyps present [34]. Regarding the second group, the use of several general descriptors has been proposed, such as wavelets in [35], local binary patterns in [36] or co-ocurrence matrices [37]. A method combining MPEG-7 texture and color descriptors was proposed in [38]. One big drawback of descriptor-based methods is that they tend to need of an exhaustive training and they are

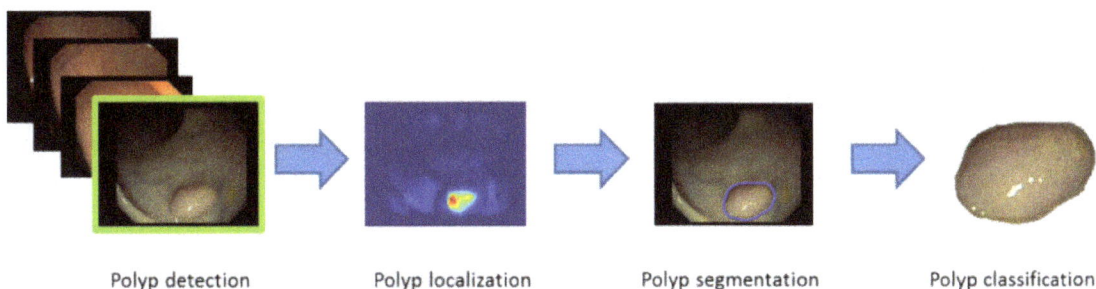

| Polyp detection | Polyp localization | Polyp segmentation | Polyp classification |

Figure 16. Example of the output of each polyp characterization group of algorithms.

very sensitive to parameter tuning. Finally the work published in [39] combines shape and texture features to build up a polyp detection method which also considers spatial and temporal adjacency information present in colonoscopy videos.

- *Polyp localization/highlighting:* These methods are focused on highlighting the area of the image more likely to contain a polyp. Considering this, they can be understood as a sub-group of polyp detection method but, in this case, with the objective to establish the area of the image where the polyp is. These methods rely on the definition of a model of polyp appearance and on the exploration of low-level features of the image –in this case, the definition of polyp boundaries in terms of valley information- in order to provide with methods that can be applied in the intervention rooms. Some examples of these methods can be found in the works of Bernal et al [13, 29].

- *Polyp segmentation:* In this case the objective is to delimit the region of the image that the polyp occupies. The majority of available works deal with polyp segmentation in CT images -such as the works depicted in [40,41] -, which can also be useful to provide further features of the polyp such as its size, although considering CT limitations regarding small polyps visibility as mentioned in Section2. Recent works on white light colonoscopy exploit the output from polyp localization methods in order to delimit the final polyp region [42], providing accurate results that could be directly applicable in the intervention room without additional radiation of the patient. Finally there are some recent works [43] that deal with polyp segmentation using narrow-band imaging; preliminary results are promising although its usefulness is restricted to the availability of this imaging modality.

- *Polyp characterization/classification*: The aim of these methodologies concerns lesion characterization according to the content of the polyp region. In this case the objective is to aid clinicians in in-vivo diagnosis and some of the existing works aim to provide automatic lesion labeling using previously-mentioned classifications such as NICE [23] or KUDO [22]. These systems would benefit from an accurate localization and segmentation of the polyp region in order to find features that best discriminate between different polyp types.

As it can be seen from the classification exposed above, a potential intelligent system with applicability in the intervention room could easily use a system from each of the four groups in order to build up a computer-aided diagnosis tool. We show in Fig. 16 a graphical example of such a system. In a first stage the system will automatically decide which frames contain a polyp and which region of the frame contains the polyp. From this, an accurate segmentation of the polyp region will be obtained in order to extract meaningful features to help in the classification process.

5.2. Luminal area

Luminal area is defined as the interior space of a tubular structure, such as the intestine. The detection of the lumen and its position can be crucial in both intervention and post-intervention time.

On the one hand, an accurate detection of the lumen region during in-vivo intervention may be useful to discard areas of the image with low visibility –Fig. 17(a) - in order to save computation time for other interesting regions of the image as proposed in [44]. Lumen detection can also be helpful to guide the clinician inside the intestine by pointing out which direction he/she should take to progress. On the other hand, lumen characterization in post-intervention can be used to discard frames for further revision: frames where the proportion of lumen out of the entire image is large can be related to the progression of the colonoscope through the gut but, conversely, frames where the amount of lumen presence is low may potentially indicate areas of the image where the physician has paid more attention. This can be useful to obtain summary videos of the whole procedure. Lumen characterization has been an active topic of research in several endoscopy image modalities such as optical –works of [45] and [46] - and virtual colonoscopy [47]. The main reasoning behind the majority of the luminal region characterization methods is the assumption that lumen is the darkest region of the image and from this seed region growing algorithms are built in order to find lumen boundaries.

5.3. Blood vessels

Blood vessels are the part of the circulatory system that transports blood through the body and they can be identified by their tree-like shape with ramifications. The characterization of these branching structures has been reported in domains such as retinal image analysis [48] or palm prints recognition [49]. Blood vessels characterization in colonoscopy images can be useful in two domains: helping in polyp localization and segmentation tasks, as it has been proven in [13, 29, 42], and as key points to be used in potential follow-up methods, as proposed in [50]. Regarding the former, a mitigation of blood vessels related valleys by using contrast properties of blood vessels contours has been proven to be useful to improve polyp localization segmentation, as in some images -Fig. 17(b)- blood vessels can be identified easier than polyp boundaries. Concerning the latter, we could think of a univocal characterization of blood vessels branching patterns using methods such as the one proposed in [51] to recognize a same region during different interventions.

5.3.1. Folds

Haustral folds represent folds of mucosa within the colon. They are formed by circumferential contraction of the inner muscular layer of the colon. In the context of intelligent systems for colonoscopy, folds characterization can play a key role in polyp characterization tasks. In this sense, we have to consider that the fold contours appearance in colonoscopy images is very similar to the one of polyps. We can observe in Fig. 17 (c) that folds and polyp contours present similar appearance but different levels of curvature; consequently, an accurate identification of folds could lead to an improvement in polyp characterization tasks. Some recent works build up advances model of polyp appearance to discriminate polyp contours from folds by considering desirable properties of polyp contours such as concavity, completeness or continuity, as proposed in [13].

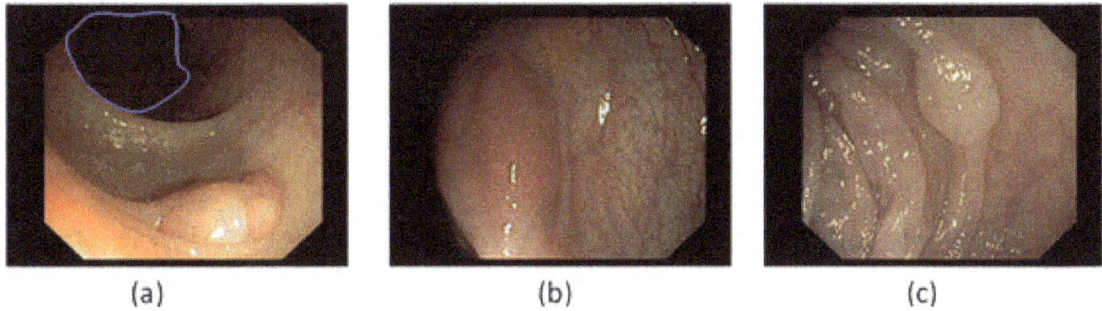

Figure 17. Effect of endoluminal scene structures in polyp characterization: (a) Luminal region (delimited by a blue mask); (b) Blood vessels and (c) Folds.

5.4. Fecal content

Apart from the elements that have already been covered, there are more elements that can appear in the endoluminal scene as a result of bad patient preparation. In this sense high presence of intestinal content is considered by clinicians as an indicator to decide whether a procedure has to be repeated or not as no clinician or computer vision method would work with very low quality images. Moreover, there are some cases when the presence of fecal content can affect the output of computer vision methods, as it was shown in [13]. Therefore an accurate identification of fecal content in colonoscopy images could be used to provide automatic indicators of the quality of patients' preparation.

6. Building up validation frameworks for intelligent systems

One of the main problems when assessing the performance of the different available intelligent systems for colonoscopy is that the majority of them are tested on private databases, which makes it difficult to observe the differences in performance between them and to extrapolate its functioning in other environments. Moreover, it is very difficult to compare performance levels of different methods as each of them proposes or uses different evaluation metrics which, for some cases, can be only used with a specific application in mind. Considering this two problems, we present in this section our proposal for a complete validation framework covering from database and ground truth creation to the definition of the metrics to be used to evaluate a given method.

6.1. Database creation

In order to validate and assess the performance of a computer vision method, this has to be tested in a set of images covering as many possible cases of study. For instance, if we want our method to be able to characterize polyps from all the types present in Paris classification our database should contain several examples from each of the classes that are defined there. Apart from the original images, a ground truth should also be provided. This ground truth will be used to assess the performance of the method and its configuration will depend on the concrete experiment. Following the same example used before, for polyp localization purposes the ground truth should consist of a binary image where pixels in white should correspond to those pixels which are part of the polyp. If the output of a given method falls in the white pixels of the image, the method will be performing as expected. As it can be seen there are two processes involved when creating databases for intelligent systems validation: the selection of the cases to be included in the database and the creation of the corresponding ground truth.

Regarding the selection of the cases, in order the use of a method can be extended outside research domain, these cases should represent the clinical variability that the clinician can find during interventions. In case we have several types of elements to be characterized, the database should contain as many different examples as possible for all the possible classes. It is important to mention than the more different the examples, the more robust will be our method and the better it will perform once a new case of study is to be analyzed. By doing this if we achieve that a given method offers good performance in our database it will be easy to extrapolate its performance in a potential clinical application.

There is one branch of computer vision known as machine learning which involves method training in a set of images and a posterior testing of this method in a different set of images, once its performance has been optimized in the training stage. Considering this, the size of the database should permit the division in training and testing examples and we should define our database in a way such representative examples of all the possible cases are present both in training and testing databases. The final size of the database should allow extracting statistically significant conclusions. In clinical trials, a variability of less of 10 % is not considered as relevant as stated in [52], being variability calculated as the inverse of the square root of the number of samples –N- in our database. Considering this, the minimum size of the database should be of 100 images.

Once database has been defined, ground truth must be created to validate the performance of the methods. The definition of this ground truth is clearly application dependent: for instance if we are developing a polyp detection method the ground truth may only consist of an excel file indicating for each frame whether there is a polyp or not in the image but for a polyp segmentation method we would need a binary image representing the structure to be segmented, as it can be seen in Fig. 18.

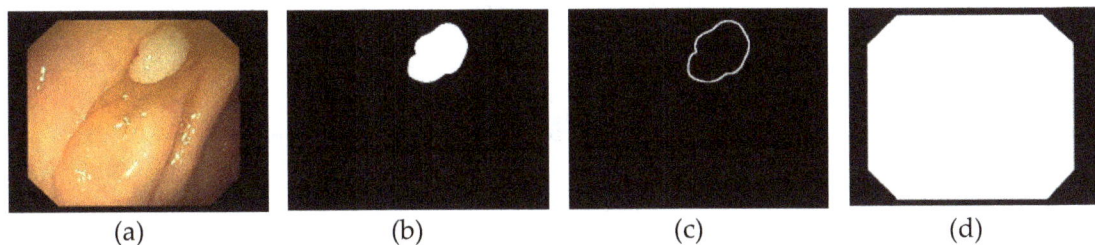

(a)   (b)   (c)   (d)

Figure 18. Possible contents of a polyp segmentation database: (a) Original image; (b) Polyp mask; (c) Polyp contour mask and (d) Black mask.

Image-based ground truth are commonly created using image editing software such as Microsoft Paint or Adobe Photoshop, although there is an increasing use of specific tools such as ImageJ [53] which allows the creation of segmentation ground truths by marking a few points in the image. Concerning ground truth creation, it should be created either by clinicians or by experts under clinicians' supervision. Having more than one ground truth per image is recommendable for validation purposes as a way to avoid possible subjectivity in ground truth creation. This allows performing statistical tests and also to assess whether the performance of a given method is within inter-observer variability. If clinical conclusions are meant to be extracted from the performance of intelligent systems, clinical metadata should be provided. For instance, if we want to assess the performance of a polyp classification method, apart from the mask representing where the polyp in the image is, clinicians should provide which is the class of the polyp (i.e., KUDO type I).

Currently there are only, up to our knowledge, three different databases related to colonoscopy image analysis: two of them consisting of still images showing a polyp - CVC-ColonDB and CVC-ClinicDB- and another - ASU-Mayo Clinic polyp database-, which consists of full colonoscopy videos with and without polyps. The first two databases are meant for the validation of model of appearance for polyps to ease polyp localization and segmentation whereas the latter has been developed for the validation of polyp detection algorithms. Currently only CVC-ClinicDB incorporates clinical metadata associated to each polyp, including information regarding polyp size, Paris classification and histological type of polyp. This allows break down of the results according clinical criteria, as exposed in [13]. We introduce the main features of each of the three databases in Table 3.

6.2. Performance metrics

The way a given intelligent system method is validated will depend greatly on what this intelligent system is for. The potential application the system is designed for will define both how database and ground truth need to be generated and the metrics used to assess the performance of the method. In this subsection we propose validation protocols for each of the four main types of intelligent systems reported in the literature.

Database	Number of frames/videos	Ground truth content
CVC-ColonDB	380 frames from 15 different sequences with a polyp	For each image with a polyp the following images are provided: 1) original image; 2) polyp mask; 3) non-informative regions mask and 4) polyp contour.
CVC-ClinicDB	612 frames from 29 different sequences with a polyp.	For each image both the original frame along with a mask covering the polyp are provided. For each polyp, clinical metadata associated is provided (size, Paris classification, histological type of polyp after biopsy) [13]
ASU-Mayo Clinic polyp database	Training set: 20 videos (10 with a polyp and 10 without polyps). Testing set: 18 videos	For each frame of the video a binary image is provided. Absence of polyp in the image can be identified by having a completely black associated image. In case of polyp presence, an approximation of polyp region is provided.

Table 3. Summary of available databases for colonoscopy image analysis

- *Polyp Detection:* A given polyp detection method should provide an output whenever a polyp is present in the image and should not provide any output if there is no polyp.

Performance metrics:

Considering this we propose the use of four different concepts (True Positive (TP), False Positive (FP), True Negative (TN) and False Negative (FN)) which are commonly used in object detection and characterization problems. We present these concepts in Table 4.

Concept	Method	Ground truth
TP	Provides an output	There is a polyp in the image
FP	Provides an output	There is no polyp in the image
TN	Does not provide an output	There is no polyp in the image
FN	Does not provide an output	There is a polyp in the image

Table 4. Explanation of polyp detection metrics

Consequently a good polyp detection method should provide with a high number of TP and TN along the lowest possible number of FN and FP. In order to allow a more clear representation of these results, four different metrics are calculated from TP, FP, TN and FN values:

- Precision, calculated as: $Prec = \frac{TP}{TP + FP}$. It represents the fraction of relevant retrieved information. Regarding polyp detection, it represents the percentage of correct alarms (frames where the method provides an output and the image has a polyp). A low precision rate will be interpreted as the system providing a high number of false alarms.

- Recall, calculated as: $Rec = \frac{TP}{TP + FN}$. Recall represents the fraction of elements to be retrieved that have been successfully retrieved. In our context, represents the fraction of polyps out of the total that have been correctly detected. Considering this, the highest recall the best the detection method.

- Accuracy, calculated as: $Acc = \frac{TP + TN}{TP + FP + TN + FN}$. This measure represents the amount of information that has been correctly labeled. It is useful in cases where positive and negative examples are balanced which is not always the case for polyp detection.

- Specificity, calculated as: $Spec = \frac{TN}{FP + TN}$. This represents how good a polyp detection method is when detecting the absence of polyps. A high number of false alarms can be interpreted as the method being less specific regarding polyp presence.

Finally, a polyp detection method will be considered as clinically useful if it can helps the clinician to detect the polyp. Considering this and assuming that a given sequence contains a polyp, the following metrics can be defined:

- Reaction time: difference in number of frames between first apparition of the polyp in the sequence and the first frame in which a given method provides detection.

- Dwell time: number of frames with a polyp in which the detection method provides detection.

Considering this two metrics, a comparison can be made between the performance of a given automatic method and clinicians, as it was presented in [13]. This can allow the assessment of the potential of a given method to be included to support clinicians in polyp detection tasks.

Ground truth:

Ground truth for polyp detection methods validation can consist in either a text file stating which frames contain a polyp or in a binary mask corresponding to each original frame. In this case the binary mask should represent polyp presence and absence (for instance, an all-black image can represent polyp absence).

- *Polyp localization:* Polyp localization methods aim to extend the information provided by polyp detection methods by not only indicating whether there is a polyp in the image or not, but also indicating where the polyp is within the image.

Performance metrics:

Considering the purpose of localization methods, we cannot use all the four concepts explained before as the use of TN does not make sense in this type of problems as there is always a polyp in the image. In this case several authors [13] propose a more direct performance referred as localization accuracy. Considering that a polyp localization method always provide a potential polyp location, we can define a good localization (GL) whenever the output of the localization method coincides with a polyp. Conversely we define false localization (FL) in the opposite case when the localization proposed by the method falls outside the polyp. Taking this into account, we define localization accuracy as:

$$LAcc = \frac{GL}{GL + FL}$$

In cases where the output of a localization image does not consists of points representing polyp locations but of energy images representing areas with more likelihood of containing a polyp –as it can be seen in Fig. 16- the use of energy concentration metrics seems useful to represent the performance of a method [13]. Considering these two metrics, LAcc and concentration, a good localization method should provide a low number of FL while concentrating the majority of the polyp presence likelihood image inside the polyp mask.

Ground truth:

Ground truth for polyp localization should consist of binary masks representing the area of the image that is occupied by the polyp, as it is shown in Figure 18.

- *Polyp segmentation:* An accurate segmentation of the region that contains the polyp can be useful for both lesion recognition tasks as well as for delimiting the area of the image to be used for lesion classification purposes.

Performance metrics:

We propose the use of common segmentation metrics such as Precision and Recall, as they were defined for polyp detection. In this case we classify each pixel as TP, FP, TN and FN considering methods' output and the ground truth (i.e. a false positive pixel is defined as a pixel in which our method states it is part of the polyp when it is not). In this context, a good polyp segmentation method should provide higher Precision and Recall results (Fig. 19 (b)); a method providing high Precision with low Recall will provide regions that cannot be used for further polyp characterization as they contain lots of non-polyp information (Fig. 19 (c)). Conversely a method providing with high Recall but low Precision values will be useful for polyp description but will leave a lot of useful polyp content out of posterior analysis (Fig. 19 (d)).

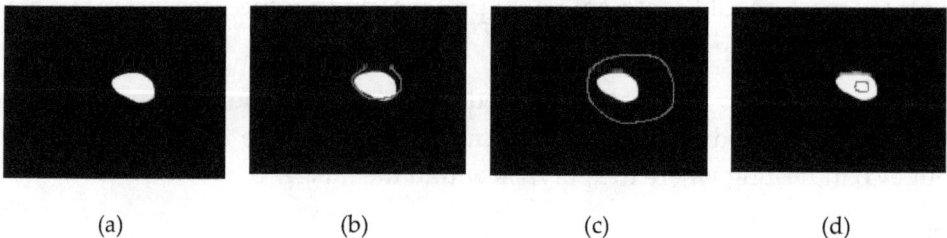

| (a) | (b) | (c) | (d) |

Figure 19. Interpretation of segmentations: (a) Original ground truth. Segmentation results with (a) good Precision and Recall values; (c) good Precision but low Recall value and (d) low Precision but good Recall value. Mask representing the output of a given method is represented in blue.

Ground truth:

As for the case of polyp localization, ground truth for polyp segmentation should consists of binary masks representing either the area of the image that is occupied by the polyp -Figure 18 (b)- or the contour of the polyp region -Figure 18 (c)-.

- *Polyp classification:* A good polyp classification method should be able to assign the polyp present in the image the same label/class that is attached to the polyp in the ground truth.

Performance metrics:

In this case we can have two different types of evaluation, depending on the number of possible classes that we define: if a polyp can only have two different classes we could evaluate our method by checking whether the output of a method coincides or not with the ground truth; in this case for each image we will have a correct (OK) or incorrect classification (NOK). The accuracy of the system will be calculated as

$$Acc = \frac{OK}{OK + NOK}$$

The second type of evaluation is related to multiclass classification; in this case we can also include studies regarding which classes are more easily identified and which classes are mostly confused over each other. In this last case we can use confusion matrices, similar to the ones presented in [54] to represent the output of a given classification method.

Ground truth:

Ground truth for polyp classification should consist of a label associated to each frame with a polyp; this label must include the given polyp in any of the possible classes defined in the problem.

7. Conclusions

Collaboration between clinicians and computer scientists is crucial for the development of intelligent systems for colonoscopy. Those systems need to be designed to solve real clinical problems if they want to be deployed in clinical environments. Considering this, apart from application development and validation, efforts must be focused on the definition of the aim of the proposed intelligent system.

We have presented in this chapter some of the problems that colonoscopy still present nowadays, being polyp miss-rate the most important of them. Additionally there is a need expressed by clinicians of systems that can allow them to have a first approach to polyp histology, which could be useful to take in-vivo decisions. Considering this we define three possible domains of application of a given intelligent system: polyp detection and localization, polyp classification and development of navigation-assisting and patient follow-up methods.

Once the clinical need is defined, computer scientists must deal with image processing in order to provide with meaningful results. In this context, we have subdivided this problem in two:

image preparation for optimal image processing and endoluminal scene description for intelligent system applications.

Regarding image preparation, one of the main objectives of this chapter was to rise up some concerns about image quality for later processing and clinicians and computer scientists must reach an agreement to obtain images that are useful for both domains. Endoluminal scene description has been proven as a challenging task due to the great variability in structures' appearance throughout different interventions. The majority of bibliographical sources are devoted to polyp characterization, although we have observed an increasing interest in the definition of other elements of the scene, as they have been proven to have an impact in polyp characterization tasks. At this point it is important to mention that there are some aspects that we have not covered in full such as patient preparation although it has a direct consequence on the output of a given intelligent system. In this case we opt to follow the same criteria that clinicians do: if patient preparation is bad neither computer vision nor clinicians would be able to distinguish anything.

The objective of the development of an intelligent system is to take profit of the synergies between clinicians and computer scientists. During the development of a given system, clinicians must provide with data in order to test different methods. We propose in this chapter a validation framework which covers topics such as database and ground truth creation as well as the definition of performance metrics. The proposal of a validation framework including database creation and management along with the definition of standard evaluation metrics can pave the way for a standardized comparison of the performance of intelligent systems which would allow in the future clinicians choose the one that fulfills better their necessities.

The main conclusion that can be extracted from this chapter is that there is indeed room and necessity for the collaboration between these two domains of research. Acknowledging the necessities of each other is meant to play a key role in the development of applicable and deployable intelligent systems for colonoscopy.

Author details

Jorge Bernal[1*], F. Javier Sánchez[1], Cristina Rodríguez de Miguel[2] and Gloria Fernández-Esparrach[2]

*Address all correspondence to: jbernal@cvc.uab.es

1 Computer Science Department at Universitat Autònoma de Barcelona and Computer Vision Center, Barcelona, Spain

2 Endoscopy Unit, Gastroenterology Department, Hospital Clínic, IDIBAPS, CIBEREHD, University of Barcelona, Barcelona, Spain

References

[1] Bratko, I., Mozetič, I., & Lavrač, N. (1990). KARDIO: a study in deep and qualitative knowledge for expert systems. MIT Press. DOI:10.1016/0933-3657(91)90006-W

[2] Wilschut, J. A., Steyerberg, E. W., van Leerdam, M. E., Lansdorp-Vogelaar, I., Habbema, J. D. F., & van Ballegooijen, M. (2011). How much colonoscopy screening should be recommended to individuals with various degrees of family history of colorectal cancer?. Cancer, 117(18), 4166-4174. DOI: 10.1002/cncr.26009

[3] Viswanath, S., Palumbo, D., Chappelow, J., Patel, P., Bloch, B. N., Rofsky, N et al. (2011, March). Empirical evaluation of bias field correction algorithms for computer-aided detection of prostate cancer on T2w MRI. In SPIE Medical Imaging (pp. 79630V-79630V). International Society for Optics and Photonics. DOI:10.1117/12.878813

[4] Bale, R., & Widmann, G. (2007). Navigated CT-guided interventions. Minimally Invasive Therapy & Allied Technologies, 16(4), 196-204. DOI:10.1080/13645700701520578

[5] Schwarz, Y., Greif, J., Becker, H. D., Ernst, A., & Mehta, A. (2006). Real-time electromagnetic navigation bronchoscopy to peripheral lung lesions using overlaid CT images: the first human study. CHEST Journal, 129(4), 988-994. DOI:10.1378/chest.129.4.988

[6] Fernández-Esparrach, G., Estépar, R. S. J., Guarner-Argente, C., Martínez-Pallí, G., Navarro, R., de Miguel, C. R et al. (2010). The role of a computed tomography-based image registered navigation system for natural orifice transluminal endoscopic surgery: a comparative study in a porcine model. Endoscopy, 42(12), 1096. DOI: 10.1055/s-0030-1255824

[7] Grbic, S., Ionasec, R., Mansi, T., Georgescu, B., Vega-Higuera, F., Navab, N., & Comaniciu, D. (2013, April). Advanced intervention planning for Transcatheter Aortic Valve Implantations (TAVI) from CT using volumetric models. In Biomedical Imaging (ISBI), 2013 IEEE 10th International Symposium on (pp. 1424-1427). IEEE. DOI: 10.1109/ISBI.2013.6556801

[8] Thomas-Gibson, S., Bassett, P., Suzuki, N., Brown, G. J., Williams, C. B., & Saunders, B. P. (2007). Intensive training over 5 days improves colonoscopy skills long-term. Endoscopy, 39(9), 818-824. DOI: 10.1055/s-2007-966763

[9] Kiesslich, R., Fritsch, J., Holtmann, M., Koehler, H. H., Stolte, M., Kanzler, S. et al. (2003). Methylene blue-aided chromoendoscopy for the detection of intraepithelial neoplasia and colon cancer in ulcerative colitis. Gastroenterology, 124(4), 880-888. DOI:10.1053/gast.2003.50146

[10] Machida, H., Sano, Y., Hamamoto, Y., Muto, M., Kozu, T., Tajiri, H., & Yoshida, S. (2004). Narrow-band imaging in the diagnosis of colorectal mucosal lesions: a pilot study. Endoscopy, 36(12), 1094-1098. DOI:10.1055/s-2004-826040

[11] Yoshida, Y., Matsuda, K., Sumiyama, K., Kawahara, Y., Yoshizawa, K., Ishiguro, H., & Tajiri, H. (2013). A randomized crossover open trial of the adenoma miss rate for narrow band imaging (NBI) versus flexible spectral imaging color enhancement

(FICE). International journal of colorectal disease, 28(11), 1511-1516. DOI:10.1007/ s00384-013-1735-4

[12] Hoffman, A., Kagel, C., Goetz, M., Tresch, A., Mudter, J., Biesterfeld, S. et al. (2010). Recognition and characterization of small colonic neoplasia with high-definition co-lonoscopy using i-Scan is as precise as chromoendoscopy. Digestive and Liver Dis-ease, 42(1), 45-50. DOI :10.1016/j.dld.2009.04.005

[13] Bernal, J., Śanchez, F. J., Ferńandez-Esparrach, G., Gil, D., Rodŕiguez, C., & Vilariño, F. (2015). WM-DOVA Maps for Accurate Polyp Highlighting in Colonoscopy: Vali-dation vs. Saliency Maps from Physicians. Computerized Medical Imaging and Graphics, 43,pp. 99-111. DOI :10.1016/j.compmedimag.2015.02.007

[14] Modlin, I. M. (2000). A brief history of endoscopy. MultiMed.

[15] Pellise, M., Fernández-Esparrach, G., Cardenas, A., Sendino, O., Ricart, E., Vaquero et al. (2008). Clinical impact of wide-angle, high-resolution endoscopy in the diagno-sis of colorectal neoplasia in a non-selected population: a prospective randomized controlled trial. Gastrointestinal Endoscopy, 67(5), AB101. DOI :10.1016/j.gie. 2008.03.119

[16] Rex, D. K., & Helbig, C. C. (2007). High yields of small and flat adenomas with high-definition colonoscopes using either white light or narrow band imaging. Gastroen-terology, 133(1), pp. 42-47. DOI :10.1053/j.gastro.2007.04.029

[17] Quintero, E., Castells, A., Bujanda, L., Cubiella, J., Salas, D., Lanas, Á. et al. (2012). Colonoscopy versus fecal immunochemical testing in colorectal-cancer screening. New England Journal of Medicine, 366(8), pp. 697-706. DOI: 10.1056/NEJMoa1108895

[18] Barclay, R. L., Vicari, J. J., Doughty, A. S., Johanson, J. F., & Greenlaw, R. L. (2006). Colonoscopic withdrawal times and adenoma detection during screening colonosco-py. New England Journal of Medicine, 355(24), pp. 2533-2541. DOI: 10.1056/ NEJMoa055498

[19] van Rijn, J. C., Reitsma, J. B., Stoker, J., Bossuyt, P. M., van Deventer, S. J., & Dekker, E. (2006). Polyp miss rate determined by tandem colonoscopy: a systematic review. The American journal of gastroenterology, 101(2), pp. 343-350. DOI:10.1111/j. 1572-0241.2006.00390.x

[20] Bretagne, J. F., Manfredi, S., Piette, C., Hamonic, S., Durand, G., & Riou, F. (2010). Yield of high-grade dysplasia based on polyp size detected at colonoscopy: a series of 2295 examinations following a positive fecal occult blood test in a population-based study. Diseases of the Colon & Rectum, 53(3), pp. 339-345. DOI: 10.1007/DCR. 0b013e3181c37f9c

[21] Samadder, N. J., Curtin, K., Tuohy, T. M., Pappas, L., Boucher, K., Provenzale, D. et al. (2014). Characteristics of missed or interval colorectal cancer and patient survival:

a population-based study. Gastroenterology, 146(4), pp. 950-960. DOI:10.1053/j.gastro.2014.01.013

[22] Kudo, S. E., Wakamura, K., Ikehara, N., Mori, Y., Inoue, H., & Hamatani, S. (2011). Diagnosis of colorectal lesions with a novel endocytoscopic classification–a pilot study. Endoscopy, 43(10), 869. DOI: 10.1055/s-0030-1256663

[23] Hayashi, N., Tanaka, S., Hewett, D. G., Kaltenbach, T. R., Sano, Y., Ponchon, T. et al. (2013). Endoscopic prediction of deep submucosal invasive carcinoma: validation of the narrow-band imaging international colorectal endoscopic (NICE) classification. Gastrointestinal endoscopy, 78(4), pp. 625-632. DOI:10.1016/j.gie.2013.04.185

[24] Fidler, J. L., Johnson, C. D., MacCarty, R. L., Welch, T. J., Hara, A. K., & Harmsen, W. S. (2002). Detection of flat lesions in the colon with CT colonography. Abdominal imaging, 27(3),pp. 292-300. DOI: 10.1007/s00261-001-0171-z

[25] Fidler, J., & Johnson, C. (2009). Flat polyps of the colon: accuracy of detection by CT colonography and histologic significance. Abdominal imaging, 34(2), pp. 157-171. DOI: 10.1007/s00261-008-9388-4

[26] Johnson, C. D., Chen, M. H., Toledano, A. Y., Heiken, J. P., Dachman, A., Kuo, M. D et al. (2008). Accuracy of CT colonography for detection of large adenomas and cancers. New England Journal of Medicine,359(12), pp. 1207-1217. DOI: 10.1056/NEJMx080041

[27] Poynton, C. (2012). Digital video and HD: Algorithms and Interfaces. Elsevier.

[28] Cambridge in Color: A Learning Community for Photographers. Sharpening: Unsharp Mask. http://www.cambridgeincolour.com/tutorials/unsharp-mask.htm. Last visit: 29/03/2015.

[29] Bernal, J., Sánchez, F. J., & Vilariño, F. (2013, July). Impact of image preprocessing methods on polyp localization in colonoscopy frames. In Engineering in Medicine and Biology Society (EMBC), 2013 35th Annual International Conference of the IEEE (pp. 7350-7354). IEEE. DOI:10.1109/EMBC.2013.6611256

[30] Sánchez, C., Bernal, J., Sánchez, F.J., Díez, M., Rosell, A. & Gil, D. (2015). Towards On-line Quantification of Tracheal Stenosis from Videobronchoscopy. International Journal of Computer Assisted Radiology and Surgery, 10(6), pp. 935-945. DOI: 10.1007/s11548-015-1196-z

[31] Krishnan, S. M., Yang, X., Chan, K. L., Kumar, S., & Goh, P. M. Y. (1998). Intestinal abnormality detection from endoscopic images. In Engineering in Medicine and Biology Society, 1998. Proceedings of the 20th Annual International Conference of the IEEE (Vol. 2, pp. 895-898). IEEE. DOI:10.1109/IEMBS.1998.745583

[32] Zhu, H., Fan, Y., & Liang, Z. (2011). Improved curvature estimation for shape analysis in computer-aided detection of colonic polyps. In Virtual Colonoscopy and Ab-

dominal Imaging. Computational Challenges and Clinical Opportunities (pp. 9-14). Springer Berlin Heidelberg. DOI: 10.1007/978-3-642-25719-3_2

[33] Tajbakhsh, N., Gurudu, S. R., & Liang, J. (2014). Automatic Polyp Detection Using Global Geometric Constraints and Local Intensity Variation Patterns. In Medical Image Computing and Computer-Assisted Intervention–MICCAI 2014(pp. 179-187). Springer International Publishing. DOI: 10.1007/978-3-319-10470-6_23

[34] Kang, J., & Doraiswami, R. (2003, May). Real-time image processing system for endoscopic applications. In Electrical and Computer Engineering, 2003. IEEE CCECE 2003. Canadian Conference on (Vol. 3, pp. 1469-1472). IEEE. DOI:10.1109/CCECE. 2003.1226181

[35] Burrus, C. S., Gopinath, R. A., & Guo, H. (1998). Introduction to wavelets and wavelet transforms (Vol. 998). New Jersey: Prentice hall.

[36] Bernal, J., Sánchez, F. J., & Vilariño, F. (2010). Feature Detectors and Feature Descriptors: Where We Are Now. Technical Report. Computer Vision Center.

[37] Ameling, S., Wirth, S., Paulus, D., Lacey, G., & Vilariño, F. (2009). Texture-based polyp detection in colonoscopy. In Bildverarbeitung für die Medizin 2009(pp. 346-350). Springer Berlin Heidelberg. DOI: 10.1007/978-3-540-93860-6_70

[38] Coimbra, M. T., & Cunha, J. S. (2006). MPEG-7 visual descriptors—contributions for automated feature extraction in capsule endoscopy. Circuits and Systems for Video Technology, IEEE Transactions on, 16(5), 628-637. DOI:10.1109/TCSVT.2006.873158

[39] Park, S. Y., Sargent, D., Spofford, I., & Vosburgh, K. G. (2012). A colon video analysis framework for polyp detection. Biomedical Engineering, IEEE Transactions on, 59(5), pp. 1408-1418. DOI: 10.1109/TBME.2012.2188397

[40] Xu, Y. R., & Zhao, J. (2014). Segmentation of haustral folds and polyps on haustral folds in CT colonography using complementary geodesic distance transformation. Journal of Shanghai Jiaotong University (Science), 19, pp. 513-520. DOI: 10.1007/ s12204-014-1534-2

[41] Van Wijk, C., Van Ravesteijn, V. F., Vos, F. M., & Van Vliet, L. J. (2010). Detection and segmentation of colonic polyps on implicit isosurfaces by second principal curvature flow. Medical Imaging, IEEE Transactions on, 29(3), pp. 688-698. DOI: 10.1109/TMI. 2009.2031323

[42] Bernal, J., Núnez, J. M., Sánchez, F. J., & Vilariño, F. (2014). Polyp Segmentation Method in Colonoscopy Videos by Means of MSA-DOVA Energy Maps Calculation. In Clinical Image-Based Procedures. Translational Research in Medical Imaging (pp. 41-49). Springer International Publishing. DOI: 10.1007/978-3-319-13909-8_6

[43] Ganz, M., Yang, X., & Slabaugh, G. (2012). Automatic segmentation of polyps in colonoscopic narrow-band imaging data. Biomedical Engineering, IEEE Transactions on, 59(8), pp. 2144-2151. DOI: 10.1109/TBME.2012.2195314

[44] Bernal, J., Gil, D., Sánchez, C., & Sánchez, F. J. (2014). Discarding Non Informative Regions for Efficient Colonoscopy Image Analysis. In Computer-Assisted and Robotic Endoscopy (pp. 1-10). Springer International Publishing. DOI: 10.1007/978-3-319-13410-9_1

[45] Arnold, M. An Image Analysis and Machine Learning Approach to Measuring the Quality of Individual Colonoscopy Procedures, PhD Thesis, (2012).

[46] Tian, H., Srikanthan, T., & Asari, K. V. (2001). Automatic segmentation algorithm for the extraction of lumen region and boundary from endoscopic images. Medical and Biological Engineering and Computing, 39(1), pp. 8-14. DOI: 10.1007/BF02345260

[47] Lu, L., Zhang, D., Li, L., & Zhao, J. (2012). Fully automated colon segmentation for the computation of complete colon centerline in virtual colonoscopy. Biomedical Engineering, IEEE Transactions on, 59(4), pp. 996-1004. DOI:10.1109/TBME. 2011.2182051

[48] Azzopardi, G., & Petkov, N. (2013). Automatic detection of vascular bifurcations in segmented retinal images using trainable COSFIRE filters. Pattern Recognition Letters, 34(8), pp. 922-933. DOI:10.1016/j.patrec.2012.11.002

[49] Pudzs, M., Fuksis, R., & Greitans, M. (2013, April). Palmprint image processing with non-halo complex matched filters for forensic data analysis. In Biometrics and Forensics (IWBF), 2013 International Workshop on (pp. 1-4). IEEE. DOI:10.1109/IWBF. 2013.6547317

[50] Núñez, J. M., Bernal, J., Ferrer, M., & Vilariño, F. (2014). Impact of Keypoint Detection on Graph-Based Characterization of Blood Vessels in Colonoscopy Videos. In Computer-Assisted and Robotic Endoscopy (pp. 22-33). Springer International. DOI: 10.1007/978-3-319-13410-9_3

[51] Núñez, J. M., Bernal, J., Sánchez, F. J., & Vilariño, F. (2015). GRowing Algorithm for Intersection Detection (GRAID) in branching patterns. Machine Vision and Applications, 26(2-3), pp. 387-400. DOI: 10.1007/s00138-015-0663-4

[52] Julious, S. A. (2009). Sample sizes for clinical trials. CRC Press. DOI: 10.1201/9781584887409

[53] Abràmoff, M. D., Magalhães, P. J., & Ram, S. J. (2004). Image processing with ImageJ. Biophotonics international, 11(7), pp. 36-43.

[54] Chapelle, O., Haffner, P., & Vapnik, V. N. (1999). Support vector machines for histogram-based image classification. Neural Networks, IEEE Transactions on, 10(5), pp. 1055-1064. DOI:10.1109/72.788646

4

Our Experience in Self-Management Support following Colorectal Cancer Treatment

Racho Ribarov

"Clinical services, systems, processes and environments must all convey to patients the message: 'You have a part to play. We are partners. We respect your role and will support you to be part of the team.'" [1]

Abstract

The aim of this chapter is to present information and data from our studies on the analysis and assessment of the necessity of self-management support and promoting the awareness of Bulgarian patients with colorectal cancer. This survey covered a total of 315 patients with stoma, making use from consultations at specialized offices in 8 Bulgarian towns. An anonymous questionnaire was conducted, covering a total of 31 questions. The chapter presents results from nonparametric analysis for the more important questions searching for statistically significant relationship with other comparable questions listed in the questionnaire. The necessity of self-management support is assessed on the basis of the received answers. The activity of the established consultation room's network is described, and information is provided concerning the realized self-management support through enhancing the patients' and health-care specialists' awareness on recent scientific achievements referring to dietary preventive and risk factors. Additional studies are needed in order to involve effectively each patient's potential in the struggle for successful disease outcome and to select the best and most effective approaches for self-management support in compliance with the individual demands of patients with colorectal cancer.

Keywords: colorectal cancer, self-management support, consultation rooms, patients' awareness, dietary factors

1. Introduction

The current diverse picture of colorectal cancer epidemiology outlines prevailing data showing systematic recent increase of the global colorectal cancer incidence rate with certain emphasis reflecting already some reduction of the prevalence characteristic only for some well-developed countries [2, 3]. In this aspect the evidence revealing synchronous growth of age and concomitant chronic disease provokes great interest. For them the predictions of the Institute for the Future, Health and Health Care are that the population aged 65+ will increase from 35 million in 2000 to 53 million in 2020 [4]. The outlined data substantiate the necessity to enhance the variety of approaches to both the prevention and treatment of colorectal cancer and particularly on the involvement of self-management. The complexity of care, intrinsic for colorectal cancer, with its personal, clinical, and social aspects outlines the necessity of self-management support. To respond to this necessity, we focused on involvement of self-management in the struggle against colorectal cancer and provision of the necessary support to achieve an effective disease outcome.

The aim of this paper was to provide information and data from our surveys on the analysis and assessment of the necessity of self-management support and improving the awareness of Bulgarian patients with colorectal cancer.

The survey covered a total of 350 patients with stoma consulted at specialized offices in eight Bulgarian towns: Sofia, Plovdiv, Varna, Burgas, Ruse, Pleven, Haskovo, and Stara Zagora. An anonymous questionnaire study was conducted with a total of 315 respondents delivering correctly completed questionnaire, and 35 questionnaires were discarded because of incorrectly supplied information. Questionnaire studies are among the most informative approaches particularly to problems depending on numerous factors such as colorectal cancer.

The questionnaire contained 31 questions, some of them with sub-questions. The questions were distributed in three main directions: sociodemographic characteristics, treatment quality and patients' satisfaction, and institutions' arrangements, public attitudes, patient's own activity, and supporting environment. The results were processed with descriptive statistical approach presented in one of our previous studies [5]. In this paper we present results from nonparametric analysis of some of the more important questions, searching for statistically significant relationship with other compatible questionnaire questions. Those achieved results were listed in relevant tables.

2. Analysis and assessment of the necessity of self-management support

The role and importance of self-management among the current diversity of measures and approaches for effective CRC treatment is more and more often emphasized. Many studies have shown that patients with colorectal cancer have to be educated to self-manage their condition and improve the quality of their physical, mental, and social life after cancer [5–7].

Self-management is identified as an approach with many benefits in the aspect of patient and economic outcomes and is set as a key element in the current health-care reforms. This approach is often defined as activities performed by the individuals and care providers for themselves, their children, their families, and other individuals in order to be in good shape and maintain good physical and mental health, to respond to social and psychological demands, to prevent disease or accidents, to take care of minor health issues and chronic health states and to maintain health and well-being. In view of patients with colorectal cancer, self-management is an important problem because of the introduction of complex therapeutic regimes often including numerous combinations of chemotherapeutic drugs, and our previous evidence has shown poor patients' awareness concerning the role and effect of administered therapeutic and preventive approaches [5, 8].

Having in mind that during the last years there is greater interest to the use of chemotherapeutics administered orally and the patients' potential to implement chemotherapy at home, there will be a necessity to further activating of self-management. Those perspectives have certain claims to self-management as they require greater responsibility of the patients and their families in the administration of chemotherapy and associated risks. The complexity of the regimes also supposes that the patients will experience potentially toxic side effects requiring quick and effective self-control in order to prevent the unfavorable effects on the treatment and life quality.

Some of our previous studies have shown the necessity to trigger the activities associated with self-management of Bulgarian patients with colorectal cancer, because inadequate awareness about the disease, the risk, and preventive factors as well as the results revealed low level of trust in the administered therapeutic and health care [5, 8]. The realization of those activities requires numerous additional studies.

Patients' mental state, their living environment, and their activity in the treatment process are the most important conditions for successful course and maximal increase of the postoperative period and for good life quality. In this respect we selected three of the questions that to the greatest extent could provide an adequate response concerning the need of patient's active involvement in the processes of treatment and prevention of the concomitant aggravations: "Are you concerned about functions and abilities?" "Is the word 'cancer' a taboo for you and your family?" "Do the people with whom you have shared your diagnosis support you?" The replies to those questions were first assessed by descriptive statistics in percent, showing the trends, without statistical significance [5], providing an assessment of the momentary opinion of the respondents. This assessment, of course, is very important, but it is equally important to reveal what has affected those opinions, in order to undertake respective corrective activities.

The tools of the nonparametric statistical analysis (Fisher's exact test) were used to investigate the effect of most questions, compatible with each of the above-listed questions. The results obtained for each of the three questions are presented in tables covering only the questions with statistically significant effect on the formation of the responses to those three questions.

Table 1 presents the relationships with the question "Are you concerned about your functions and abilities?"

Analyzing the data in the table, the effect of patient's satisfaction with medical care as a significant factor is clearly highlighted (p<0.005). The assessment of the professionalism of

Independent variable	p <
How would you evaluate as a whole your satisfaction with the medical services you experienced by now?	0.005
Doctors' professionalism/competence in diagnostics and treatment	0.02
Doctors' attitude to the patients	0.05
Observing the confidentiality, discreetness, and keeping the disease secret	0.003
Information about the disease course and treatment results	0.003
Provision of psychological consultations	0.02
What do you think about the current scheme of prescribing the necessary drugs?	0.0001
Do you meet difficulties in finding the necessary medical specialist?	0.0001
To what extent are you informed about the character of your disease, and do you think you have chances to overcome the disease?	0.001
Do you know the effect of the prescribed treatment and what could be expected from it?	0.0001
Do you think that the state policy is sufficiently beneficial for cancer patients?	0.0001
Do you think that cancer patients should work in alleviated working conditions?	0.02
How do you envisage the future?	0.001

Table 1. Are you concerned about your functions and abilities? (Dependent variable).

the medical doctors engaged in the treatment process is also a factor for overcoming the patients' concern ($p < 0.02$) as their trust in the positive health outcome is to a great extent based on the doctor's knowledge and skills. The good attitude together with understanding of the patient's state contributes to overcome the concern ($p < 0.05$) and increases the extent of trust in the treatment process and associated health care. Observing confidentiality and discreetness and keeping the disease secrets by the medical specialists are also important factors ($p < 0.003$) to cope with patients' concern. In fact this result could be regarded as patient's confidence in the positive outcome of the disease in the future when the present disease will possibly not be commented. A very important requirement for self-management is the patients' awareness of the disease course and treatment results ($p < 0.003$). The clarification of the disease course and the role of implemented treatment approaches causes marked decrease of patients' concern. The poorly informed patients will have, respectively, the greatest extent of concern. The difficulties in finding the necessary medical specialist affect significantly ($p < 0.0001$) the patients' concern about their functions and abilities. In this aspect it is necessary to clarify the possible ways to realize specific medical consultations complying with the cultural competence of the individual patient that is an accent on self-management support.

The closer and better psychological consultations are an important factor for overcoming the patients' anxiety and raising their trust in the further disease development and outcome ($p < 0.001$). The knowledge on the effect of the administered treatment and the expected results helps significantly ($p < 0,001$) to relieve patients' anxiety.

One of the main components of the psychological status of the colon cancer victim is confidentiality, focusing on one side on the consciousness about the vicious character of the disease and, on the other side, giving hope, though small, for a positive outcome.

Table 2 presents the relationships between patients' answers referring to their requirement for confidentiality ("Is the word 'cancer' taboo for you and your family?"). This table also clearly outlines the significant relationships between the answer to the question and the patients' assessment of doctor's competence and professionalism ($p < 0.02$), substantiating their trust and possibility to overcome the "disease taboo." From emotional point of view, the personal attitude of the doctor to the patient as to an ill person but also as to a personality is of particular importance ($p < 0.05$). The patient's demand to accomplish the doctors' professionalism with sympathy and personal approach to the victim is clearly manifested. This table, like the previous one, shows the necessity of psychological consultations which is a focus for self-management support for the studied patients.

In many cases of grave diseases, the patients do not want the people around them to be informed about their status, a standpoint particularly characteristic for cancer patients. This discreetness means that they do not want to be considered doomed, as their hope for getting well is stronger than the feeling of hopelessness.

The defeatist thinking is characteristic for most ill people, but it is most clearly expressed in cancer patients. The causes are as follows: the disease is incurable in an advanced stage, and even in an initial stage, there is no guarantee that the remission will not be followed by disease recurrence. That is why the doomed thinking and the constant stay at hospitals, resection of some parts of the body, lead to disturbed normal life rhythm and make patients dependent on drugs and time without a clear view whether they could plan—even for a short period of time—their life activities. All that leads to a second-rate life when the patients look mainly for information that makes things more optimistic for them. That is why, besides their own awareness, they need the information and discussion with the monitoring physician that should be provided by the self-management support.

Independent variable	p <
How did you choose the respective hospital establishment?	0.001
How would you evaluate as a whole your satisfaction with the medical services you experienced by now?	0.005
Provision of psychological consultations	0.02
What do you think about the current scheme of prescribing the necessary drugs?	0.0001
To what extent are you informed about the character of your disease and do you think you have chances to overcome the disease?	0.001
What do you think about your obligation to visit the hospital once per month for treatment?	0.002

Table 2. Is the word "cancer" a taboo for you and your family? (Dependent variable).

Independent variable	p <
Doctors' professionalism/competence in diagnostics and treatment	0.02
How would you evaluate as a whole your satisfaction with the medical services you experienced by now?	0.005
If you do not succeed to visit the doctor for treatment every month, what are the reasons for that?	0.02
Please, share with us whether you have problems during the visit to the outpatients' and what they are	0.0001
Provision of psychological consultations	0.02
Doctors' attitude to the patients	0.05

Table 3. Are you supported by the people with whom you have shared about your diagnosis? (dependent variable).

The data from the analysis of the answers to the question whether patients get support are presented in **Table 3**.

Social support is very important in the case of chronic diseases—it is a tool to collect information associated with the disease and sufferings, to reduce uncertainty—with chronic diseases there is always uncertainty about who will administer the treatment and how and what the patient's future will be, to establish a sense of certainty. Social support is effective when the chronically ill individual assesses it as adequate and is satisfied with it.

The psychological ban to use the word "cancer" is usually imposed by the victim or the people he/she lives with. The most frequent case is that his close relatives do not want to suggest him/her that he/she is ill and that the probability for a lethal exit is quite high. At the same time, the patient himself does not want to feel inferior, and in this aspect, he/she rejects talking about his disease, accepting his/her state as natural.

The patient prefers to talk about this topic only with people with the same diagnosis. They want to hear how other people who have been in the same situation have overcome the situation successfully. Only a person who has had cancer can understand the experience carried by the diagnosis, illness, and treatment. The strongest support is usually provided by their closest relatives, but in this case, there are many embarrassing facts depending on the victim's state that could impede his sincerity to his relatives.

3. Self-management support through establishing consultation rooms

Considering the difficulties experienced by each patient with colorectal cancer, we primarily started organizing consultations on the use of anus praeter pouches after surgical intervention. During those consultations it was established that the patients needed not only practical training but also support in various aspects: information about the disease itself, about the treatment course and disease development, the effect of administered drugs and therapeutic approaches, the importance of self-management, and role of psychological control.

Our consultation activities started with the first office in Sofia, followed in the subsequent years by similar consultation rooms in the towns: Plovdiv, Varna, Burgas, Pleven, Ruse, Stara Zagora, and Haskovo. The consultations are held by a doctor, a pharmacist, or a nurse—specially trained to work with patients with stoma. The Sofia office has employed the largest staff of consulting specialists followed by Varna and Plovdiv offices employing two different specialists. The offices at the other towns have only one consultant. The total number of patients who have visited the consultation rooms exceeds 5000, unevenly distributed in the years with a marked trend to increase during the recent years. Thus, at this stage the number of patients who have visited the consultation offices exceeds 1500 per year. The expectations envisage significant increase in compliance with the current data from epidemiological studies on colorectal cancer incidence rate. The preoperative consultations cover informing the patient about the necessity of specific tests aiming at precise diagnosis, eventually surgical intervention, revealing the particular options to delay the disease development process or the disease outcome. The patient is introduced to the possibilities of the postoperative therapeutic approaches focusing on handling the stoma bag. The matter is visualized by specially prepared brochures, photos, films, stoma model, and products for servicing the stoma, though without detailed training. The postoperative consultations mainly refer to handling the stoma through the use of various products, cosmetics, and accessories facilitating the patient's work. The patients participate in training courses, and in the majority of cases, their relatives are also trained because after the surgery, most of the patients cannot perceive correctly the recommendations due to the stress they are experiencing. This state is about new products and accessories. The patients are also advised about the procedures to reimburse the products. The role of the consultant who must help the patient in the postoperative recovery period is particularly important. That type of patients, especially the younger ones, is to be resocialized as quickly as possible, to go back to work, to have the same engagements as before the intervention. They must be sure that there is no difference between them and the other people and to have normal lifestyle. This is particularly valid for their sexual life due to the embarrassing presence of the stoma. The so-called "emotional self-care" incorporates approaches associated with clarification and enrichment of the information about the therapeutic interventions in order to comprehend their effect on the patient's physical and mental well-being and to help him to rationalize the effect of the comprehensive treatment process. The consultations affected the normalization of the patients' lifestyle and strengthened their sense of identity. In all above aspects, the patients get the necessary advice and current scientific information. Thus their awareness, respectively, the effectiveness of the self-management, is enhanced, achieving successful risk management. In addition to the basic consultation activity of the offices established in the towns, medical nurses were employed by contracts for home visits. Those visits are postoperative, and each patient is entitled to two free visits, paid by us. The office staff also organizes lectures engaging leading specialists in nutrition because of the particular patients' interest associated with possibilities and changes in their dietary regime, suggested by the disease. The series of activities provided by the specialists at the consultation offices substantiates the effectiveness of risk management at colorectal carcinoma. Although the importance of self-management is widely acknowledged and the patients are actively encouraged to take greater responsibility for their self-care, the scientific publications show that there is little empirical evidence and self-care is not in the patients' center of attention [9].

We would like to underline, listing the results of this survey, that the understanding of the meaning, content, and importance of self-management and self-management support, concerning particularly Bulgarian patients treated for colorectal cancer, is still insufficient. We would accentuate on the recommendations for broader scope of self-management upgrading it with the psychological and emotional aspects of health care and health management, facilitating it with appropriate effective self-management support.

4. Self-management support through promoting the awareness of colorectal cancer patients

The quick development of science provides many interesting data and facts that have to be clear not only to the therapist, manager, and health-care specialists but also to the patients and individuals at risk. In this aspect we attempted to introduce to our patients certain topics that we shall present briefly in this paper. The topics that were discussed with the patients and health-care specialists were intake of vitamins, antioxidants, and fibers as they are implemented broadly even without being prescribed by a doctor in the diet of cancer patients. The most frequent questions during the consultations were focused on those topics. Patients' awareness in this respect is recommendable not only for the self-management of the individual patient but also for the effective health management and health care.

4.1. Thiamine (vitamin B_1): colorectal cancer

The reason to focus on this problem is the patients' question "Why must we not intake vitamins of the group B?" as well as the growing amount of data showing a relationship between thiamine deficiency and the low extent of cancer incidence. Very often the recent recommendations for the nutrition of cancer patients include the recommendation to avoid the intake of vitamins of the group B and particularly vitamin B1 [10–12]. It is necessary to make it clear to patients that one and the same compound could be essential for the normal functioning of the organism and a risk factor at the same time. Are those facts due to the chemical nature of the vitamin itself or to the processes it is involved in? In this aspect many researchers are striving to find the exact answer, but there are still disputable items.

Thiamine is an essential, water-soluble vitamin, necessary for supporting the carbohydrate metabolism. It is essential for the activity of four key enzymes: pyruvate dehydrogenase, alpha-ketoglutarate dehydrogenase in the pathway of the tricarbonic acids, transketolase in the pentose-phosphate pathway, and branched chain alpha-keto acids—dehydrogenase complex, engaged in the amino acid catabolism.

The importance of thiamine for cancer cell proliferation has been proven with the use of the thiaminase enzyme. It has been confirmed that adding thiamine to a cell culture containing thiamine has a significant suppressing effect on the growth of cancer cells. Thiaminase causes reduction of ATP in the cancer cells underlining the key role of thiamine in maintaining the bioenergetic status of cancer cells. The role of thiamine was most clearly studied through using its analogue—oxythiamine. It can suppress tumor growth both in vivo and in vitro. Transketolase inhibition by oxythiamine causes reduction of DNA and RNA synthesis through reduction of riboso-5-phosphate. This pentose is involved in the synthesis of all nucleotides. It has also been proven that oxythiamine is involved in apoptosis initiation in an experimental study on rats [13–15].

Together with those announcements come very interesting data from epidemiological studies showing a mono-directional relationship between low thiamine intake and very low level of cancer disease incidence rate [3, 12, 16]. It is accepted that the low dietary intake of vitamin B1 can be due both to its low content in the dietary foods and the high content of the thiaminase enzyme, decomposing thiamine. In the Asian and African countries, many food products characteristic for the local population diet contain thiaminase in higher amounts (fish, vegetables, nuts, seeds, and insects) that is the reason for the low dietary import of the vitamin. In this respect the clearest data are obtained by epidemiological studies, conducted in Gambia and Nigeria where the seasonal thiamine deficiency is a well-known health problem [10]. According to the reports of the National Cancer Register in America, providing data at global level as well, the lowest extent of prevalence of colorectal cancer, prostate cancer, and breast cancer is just in those countries (Gambia and Nigeria). Compared to them the prevalence of those cancer diseases in the Western countries is 50–100 times greater [3, 14, 15]. The exact mechanism of thiamine involvement in carcinogenesis processes is still disputable, but the epidemiological data are sufficient to make us cautious when administering vitamins of group B to population groups at risk for colorectal cancer.

It should be outlined that the scientific publications have reported data that did not reveal such relationship between thiamine deficiency and carcinogenesis [17, 18]. The relationship between changes in the thiamine status and the enhanced proliferation of the cancer tissue directs the scientific research efforts to a more detailed investigation of the role of thiamine and its involvement in the biochemical mechanisms of carcinogenesis [14, 16, 19]. The analysis of recent scientific publications proves that, in spite of the relatively small number of studies on the dependence between thiamine diet supplementation and the occurrence of cancer diseases, the majority of them confirm that thiamine deficiency in the organism could be accepted as a preventive factor against the development of various cancer diseases. The metabolic investigations reveal the dependence of cancer cells on the availability of thiamine-dependent enzymes for the processes of anabolism and proliferation and for their existence as a whole.

4.2. Antioxidants: colorectal cancer

The second aspect of the application of scientific achievements refers to the role of antioxidants. Antioxidants are a subject of comprehensive research of cancer diseases as the oxidative stress is the first step involved in the mutagenesis and carcinogenesis processes, confirmed by numerous studies [20–22]. A detailed analysis and evaluation of the recent scientific evidence concerning antioxidant effect in the case of colorectal cancer are presented in our previous works [23].

According to the "antioxidant hypothesis," the reduction agents protect the organism against oxidative damage, and their higher level is a warranty to reduce the risk for development of many diseases. Oxidative stress plays an important role in the pathogenesis of cancer diseases as it is a disbalance between the effect of active oxygen radicals and that of the antioxidant's defense system. Because of the substantial increase of colorectal cancer incidence rate and the associated elevated mortality rate in the last decades, a number of studies have been dedicated to the role of antioxidants in the diet of patients with colorectal cancer [20, 24, 25]. The spectrum of those compounds contains a broad variety of vitamins, amino acids, minerals, and bioactive compounds—flavonoids, carotenoids, glucosinolates, etc.

The general antitumor therapies such as surgical intervention and chemo- and radiation therapy have been and still are subjected to improvements, but it is still necessary to develop innovative approaches for the effective cancer therapy as well as for provision of healthy life style. One of the promising more recent approaches is associated with the administration of antioxidants; thus, during the last years, their chemopreventive potential was analyzed in-depth and implemented successfully in a number of cases [26, 27]. New, particular information is needed, characterizing the rich variety of antioxidant-active compounds as well as information about the approaches and specificity of their administration. It is a mass practice nowadays that patients, upon their desire, without doctor's advice or prescription use various antioxidants that challenges the medical science to clarify those issues. Because of the existing numerous, different standpoints concerning antioxidant implementation in primary and secondary prevention of cancer diseases, it is necessary that the patients receive particular information from their doctor and dietician complying with their health status.

Numerous research studies have confirmed that the high consumption of fruits and vegetable has a certain preventive role against the development of cancer diseases that is associated with their rich content of various antioxidants [28, 29]. Having in mind that the main route of intake of exogenous antioxidants is with food which undergoes different metabolic processes in the digestive system, it is logical to assume their direct effect on the particular organs building that system. The diet for cancer diseases depends to a large extent on the involved organ determining its specificity. The most frequently applied diets are those rich in vitamins and minerals, and recently, their spectrum was enhanced with some bioactive compounds contained in the foods and food supplements [2, 25].

After the culmination of data and information about the positive effect of antioxidant implementation against the development of various cancer diseases, other evidence, not confirming similar effects, were communicated [24, 26]. Differences were outlined in the positive results from experimental studies and those from and clinical studies revealing negative effects.

Antioxidant intake is not recommended during chemo- and radiation therapy courses in order to prevent reduction of their power. In the case of diagnosed colorectal cancer after surgery and chemo- and radiation therapy, very high doses of individual antioxidants or combinations of synergically acting bioactive compounds with antioxidant activity must be administered depending on the patient's status. In risk groups, with family history it is recommendable to include high antioxidant doses in the primary prevention programs. The successful health management requires the administration of high doses of antioxidants also in the secondary prevention of colorectal cancer in the form of a cocktail of several antioxidants with upgrading activity.

4.3. Fibers: colorectal cancer

The third aspect of scientific evidence covers the clarification of the role of dietary fibers as the knowledge in this respect undergoes serious changes proven by scientific research [30, 31].

The necessity to know the evolution of knowledge on risk factors on one side and their contradistinction with relevant preventive factors on the other are important elements of health management in the case of colorectal cancer. Logically, serious attention is given to food which, following its metabolic pathways, has direct effect on the gastrointestinal system as well as systemic effect through the nutrients and bioactive compounds contained in it. Many scientific investigations associated with the analysis and assessment of risk and preventive factors are focused on fibers. In one of our publications, we have presented very detailed information and analysis of existing scientific views on the "fibers and colorectal cancer" issue [32]. We have presented the assessment of the scientific information in two major aspects: mechanisms of fibers activity and studies on patients with colorectal cancer.

The general classic explanations of the biological activity of fibers are establishment of a larger area for development of intestinal microflora, activation of the peristaltic, and creation of a sensation of satiety. In relation to oncogenesis and colorectal cancer in particular, those explanations have their specificity determined by the anatomy and physiology of the colon. Of particular importance are the fibers' composition, their solubility, and ability to ferment, to modify the acid-alkaline balance, and to participate indirectly in the transformation of bile acids. An important factor is also the direct physical effect on the inner lining of the colon, a fact that must not be neglected especially after surgical intervention.

Almost all studies reveal the lack of consensus on the issue and need of further studies in order to provide a particular explanation of the mechanisms involved by fibers to realize their preventive effect against colorectal cancer. The recommendations for consumption of dietary fibers after surgery should be particularly careful because of their direct effect on the colon. The lack of unified test models, the significant methodological errors in the assessment of the diet of the investigated patients, as well as the differences between the experimental and clinical trials seriously challenge the science to plan further comprehensive studies covering all dimensions of the problem dietary fibers—carcinogenesis.

5. Conclusion

This survey on the necessity of activating the self-management of patients with colorectal cancer shows a definite need to promote patients' awareness on the etiopathogenesis of the disease, individual disease course, the role and importance of the administered drug treatment, and implementation of various therapeutic approaches and health care.

The repeating of the relationships between the discussed questions is identified as a primary task in the orientation of the patients to doctors and health-care specialists with proven professionalism with cultural competence allowing particular personal attitude to each patient.

The presented data reveal the need to conduct studies at individual level as each patient is characterized by the specificity of the disease course, awareness, psychological status, and cultural competence. Those diverse characteristics require also different self-management support in order to encourage the patients with colorectal cancer to improve and maintain a healthy lifestyle.

Author details

Racho Ribarov

Address all correspondence to: r.ribarov@rsr-bg.com

Faculty of Public Health, Medical University – Sofia, Sofia, Bulgaria

References

[1] Grazin N. Long-term conditions: Help patients to help themselves. The Health Service Journal. 2007;**117**:28-29

[2] Tarraga P, Solera J, Rodriguez-Montes J. Primary and secondary prevention of colorectal cancer. Clinical Medicine Insights: Gastroenterology. 2014;**7**:33-46

[3] Ribarov R. Interesting facts related to colorectal cancer epidemiology. Archives of the Balkan Medical Union. 2015;**50**(1):45-49

[4] Bodenheimer T, Loring K, Holman H. Patient self-management of chronic disease in primary care. Journal of the American Medical Association. 2002;**288**(19):2469-2475. DOI: 10.1001/jama.288.19.2469

[5] Ribarov R, Tz V, Ivanov A, Ivanova N. Necessity of self-management support following colorectal cancer treatment. Archives of the Balkan Medical Union. 2017;**52**(3):285-291

[6] Foster C, Fenlon D. Recovery and self-management support following primary cancer treatment. British Journal of Cancer. 2011;**105**:S21-S28

[7] Kidd LA. Consequences, control and appraisal: Cues and barriers to engaging in self-management among people affected by colorectal cancer-A secondary analysis of qualitative data. Health Expectations. 2014;**17**(4):565-578

[8] Ribarov R. Study on the awareness of patients with colorectal cancer. The 33 Balkan medical week, 8-11 October, 2014, Bucharest, Romania. Archives of the Balkan Medical Union. 2014;**49**(1):A119-A120

[9] Kidd L, Kearney N, O'Carroll R, Hubbard G. Experiences of self-care in patients with colorectal cancer: A longitudinal study. Journal of Advanced Nursing. 2008;**64**(5): 469-477

[10] Boros L. Population thiamine status and varying cancer rates between Western, Asian and African counters. Anticancer Research. 2000;**20**:2248

[11] Cascante M, Centelles J, Velch R. Role of thiamin (vitamin B1) and trans ketolase in tumor cell proliferation. Nutrition and Cancer. 2000;**36**(2):150-154

[12] Lee B, Yanamandra K, Bocchini J. Thiamin deficiency: A possible major cause of some tumors? Oncology Reports. 2005;**14**:1589-1592

[13] DeBorardinis R, Lum J, Hatzivassillon G, Thompson C. The biology of cancer & metabolic reprogramming fuels cell growth and proliferation. Cell Metabolism. 2008;**7**:11-20

[14] Yang CM, Liu YZ, Liao JW, ML H. The in vitro and in vivo anti-metastatic efficacy of oxythiamine and the possible mechanisms of action. Clinical & Experimental Metastasis. 2010;**27**:341-349

[15] Daily A, Liu S, Bhatnagar S, Karabakhtsian RG, Moscow JA. Low-thiamine diet increases mammary tumor latency in FVB/N-Tg(MMTVneu) mice. International Journal for Vitamin and Nutrition Research. 2012;**82**:298-302

[16] Zastre J, Sweet L, Hanberry B, Ye S. Linking vitamin B1 with cancer cell metabolism. Cancer Metabolism. 2013;**1**:1-16

[17] Kabat G, Miller A, Rohan T. Dietary intake of selected B vitamins in relation to risk of major cancers in women. British Journal of Cancer. 2008;**99**:816-821

[18] Liu S, Monks NR, Hanes JW, Begley TP, Yu H, Moscow JA. Sensitivity of breast cancer cell lines to recombinant thiaminase I. Cancer Chemotherapy and Pharmacology. 2010;**66**:171-179

[19] Willett WC. Diet and cancer: An evolving picture. Journal of the American Medical Association. 2005;**293**:233-237

[20] Papaioannou D, Cooper K, Carroll C. Antioxidants in the chemoprevention of colorectal cancer and colorectal adenomas in the general population: A systematic review and meta-analysis. Colorectal Disease. 2011;**13**(10):1085-1099

[21] WCRF: World Cancer Research Fund and American Institute for Cancer Research. Colorectal Cancer Report. Food, Nutrition, Physical Activity, and the Prevention of Colorectal Cancer. 2010. http://www.wcrf.org

[22] Zhang R, Kang K, Kim K. Oxidative stress causes epigenetic alteration of CDX1 expression in colorectal cancer cells. Gene. 2013;**524**(2):214-219

[23] Ribarov R. Antioxidants and colorectal cancer. Journal of Contemporary Medical Problems. 2015;**3**:5-11

[24] Pais R, Dumitrascu D. Do antioxidants prevent colorectal cancer ? A meta-analysis. Romanian Journal of Internal Medicine. 2013;**51**(3-4):152-163

[25] Saud S, Young M, Jones-Hall Y. Chemopreventive activity of plant flavonoid isorhamnetin in colorectal cancer is mediated by oncogenic Src and beta-catenin. Cancer Research. 2013;**73**(17):5473-5484

[26] Bjelakovic G, Nagorny A, Nikolowa D. Meta-analysis: Antioxidant supplements for primary and secondary prevention of colorectal adenoma. Alimentary Pharmacology & Therapeutics. 2006;**15**(24):281-291

[27] Wang Z, Ohnaka K, Morita M. Dietary polyphenols and colorectal cancer risk: the Fukuoka colorectal cancer study. World Journal of Gastroenterology. 2013;**19**(17):2683-2690

[28] Hou N, Huo D, Dignam J. Prevention of colorectal cancer and dietary management. Chinese Clinical Oncology. 2013;**2**:13-26

[29] Royston K, Tollefsbol T. The epigenetic impact of cruciferous vegetables on cancer prevention. Current Pharmacology Reports. 2015;**1**(1):46-51

[30] Peters U, Sinha R, Chatterjee N. Dietary fibre and colorectal adenoma in a colorectal cancer early detection programme. Lancet. 2003;**361**:1491-1495

[31] Schatzkin A, Mouw T, Park Y. Dietary fiber and whole–grain consumption in relation to colorectal cancer in NIH-AARP diet and health study. The American Journal of Clinical Nutrition. 2007;**85**:1353-1360

[32] Ribarov R, Tz V, Ivanov A. Dietary fibers and colorectal cancer. Archives of the Balkan Medical Union. 2015;**50**(3):410-413

5

Screening and Surveillance Colonoscopy

Rotimi R. Ayoola, Hamza Abdulla, Evan K. Brady, Muhammed Sherid and Humberto Sifuentes

Abstract

Colorectal cancer is a major cause of worldwide morbidity and mortality. As such, there are many guidelines and recommendations set forth by various medical societies regarding colonoscopy for screening and surveillance. The universal goal of these guidelines is to reduce colorectal cancer prevalence and mortality. Recommendations for colorectal cancer screening and surveillance using colonoscopy vary slightly between medical society guidelines and are often dictated by some combination of age, known disease severity, length of time since last study, family history, and comorbid conditions.

Keywords: Screening, surveillance, colonoscopy, recommendations, colorectal cancer

1. Introduction

Colorectal cancer is the second leading cause of death from cancer in the United States, as well as the fourth most common cause of cancer-related death, and the third most diagnosed cancer worldwide.[1, 3] In 2008, there were an estimated 1.2 million newly diagnosed cases of colorectal cancer worldwide and an estimated 609,000 colorectal cancer-related deaths.[3] In 2014, it was estimated that there were 136,830 newly diagnosed cases of colorectal cancer and nearly 50,310 deaths associated with this disease in the Unites States alone.[4] The age-adjusted incidence of colorectal cancer in the United States was 43.7 cases per 100,000 population among men and women based on reported cases from 2007 to 2011.[4] In 2011, there were an estimated 1,162,426 people living with colon and rectum cancer in the United States.[4] Screening of those at average risk may result in lower mortality rates by detecting cancers at earlier and more curable stages. Also, detection of cancer-precursor lesions may reduce the incidence of colorectal cancer if removed on endoscopic screening tests.[5, 6] The incidence and mortality of colorectal cancer have declined from 2002 to 2010 in the United States,[7] possibly due to improvement in the adherence to screening and surveillance guidelines.

2. Colorectal cancer screening

2.1. Prevention strategies

Recommended strategies for colorectal cancer screening can be divided into two categories: stool tests (occult blood and DNA tests) and structural examinations (flexible sigmoidoscopy, colonoscopy, double contrast barium enema, capsule endoscopy, and computed tomographic colonography). Each screening method has its own advantages and disadvantages, which are summarized in Table 1. Screening is currently recommended beginning at 50 years of age in average-risk populations, and varies in populations with increased risks.[6, 8]

Test	Advantages	Disadvantages
Sensitive guaiac fecal occult blood test	Inexpensive, easily done at home	Low sensitivity, annually repeated, lack of compliance
Fecal immunochemical test	Inexpensive, easily done at home	More expensive than guaiac fecal occult, annually repeated, unknown adherence, low sensitivity for advanced adenomas
Stool DNA	More accurate than blood detection; easily done at home	Expensive, sensitivity and specificity unknown, uncertain screening intervals
CT Colonography	High sensitivity of lesions >10 mm in diameter; not invasive	Not been proven to reduce incidence or mortality, bowel prep needed, unknown management of polyps <6 mm in diameter, radiation exposure
Sigmoidoscopy	Can be done in office without sedation, 60% reduction in mortality from cancer of the distal colon	Proximal colon cancer may be missed
Colonoscopy	90% sensitivity for lesions >10 mm in diameter, 53-72% reduction in incidence and 31% reduction in mortality from colorectal cancer, lesions can be detected and removed during one examination	Bowel preparation and expertise needed, expensive, invasive with possible complications

**Data from Lieberman[6], Baxter, et al.[9], Muller, et al.[10], and Singh, et al.[11]

Table 1. Advantages and disadvantages of screening tests

Strategies used to identify patients at an increased risk for developing colorectal cancer should be started early. Before determining the best screening tool, clinicians should determine a patient's level of risk. The most common indicator of increased risk is a first-degree relative with colorectal cancer. Diagnosis of colorectal cancer in a first-degree relative before 50 years of age is concerning for hereditary gastrointestinal cancer syndromes such as Lynch syndrome, familial adenomatous polyposis (FAP), attenuated familial adenomatous polyposis (AFAP), and MUTYH-associated polyposis (MAP). Patients with hereditary gastrointestinal cancer syndromes require a special timing for endoscopic screening and surveillance. Colonoscopy is the preferred screening test in these persons, which should be initiated at 40 years of age or 10 years younger than the age at which the family member was diagnosed with colorectal cancer, whichever comes first.[6, 8] Patients with chronic ulcerative colitis or colitis due to Crohn's disease are at increased risk for colorectal cancer and should undergo a screening colonoscopy after 8-10 years.[6, 8] Prior colorectal cancer or polyps also increases the risk of colorectal cancer, especially if polyps are large, or have villous architecture.[12]

2.2. Identifying high-risk individuals

The risk of developing colorectal cancer is largely multifactorial. The factors associated with an increased risk of colorectal cancer include lack of physical activity, obesity, high-fat and low-fiber diets, tobacco use, gender, ethnicity, and genetics. There is limited evidence to suggest that lifestyle modification alone in adults will reduce the risk of this cancer.[6, 13] Aspirin, nonsteroidal anti-inflammatory drugs, and hormone-replacement therapy can decrease the risk of adenomas or colorectal cancer but are not recommended in prevention of colorectal cancer because the possible adverse effects are higher than the potential benefits.[6, 14, 15]

2.3. Screening modalities

Multiple tests are used as options for colorectal cancer screening. Stool-based tests can improve disease prognosis by detecting early cancers. Endoscopic or radiologic tests can visualize the bowel mucosa and detect polyps that can be removed before malignant transformation. Sensitivities of various screening modalities (Table 2) and screening guidelines (Table 3) can be very useful when choosing the most appropriate screening test.

Test	Sensitivity		References
	Cancer Detection	Advanced Adenoma* Detection	
Standard guaiac fecal occult blood test (three stool samples)	33-50%	11%	Mandel et al.[16], Hardcastle et al.[17], Kronborg et al.[18], Imperiale TF.[19], Ahlquist.[20]

Test	Sensitivity		References
Sensitive guaiac fecal occult blood test (three stool samples)	50-75%	20-25%	Allison et al.[15], Levin et al.[21], Whitlock et al. [22], Ahlquist et al.[20]
Immunochemical fecal occult blood test (one-three stool samples)	60-85%	20-50%	Levin et al.[21], Whitlock et al.[22]
Old stool DNA test (one stool sample)	51%	18%	Imperiale et al.[19]
New stool DNA test (one stool sample)	≥80%	40%	Allison et al.[15], Itzkowitz et al.[23]
CT Colonography	Uncertain; probably >90%	90% (if ≥10 mm diameter)	Johnson et al.[24]
Sigmoidoscopy	>95% (for distal colon)	70%	Lieberman[6], Shelby et al.[25]
Colonoscopy	>95%	88-98%	Lieberman[6], Imperiale et al.[19], Schoenfeld et al.[26], Lieberman et al.[27], Pickhardt et al.[28], Cotton et al.[29], Rockey et al.[30]

*Advanced adenoma is defined as tubular adenoma that is ≥10 mm in diameter or with villous histologic features or high-grade dysplasia.

Table 2. Sensitivity of one-time colorectal cancer screening tests

Screening Test	ACS-MSTF-ACR	USPSTF	Recommended Interval for Rescreening
Sensitive guaiac fecal occult blood test	Recommended if "/>50% sensitivity for colorectal cancer	Recommended	1 yr
Fecal immunochemical test	Recommended if >50% sensitivity for colorectal cancer	Recommended; high-sensitivity test only	1 yr
Stool DNA test	Recommended if >50% sensitivity for colorectal cancer	Not Recommended (insufficient evidence to assess sensitivity and specificity of fecal DNA)	Uncertain

Screening Test	ACS-MSTF-ACR	USPSTF	Recommended Interval for Rescreening
Flexible sigmoidoscopy	Recommended if sigmoidoscope is inserted to 40 cm of the colon or to the splenic flexure	Recommended; with guaiac fecal occult blood test every 35 yr yr	
Barium enema Examination	Recommended, but only if other tests not available	Not recommended	5 yr
CT colonography	Recommended, with referral for colonoscopy if polyps ≥6 mm in diameter detected	Not recommended (insufficient evidence to determine risk-benefit ratio)	5 yr
Colonoscopy	Recommended	Recommended	10 yr

* Data from Lieberman[6], Preventive Services Task Force[14], Levin et al.[21], Preventive Services Task Force[14], and Whitlock et al.[22]; ACS-MSTF-ACR denotes American cancer Society, US Multisociety task force on Colorectal Cancer, and American College of Radiology; and USPSTF denotes US Preventive services Task Force.

Table 3. US colorectal cancer screening guidelines, 2008*

2.3.1. Fecal screening tests

Fecal screening tests use small stool samples to help determine the presence of colorectal cancer. Fecal screening tests include Guaiac-based fecal occult blood test, immunochemical-based fecal occult blood test, also known as fecal immunochemical test (FIT), and Cologuard (fecal DNA testing, combined with hemoglobin and DNA methylation assays). These tests are easily performed at home or in a clinical office, are noninvasive, inexpensive, without direct adverse health effects, and require few specialized resources. One disadvantage of fecal testing is that positive results require colonoscopy evaluation to confirm or exclude the diagnosis of colorectal cancer.

Guaiac fecal occult blood tests detect hemoglobin peroxidase activity and turn guaiac-impregnated paper blue, but are not specific for human blood. Three separate stool samples per test are preferred for better sensitivity.[21] The fecal occult blood test is associated with significant false-positive results, which may lead to unnecessary follow-up colonoscopies. In the Minnesota trial, false-positive test results were found in almost 9% of fecal occult blood testing.[3] The cost-effectiveness of colorectal cancer screening with an annual or biennial fecal occult blood test varied from US$ 5,691 to US$ 17,805 per life-year gained.[31] Randomized, controlled trials in which standard guaiac tests were administered annually or biennially have shown that cancers are detected at an earlier and more curable stage when compared with no regular screening. Over a period of 10-13 years, regular guaiac screening tests result in a reduction of colorectal cancer mortality by 15-33%.[6, 8, 32]

FIT uses antibodies specific to hemoglobin to screen for colorectal cancer. It is more accurate than the guaiac test.[33, 37] As a result, FIT is now recommended as the first-choice fecal occult blood test in colorectal cancer screening.[38] FIT has sensitivity for detecting cancer of 60-85%

with the use of one to three stool samples.[4, 6, 22] Cologuard is a screening modality that tests stool DNA for specific mutations that are associated with colorectal cancer. These specific segments of cellular DNA are excreted in stool and can be detected with the use of polymerase chain reaction (PCR) amplification. Newer versions of the test are currently being developed; however, overall performance, utility, and cost-effectiveness has not been well studied.

2.3.2. Structural examinations of the colon

Colorectal cancers can be detected through physical exams with a digital rectal examination, but there is little evidence to support the effectiveness of digital rectal exam in the detection of colorectal cancer and, therefore, it is not recommended in the current screening guidelines (Table 3).

Anatomical examination of the colon is effective in detection of early cancer and precancerous lesions. Radiography imaging such as barium enema and computed tomographic (CT) colonography can be used to detect lesions. In clinical studies of CT colonography for polyp detection with expert radiologists, 90% of polyps 10 mm or larger in diameter were identified correctly, with a false-positive rate of 14%.[6] CT colonography is not as sensitive for polyps less than 6 mm. There are currently no conclusive studies supporting appropriate screening intervals for negative results or suitable next steps for polyps less than 6 mm. While radiation exposure during CT colonography is considered minimal, the cumulative radiation exposure puts people at increased risk for developing other types of radiation-related cancers. Additionally, cost-effectiveness of CT colonography has not been thoroughly studied in comparison to other modalities.

Before colonoscopy became available, barium enema was the primary means of detecting polyps, and their removal required surgical colostomy.[39] Barium enema examination is not the best test for identifying precancerous lesions and is rarely used for colorectal-cancer screening in current practice.[6] Double-contrast barium enema is another screening modality that involves the patient drinking contrast, which coats the intestinal mucosa with barium. Then, the colon is insufflated with air and multiple radiographs are taken under fluoroscopy. Double-contrast barium enema detects about half of adenomas larger than 1 cm and 39% of all polyps.[40] Retrospective studies have found that double-contrast barium enema failed to diagnose 15-22% of colorectal cancers.[41] If an abnormality is found, then colonoscopy evaluation should follow. False-positives or inconclusive results can be a result of stool, mucosal irregularities, or air. Barium enemas are safe and typically do not require sedation, but may cause the patient discomfort during the procedure. The usage rates of double contrast barium enema for colorectal cancer screening recently declined with improved screening tools, but may be useful where colonoscopy is not readily available.[42]

Endoscopic screening is more sensitive than fecal testing for the detection of adenomatous polyps.[37, 43, 45] In the United Kingdom, one-time screening with flexible sigmoidoscopy significantly reduced the incidence of colorectal cancer by 23% and cancer-related mortality by 31%.[45, 46] Studies, with the use of screening colonoscopy, have shown that more than 30% of patients with advanced neoplasia have proximal lesions that would not be identified with sigmoidoscopy alone.[47, 48]

The most performed indication for colonoscopy in the United States is for screening and surveillance purposes. Colonoscopy can detect a wide range of colon pathologies including polyps, angiodysplasias, hemorrhoids, and cancer. Colonoscopy also permits therapeutic interventions. The procedure is highly feasible and relatively safe. The quality of the procedure depends on an adequate bowel preparation. The patient is typically sedated throughout the procedure. Colonoscopy can reduce the incidence and the mortality of colorectal cancer.[9, 27, 49] Endoscopic procedures may be uncomfortable for patients and carry the risks of perforation and bleeding, especially when polypectomy is performed. The risk of serious adverse events is 3-5 events per 1000 colonoscopies.[6]

Capsule endoscopy has the potential to become a useful screening tool. A camera, in the size and shape of a pill, is swallowed to help visualize the gastrointestinal tract. Reductions of incidence and mortality have not yet been studied using this modality. Capsule endoscopy does not require sedation or radiation. However, accuracy data show inferior screening performance compared to colonoscopy.[3] Despite all these available methods, colorectal cancer screening rates are still suboptimal. In a National Health Interview Survey in 2010, the rate of screening was only 58.6%.[39]

2.4. Screening guidelines

Two major guidelines, from the US Preventive Services Task Force (USPSTF) and a joint guideline from the American Cancer Society, the US Multi-Society Task Force on Colorectal Cancer, and the American College of Radiology (ACS-MSTF), were released in 2008 regarding colorectal cancer screening in the United States (Table 3). The joint guidelines recommend structural examinations for cancer prevention. The ACS-MSTF recommends offering screening beginning at age 50 years for average-risk patients, and continued surveillance every 10 years, if negative. In average-risk patients, CT colonography should be performed every 5 years, flexible sigmoidoscopy every 5 years, and double-contrast barium enema every 5 years. The joint guidelines recommend fecal occult blood testing with sensitive guaiac method or fecal immunochemical-based test every year for screening. Screening should be terminated if a patient's life expectancy is less than 10 years.[21] Prior to screening, patients should under stand that a positive test indicates a need for colonoscopy. There are no specific guidelines regarding colorectal cancer screening for sex or ethnicity but the American College of Gastroenterology supports initiation of screening in African Americans at 45 years of age.[8]

The US Preventive Services Task Force does not recommend CT colonography or stool DNA testing. The USPSTF recommends three screening options for adults 50-75 years old: sensitive fecal occult blood testing annually, flexible sigmoidoscopy every 5 years with sensitive fecal occult blood test every 3 years, and colonoscopy every 10 years. Screening for patients older than 75 is not routinely recommended by the USPSTF, and recommends against screening over the age of 85 years.[14] Colorectal cancer screening in older patients who have never undergone formal screening is controversial and there are currently no guidelines regarding appropriate screening in these scenarios. The risk of colorectal cancer and advanced polyps continues to increase in age even after 75 years. Thus, the decision to screen between the ages of 75 and 85 years should be discussed with and individualized to each patient depending on health status and other comorbidities.

In Europe, fecal occult blood testing is implemented at higher rates than in the United States. The fecal occult blood test for individuals aged 50-74 years at average-risk has been recommended to date by the European Union guidelines for colorectal screening, annually or biennially.[15]

The British Society of Gastroenterology (BSG) and the Association of Coloproctology for Great Britain and Ireland (ACPGBI) aimed to provide guidance on the appropriateness, method, and frequency of screening for people at moderate- and high-risk for colorectal cancer.[50]

3. Colorectal cancer surveillance

Surveillance colonoscopy refers to colonoscopy examination performed in asymptomatic individuals with previously identified cancerous or precancerous lesions. Colonoscopy surveillance is used to identify any recurrent or new neoplasia in these individuals.[51] High adenoma detection rate on follow-up colonoscopy (30-50%) provides the rationale for surveillance colonoscopy.[52, 56] There is strong evidence that surveillance colonoscopy decreases colorectal cancer incidence and colorectal cancer-related mortality.[57]

The timing of subsequent surveillance is crucial. Studies demonstrate both the protective effect and cost-effectiveness of performing surveillance colonoscopy on high-risk populations.[58] The overall impact of surveillance is not well defined and may be decreased by an inappropriate utilization of resources and nonadherence to published guidelines.[59]

3.1. Recommendations for surveillance colonoscopy

Guidelines from Gastrointestinal societies in the United States, the United Kingdom, and the European Union follow a risk stratification policy to time their surveillance intervals.

The US Multisociety Task Force (US MSTF) guidelines were published in 2008 and categorize patients into two major risk groups based on the likelihood of development of advanced neoplasia (Table 4). In 2012, the US MSFT updated their guidelines to address the role of serrated polyps, risk of interval colorectal cancer, and proximal colorectal cancer (Table 5).

The European Society of Gastrointestinal Endoscopy (ESGE) updated their guidelines in 2013 and formulated a risk stratification and surveillance strategy similar to the United States (Table 4 and Table 5). A new recommendation was to increase the interval from 3 years to 5 years after a normal follow-up colonoscopy in the high-risk group (3-4 adenomas, villous features or high-grade dysplasia, or ≥10 mm in size).

The UK guidelines are based on adenoma size and number without incorporating histological findings. It stratifies patients into low-, moderate-, and high-risks groups. It also recommends a "single clearing examination" at 1 year for high-risk patients (≥5 small adenomas or ≥3 adenomas, at least 1 of which is ≥1 cm).

	United States Multisociety Task Force (US MSTF)	European Society of Gastrointestinal Endoscopy (ESGE)	British Society of Gastroenterology (BSG)
Risk			
Low	1-2 tubular adenomas <10 mm	1–2 tubular adenomas <10 mm with low-grade dysplasia; serrated polyps < 10 mm and no dysplasia	1–2 adenomas <10 mm
Moderate	-	-	3–4 adenomas <10 mm or at least one adenoma >1cm
High	Adenoma with villous histology or high-grade dysplasia or ≥10 mm or ≥3 adenomas	Adenoma with villous histology or high-grade dysplasia or ≥ 10 mm in size, or ≥3 adenomas; serrated polyps ≥ 10 mm or with dysplasia	>5 small adenomas or at least 3 adenomas >1cm

Table 4. Risk stratification criteria

	United States Multisociety Task Force (US MSTF)	European Society of Gastrointestinal Endoscopy (ESGE)	British Society of Gastroenterology (BSG)
Risk			
Low	5-10 years	10 years	No surveillance or 5 years
Moderate	-	-	3 years
High	**3 years**	3 years	1 years

Table 5. Surveillance interval recommendation

A recently published study, which analyzed 3226 post-polypectomy patients, compared the US MSTF guidelines with the British Society of Gastroenterology (BSG) guidelines. The study showed that the application of the UK guidelines into the US population reclassified 26.3% of patients from high-risk to a higher-risk category and 7% to a lower-risk category.[60] The study also showed a net 19% of patients benefiting from detection 2 years earlier without substantially increasing rates of colonoscopy.[60]

3.2. Sessile serrated adenomas/polyps and surveillance colonoscopy

Sessile serrated adenoma/polyp (SSA/P) is a term used to describe polyps or adenomas characterized by the presence of a sawtooth appearance to crypt contour with prominent dilatation, serrations, and lateralization at the crypt base.[51] The discovery of the serrated adenoma/polyp pathway and the development of colorectal cancer has led to increased interest and focus on the understanding of the histological and molecular changes that lead to CRC. Hypermethylation of genes in serrated lesions leads to microsatellite instability and rapid development of colorectal cancer.[61]

Endoscopically, serrated lesions have a similar appearance to hyperplastic polyps and are often misdiagnosed as such. A recent study showed that as high as one-third of recently diagnosed hyperplastic polyps ≥5 mm were reclassified into SSA/P after a second pathology review.[62] The CARE study found that serrated lesions were five times more likely to be incompletely resected by polypectomy compared to conventional adenomas.[63] Serrated polyps larger than 1 cm or with a dysplastic component are considered advanced polyps.[63]

Surveillance recommendations for serrated adenomas/polyps are inconsistent among researchers and gastrointestinal societies and long-term studies evaluating SSA/P are limited. US MSTF and ESGE classifies serrated polyps <10 mm with no dysplasia as low-risk and serrated polyps ≥10 mm or those with dysplasia as high-risk. Both societies recommend surveillance colonoscopy in 3 years in high-risk. For low-risk lesions, ESGE recommends 10-year follow-up, whereas US MSTF recommends 5-year follow-up.[14, 50, 64]

3.3. Serrated polyposis syndrome

The World Health Organization defines serrated polyposis syndrome by either the presence of five or more serrated polyps proximal to the sigmoid colon (at least two of which must be ≥10 mm) or 20 or more serrated polyps of any size distributed throughout the colon.[65] US MSFT and ESGE recommend one-year follow-up surveillance in this patient population. [14, 66] ESGE also recommends referral for genetic counseling.[14, 66]

3.4. Effect of positive family history on surveillance intervals

Patients with a family history of colorectal carcinoma are at higher risk of developing high-risk adenoma and colorectal carcinoma. US MSTF recommends shortening the surveillance interval from 10 years to 5 years in patients with low-risk findings on colonoscopy and a first-degree relative with colorectal cancer prior to the age of 60.[14] US MSTF also recommends surveillance with colonoscopy as the preferred method.[14]

3.5. Surveillance colonoscopy in the elderly

There is a significant increase in incidence of both CRC and adenomas with increasing age.[14] The age at which screening colonoscopy should be performed remains controversial. Studies that examined the role of age in surveillance colonoscopy found no association with increasing age and polyp recurrence and concluded it was not necessary to tailor surveillance guidelines by age.[5, 67, 70] Retrospective studies have also shown that comorbidities reduce the benefits of CRC screening. The US MSTF does not give a specific age at which screening can be ceased, but recommends that competing comorbidities and life expectancy should be considered before ordering cancer screening at any age.[14]

3.6. Surveillance colonoscopy and physician nonadherence to guidelines

Nonadherence to guidelines remains a major problem in healthcare policy. The overuse of resources could lead to increased demand for colonoscopy, shifting resources from screening, and thus decreasing the cost-effectiveness of CRC screening program by increasing the unnecessary costs and possibility of adverse events. Alternatively, underuse of colonoscopy in surveillance may lead to suboptimal prevention of colorectal cancer. Schohen, et al. retrospectively evaluated 3,627 screening patients with a history of adenoma removal and found overuse of endoscopy in low-risk patients and underuse in high-risk patients.[71] The reasons for guideline nonadherence include lack of strong evidence to support the surveillance intervals, having multiple guidelines with inconsistent recommendations, lack of awareness of current evidence, fear of legal implication, suboptimal bowel preparation, financial incentive for performing the procedure, and miscommunication between gastroenterologist and primary care providers.[72] Measures to improve adherence to guidelines include continued medical education; written recommendations by endoscopist regarding the follow-up interval after the pathology report; quality improvement interventions such as reminder devices; improvement of bowel preparation quality; automated electronic alerting system[72, 73]; and continuous quality improvement process for colonoscopy (education, monitoring, audits, and financial incentives/penalties).[74]

4. Conclusion

Colorectal cancer screening and surveillance have been shown to provide many benefits. The associated risks are relatively minor and vary greatly on the particular screening test, and surveillance regimen. Patients should be informed that screening and surveillance reduce the risk of colorectal cancer, but may require additional tests and/or procedures to diagnose and manage the pathologic findings. Colorectal cancer screening rate is still suboptimal in the United States and this rate could be improved by dedicated patients and clinician reminders, patients' education, outreach, and follow-up. Screening and surveillance must be targeted to appropriate patients and occur at recommended intervals to ensure proper prevention.

Author details

Rotimi R. Ayoola*, Hamza Abdulla, Evan K. Brady, Muhammed Sherid and Humberto Sifuentes*

*Address all correspondence to: rayoola@gru.edu

Georgia Regents University, Augusta, GA, USA

References

[1] Seigel R, Ward E, Brawley O, Jemal A. Cancer statistics, 2011: the impact of eliminating socioeconomic and racial disparities on premature cancer deaths. *CA Cancer J Clin*. 2011;61:212-36.

[2] Ferlay J, Shin HR, Bray F, Forman D, Mathers C, Parkin DM. Estimates of worldwide burden of cancer in 2008: GLOBOCAN 2008. *Int J Cancer*. 2010;127:2893-2917.

[3] Segnan N, Patnick J, von Karsa L (eds.). *European guidelines for quality assurance in colorectal cancer screening and diagnosis*. 1st edn. Belgium: European Union; 2010. p. 386. DOI: 10.2772/15379

[4] National Cancer Institute. SEER Stat Fact Sheets: Colon and Rectum Cancer [Internet]. 2011. Available from: http://seer.cancer.gov/statfacts/html/colorect.html [Accessed: Feb 2015]

[5] Winawer SJ, Zauber AG, Ho MN, et al. Prevention of colorectal cancer by colonoscopic polypectomy. *N Engl J Med*. 1993;329:1977-81.

[6] Lieberman DA. Screening for colorectal cancer. *N Engl J Med*. 2009;361:1179-87. DOI: 10.1056/NEJMcp0902176

[7] Centers for Disease Control and Prevention (CDC). Vital signs: colorectal cancer screening, incidence, and mortality, 2002-2010. *Morb Mortal Wkly Report*. 2011;60:884.

[8] Winamer S, Fletcher R, Rex D, et al. Colorectal cancer screening and surveillance: clinical guidelines and rationale--update based on new evidence. *Gastroenterology*. 2003;124:544-60.

[9] Baxter NN, Goldwasser MA, PAszat LF, Saskin R, Urbach DR, Rabeneck LA. Association of colonoscopy and death from colorectal cancer. *Ann Int Med*. 2009;150:1-8.

[10] Muller AD, Sonnenberg A. Prevention of colorectal cancer by flexible endoscopy and polypectomy: a case-control study of 32,702 veterans. *Ann Int Med*. 1995;123:904-10.

[11] Singh H, Turner D, Xue L, Targownik LE, Bernstein CN. Risk of developing colorectal cancer following a negative colonoscopy examination: evidence for a 10-year interval between colonoscopies. *JAMA*. 2006;295:2366-73.

[12] Atkin WS, Morson BC, Cuzick J. Long-term risk of colorectal cancer after excision of rectosigmoid adenomas. *N Engl J Med*. 1992;326:658.

[13] Hawk ET, Umar A, Viner JL. Colorectal cancer chemoprevention--an overview of the science. *Gastroenterology*. 2004;126:1423-47.

[14] Preventative Services Task Force. Screening for colorectal cancer: US Preventative Services Task Force recommendation statement. *Ann Int Med*. 2008;149:627-37.

[15] Allison JE, Sakoda LC, Levin TR, et al. Screening for colorectal neoplasms with new fecal occult blood tests: update on performance characteristics. *J Natl Cancer Inst.* 2007;99(19):1462-70.

[16] Mandel JS, Bond JH, Church TR, et al.. Reducing mortality from colorectal cancer by screening for fecal occult blood. *N Engl J Med.* 1993;328:1365-7.

[17] Hardcastle JD, Chamberlain JO, Robinson MH, et al. Randomized controlled trial of faecal-occult blood screening for colorectal cancer. *Lancet.* 1996;348:1472-77.

[18] Kronborg O, Fenger C, Olsen J, Jorgensen OD, Sondergaard O. Randomized study of screening for colorectal cancer with faecal-occult blood test. *Lancet.* 1996;348:1467-71.

[19] Imperiale TF, Wagner DR, Lin CY, Larkin GN, Rogge JD, Ransohoff DF. Risk of advanced proximal neoplasms in asymptomatic adults according to the distal colorectal findings. *N Engl J Med.* 2000;343:169-74.

[20] Ahlquist DA, Sargent DJ, Loprinzi CL, et al. Stool DNA and occult blood testing for screen detection of colorectal neoplasia. *Ann Int Med.* 2008;149:441-50.

[21] Levin B, Lieberman DA, McFarland B, et al. Screening and surveillance for early detection of colorectal cancer and adenomatous polyps, 2008: a joint guideline from the American Cancer Society, the US Multi-Society Task Force on Colorectal Cancer, and the American College of Radiology. *Gastroenterology.* 2008;134:1570-95.

[22] Whitlock EP, Lin JS, Liles E, Beil TL, Fu R. Screening for colorectal cancer: a targeted, updated systematic review for US Preventative Task Force. *Ann Int Med.* 2008;149:638-65.

[23] Itzkowitz SH, Jandorf L, Brand R, et al. Improved fecal DNA test for colorectal cancer screening. *Clin Gastroenterol Hepatol.* 2007;5:111-7.

[24] Johnson CD, Chem MH, Toledano AY, et al. Accuracy of CT colonography for detection of large adenomas and cancers. *N Engl J Med.* 2008;359:1207-1

[25] Shelby JV, Friedman GD, Quesenberry CP Jr, Weiss NS. A case-control study of screening sigmoidoscopy and mortality from colorectal cancer. *N Engl J Med.* 1992;326:653-7.

[26] Schoenfeld P, Cash B, Flood A, et al. Colonoscopic screening of average-risk women for colorectal cancer. *N Engl J Med.* 2005;352:2061-8.

[27] Lieberman DA, Holub JL, Moravec MD, Eisen GM, Peters D, Morris CD. Prevalence of colon polyps detected by colonoscopy screening in asymptomatic black and white patients. *JAMA.* 2008;300:1417-22.

[28] Pickhardt PJ, Choi R, Hwang I, et al. Computed tomographic virtual colonoscopy to screen for colorectal neoplasia in asymptomatic adults. *N Engl J Med.* 2003;349:2191-200.

[29] Cotton PB, Durkalski VL, Pineau BC, et al. Computed tomography (virtual colono-scopy): a multicenter comparison with standard colonoscopy for detection of colorec-tal neoplasia. *JAMA*. 2004;291:1713-9.

[30] Rockey DC, Paulson E, Neidzwiecki D, et al. Analysis of air contrast barium enema, computer tomographic colonography and colonoscopy: prospective comparison. *Lancet*. 2005;365:305-11.

[31] Pignone M, Saha S, Hoerger T, Mandelblatt J. Cost-effectiveness analyses of colorec-tal cancer screening: a systematic review for US Preventive Services Task Force. *Ann Int Med*. 2001;137(2):96-104.

[32] Lasa JS, Moore R, Peralta AD, Dima G, Zubiaurre I, Arguello M, et al. Impact of the endoscopic teaching process on colonic adenoma detection. *Revista de Gastroenterol de Mexico* (Engl Ed). 2014;79:155-8.

[33] Hol L, Wilschut JA, van Ballegooijen M, et al. Screening for colorectal cancer: random comparison of guaiac and immunochemical faecal occult blood testing at different cut-off levels. *Br J Cancer*. 2009;100:1103-10.

[34] Parra-Blanco A, Gimeno-Garcia AZ, Quintero E, et al. Diagnostic accuracy of immu-nochemical versus guaiac faecal occult blood tests for colorectal screening. *J Gastroen-terol*. 2010;45:703-12.

[35] Van Rossum LG, van Rijn AF, Laheij RJ, et al. Random comparison of guaiac and im-munochemical fecal occult blood tests for colorectal cancer in screening population. *Gastroenterology*. 2008;135:82-90.

[36] Levi Z, Birkenfeld S, Vilkin A, et al. A higher detection rate for colorectal cancer and advanced adenomatous polyp for screening with immunochemical fecal occult blood test than guaiac fecal occult blood test, despite lower compliance rate: a prospective, controlled, feasibility study. *Int J Cancer*. 2011;128:2415-24.

[37] Quintero E, Castells A, Bujanda L, Cubiella J, Salas D, Lanas A, et al. Colonoscopy versus fecal immunochemical testing in colorectal cancer screening. *N Engl J Med*. 2012;366(8):697-706. DOI: 10.1056/NEJMoa1108895

[38] Yang DX, Gross CP, Soulos PR, Yu JB. Estimating the magnitude of colorectal cancers prevented during the era of screening. *Cancer*. 2014;120(18):2893-901.

[39] Wolf WI, Shinya H. Polypectomy via the fiberoptic colonoscope: removal of neo-plasms beyond the reach of the sigmoidoscope. *N Engl J Med*. 1973;288:329-32.

[40] Winawer SJ, Stewart ET, Zauber AG, et al. A comparison of colonoscopy and double-contrast barium enema for surveillance after polypectomy. *N Engl J Med*. 2000; 342:1766-72

[41]   Toma J, Paszat LF, Gunraj N, Rabeneck L. Rates of new or missed colorectal cancer after barium enema and their risk factors: a population-based study. *Am J Gastroenterol*. 2008;103:3142.

[42]   Centers for Disease Control and Prevention (CDC). Vital signs: colorectal cancer screening test use – United States, 2012. *Morb Mortal Wkly Rep*. 2013;62:881.

[43]   Weissfeld JL, Schoen RE, Pinsky PF, et al. Flexible sigmoidoscopy in the PLCO cancer screening trial: results from the baseline screening examination of a randomized trial. *J Natl Cancer Inst*. 2005;97:989-97.

[44]   Atkin WS, Edwards R, Kralj-Hans I, et al. Once-only flexible sigmoidoscopy screening in prevention of colorectal cancer: a multicentre randomized controlled trial. *Lancet*. 2010;375:1324-33.

[45]   Schoen RE, Pinsky PF, Weissfeld JL. Colorectal-Cancer Incidence and Mortality with screening Flexible Sigmoidoscopy. *N Engl J Med*. 2012: 366:2345-2357

[46]   Waye JD, Aisenberg J, Rubin PH. Indications and contraindications for colonscopy. In: *Practical Colonscopy*. Oxford, UK: Blackwell Publishing; 2013. p. 24-9. DOI: 10.1002/9781118553442

[47]   Wang YR, Cangemi JR, Loftus EV, Picco MF. Risk of colorectal cancer after colonoscopy compared with flexible sigmoidoscopy or no lower endoscopy among older patients in the United States, 1998-2005. *Mayo Clinic Proc*. 2013;88:464-70.

[48]   Evans WK, Wolfson MC, Flanagan WM, Shin J, Goffin J, Miller AB, et al. Canadian cancer risk management model: evaluation of cancer control. *Int J Tech Assess Health Care*. 2013;29:131-9.

[49]   Jemal A, Seigel R, Ward E, Hao Y, Xu J, Thun MC. Cancer statistics, 2009. *CA Cancer J Clin*. 2009;59:225-249.

[50]   Cairns SR, Scholefield JH, et al. Guidelines for colorectal cancer screening and surveillance in moderate and high risk groups (update from 2002). *Gut*. 2010; 59:666-690.

[51]   Baron TH, Smyrk TC, Rex DK. Recommended intervals between screening and surveillance colonoscopies. *Mayo Clin Proc*. 2013;88(8):854-8. DOI: 10.1016/j.mayocp. 2013.04.023

[52]   Waye J, Braunfeld S. Surveillance intervals after colonoscopic polypectomy. *Endoscopy*. 1982;14(3):79-81.

[53]   Winawer S, Zauber A, O'Brien M, et al. Randomized comparison of surveillance intervals after colonoscopic removal of newly diagnosed adenomatous polyps. *N Engl J Med*. 1993;328:901-6.

[54]   Atkin W, Williams C, Macrae F, et al. Randomized study of surveillance intervals after removal of colorectal adenomas at colonoscopy. *Gut*. 1992;33:S52.

[55] Neugut A, Jacobson J, Ashan H, et al. Incidence and recurrence rates of colorectal adenomas--a prospective study. *Gastroenterology*. 1995;108:402-8.

[56] Atkin WS, Saunders BP. Surveillance guidelines after removal of colorectal adenomatous polyps. *Gut*. 2002;51 (Suppl. V):v6-vv9.

[57] Nishihara R, Wu K, Lochhead P, Morikawa T, Liao X, Qian ZR, et al. Long-term colorectal cancer incidence and mortality after lower endoscopy. *N Engl J Med*. 2013;369(12):1095-105. DOI: 10.1056/NEJMoa1301969

[58] Saini SD, Schoenfeld P, Vijan S. Surveillance colonoscopy is cost-effective for patients with adenomas who are at high risk of colorectal cancer. *Gastroenterology*. 2010;138(7): 2292-9. DOI: 10.1053/j.gastro.2010.03.004

[59] Murphy CC, Lewis CL, Golin CE, Sandler RS. Underuse of surveillance colonoscopy in patients at increased risk of colorectal cancer. *Am J Gastroenterol*. Forthcoming. DOI: 10.1038/ajg.2014.344

[60] Martinex ME, Ahnen D, Greenberg ER. One-year risk for advanced colorectal neoplasia. *Ann Int Med*. 2013;158(8):639. DOI: 10.7326/0003-4819-158-8-201304160-00019

[61] Rex DK, Ahnen DJ, Baron JA, Batts KP, Burke CA, Burt RW, et al. Serrated lesions of the colorectum: review and recommendations from an expert panel. *Am J Gastroenterol*. 2012;107:1315-29. DOI: 10.1038/ajg.2012.161

[62] Tinmouth J, Henry P, Hsieh E, Baxter NN, Hilsden RJ, Elizabeth McGregor S, et al. Sessile serrate polyps at screening colonoscopy: have they been underdiagnosed? *Am J Gastroenterol*. 2014;109(11):1698-704. DOI: 10.1038/ajg.2014.78

[63] Pohl H, Srivastava A, Bensen SP, Anderson P, Rothstein RI, Gordon SR, et al. Incomplete polyp resection during colonscopy--results of the complete adenoma resection (CARE) study. *Gastroenterology*. 2013;144(1):74-80. DOI: 10.1053/j.gastro.2012.09.043

[64] Hassan C, Quientero E, Dumonceau JM, Regula J, Brandao C, Chaussade S, et al. Post-polypectomy colonoscopy surveillance: European Society of Gastroenterology Endoscopy (ESGE) guideline. *Endoscopy*. 2013;45:842-51. DOI: 10.1055/s-0033-1344548

[65] Bosman FT, Carniero F, Hruban Rh, Theise ND (eds.). WHO classification of tumours of digestive system. 4th edn. Geneva, Switzerland: WHO/IARC Press; 2010. p. 417.

[66] Kaminski MF, Hassan C, Bisschops R, Pohl J, Pellise M, Dekker E, et al. Advanced imaging for detection and differentiation of colorectal neoplasia: European Society of Gastroenterology Endoscopy (ESGE) guideline. *Endoscopy*. 2014;46:435-49. DOI: 10.1055/s-0034-1365348

[67] Day LW, Walter LC, Velayos F. Colorectal cancer screening and surveillance in the elderly patient. *Am J Gastroenterol*. 2011;106(7):1197-206. DOI: 10.1038/ajg.2011.128

[68] Noshirwani KC, van Stolk RU, Rybicki LA, et al. Adenoma size and number are pre-
      dictive of adenoma recurrence: implications for surveillance colonoscopy. *Gastroint-
      est Endosc*. 2000;51(4):433-7.

[69] Harewood GC, Lawlor GO. Incident rates of colonic neoplasia according to age and
      gender: implications for surveillance colonoscopy intervals. *J Clin Gastroenterol*.
      2005;39(10):894-9.

[70] Harewood GC, Lawlor GO, Larson MV. Incident rates of colonic neoplasia in older
      patients: when should we stop screening? *J Gastroenterol Hepatol*. 2006;21(6):1021-5.

[71] Schoen RE, Pinsky FP, Weissfeld JL, Yokochi LA, Reding DJ, Hayes RB, et al. Utiliza-
      tion of surveillance colonoscopy in community practice. *Gastroenterology*. 2010;138(1):
      73-81. DOI: 10.1053/j.gastro.2009.09.062

[72] Sarfaty M, Wender R. How to increase colorectal cancer screening rates in practice.
      CA Cancer J Clin. 2007;57(6):354-66.

[73] Leffler DA, Neeman N, Rabb JM, Shin JY, Landon BE, Pallav K, et al. An alerting sys-
      tem improves adherence to follow-up recommendations for colonoscopic examina-
      tions. *Gastroenterology*. 2011;140:1166-73. DOI: 10.1053/j.gastro.2011.01.003

[74] Rex DK, Petrini JL, Baron TH, Chak A, Cohen J, Deal SE, et al. Quality indicators for
      colonoscopy. Am J Gastroenterol. 2006;101(4):873-85.

6

Liquid Biopsy for Colorectal Cancer Screening: A Modern Approach for Patients Stratification and Monitoring

Octav Ginghina and Cornelia Nitipir

Abstract

Despite great advances have been made in oncologic approaches, the morbidity and mortality caused by colon cancer are still overwhelming. Particularly, the intra- and inter-tumour heterogeneity makes accurate sampling challenging and often leads to failure of even modern therapeutic strategies. Moreover, tumour molecular genotype can suffer alterations over time, triggering suboptimal therapeutic outcomes as a result of irrelevant information provided by histological biopsies. Daily, tumour cells shed into the bloodstream at the early stages of the disease. These circulating tumour cells (CTCs) can be detected and analysed after enrichment, providing this way valuable information in real time. Furthermore, apoptotic and/or necrotic tumour cells discharge DNA fragments into the circulating bloodstream. Elevated levels of these so-called circulating tumour DNA (ctDNA) fragments can be identified in the peripheral blood of patients as compared to healthy individuals. In this view, the detection and characterization of the CTCs and ctDNA are a real-time "liquid biopsy" that has been developed for accurate tumour monitoring and molecular characterization. This modern non-invasive analytical approach allows consecutive sampling to monitor CTC number and tumour genetic changes over time without the need of tissue biopsy. Consequently, "liquid biopsies" can be used to screen for cancer, stratify patients to the optimum treatment and to monitor the patient's response to treatment or identify treatment resistance. This chapter offers an overview of the following approaches with respect to liquid biopsies: CTCs and ctDNA. Some of the analytical techniques and challenges in the detection of these rare events will also be presented here.

Keywords: colorectal cancer, liquid biopsy, circulating tumour cells, ctDNA, tumour heterogeneity

1. Introduction

Uncontrolled division and growth of human cells and subsequent invasion to other tissue via the circulatory and the lymphatic systems are commonly known as cancer.

One of the cancer types known to affect the gastrointestinal (GI) tract and rated third most commonly diagnosed form irrespective of gender is colorectal cancer (CRC).

In a context outlined by alarming figures of both prevalence (with a lifetime CRC risk of 5.1%) and high mortality rate, CRC being second in line among cancer-related causes of deaths in both genders, advances in therapy have become particularly significant; thus, in addition to established liver resection, outcomes in survival rate have been greatly improved in recent years due to better means for earlier detection, advances in chemotherapy and therapies based on biological agents.

Largely studied nowadays, factors influencing the likelihood of developing CRC are a close family history of genetic changes in that respect (20% of cases), notably associated with certain genetic syndromes such as the Lynch syndrome (hereditary nonpolyposis colorectal cancer, HNPCC) in ca. 3% of cases [1] and familial adenomatous polyposis with its variant the Gardner syndrome (in a further ca. 1% of CRC instances).

HNPCC-related CRC risk factors include early onset (ca. 44 average age) triggered by an autosomal dominant inheritance, development in 70% of cases in splenic flexure proximity as well as a surplus of synchronous (18% of all patients) and metachronous CRC (45% of patients) following segmental resection or hemicolectomy. In addition to a CRC cause, Lynch syndrome frequently also results in other carcinoma types such as ovary and endometrial, other gastrointestinal location (stomach, small intestine), pancreas as well as transitional carcinoma in the renal pelvis and the ureter [2].

This high metastatic disease potential is the main cause of CRC lethal outcome and may be attributed to the contribution of a specific gene (I(MACCI)); already isolated [3], this is a transcriptional factor able to influence the expression of the hepatocyte growth factor and therefore associated with proliferation of CRC cells, scattering and new tissue invasion and further tumour growth and metastasis, as shown in cell cultures and animal studies in mice. MACCI close involvement as contributor to occurrence of metastasis makes it a novel target for CRC approach, which needs confirmation by further studies and clinical trials [4].

Contribution of genetic factors in CRC development combines with action of epigenetic ones at cell level.

However important the role of genetic features, most CRC may rather be the outcome of chronic intestinal inflammation preceding tumour development, gut microbiota and such environmental factors as life style (diet included) and food and environmental-borne mutagens [5, 6].

Among chronic intestinal inflammations responsible for CRC risk, inflammatory bowel disease (under 2% of CRC cases every year [7]), Crohn's disease and ulcerative colitis need special mention for being the frequent cause of tumour growth [8], the risk growing with the severity of inflammation and the duration of the disorder [9]. Statistically, in that respect, 10 years' duration of Crohn's disease results in CRC in 2% of patients, and the risk increases four times and nine times for 20 and 30 years' durations, respectively [7]. On the other hand, a history of over 30 years of ulcerative colitis results in development of some type of cancer precursor or CRC in ca. 16% patients [7].

2. Tumour progression

As regards CRC development, it typically originates in benign, premalignant or malignant polyps occurring at the level of the colon or rectum epithelial lining (as, for instance, hyperplastic polyps, tubular adenoma or colorectal adenocarcinoma, respectively). Such abnormalities are the result of inherited or acquired oncogenic and inactivating mutations revealed by complex genome scale analysis, which has shown the existence of hypermutated and non-hypermutated CRC tumour categories [10].

Among non-hypermutated types, one commonly occurring mutation affects the Wnt signalling pathway, leading to increased signalling activity and emerging at the level of the intestinal crypt stem cell [11].

Most frequently, the mutated CRC-related gene is the *APC* gene. APC protein prevents β-catenin protein accumulation. The absence of APC leads to β-catenin accumulation and translocation to the cell nucleus, where it binds to the DNA, thus activating transcription of proto-oncogenes. Although normally playing an important role in stem cell renewal and differentiation, when inappropriately expressed and highly accumulated, these proto-oncogene products can induce cancer.

In addition to the absence of the APC protein, high β-catenin-related CRC may also be determined by β-catenin (CTNNB1) mutation, blocking its very own breakdown, or occurrence of mutations in other APC similarly operating genes (e.g., AXINI, AXIN2, NKDI, TCF71.2) [12].

Besides deficient Wnt signalling pathways, realization of the cancer potential requires additional mutations. Usually, action of Wnt pathway defects is prevented by intervention of the cell division monitoring p53 protein, a product of the TP53 gene, which normally eliminates flawed cells. Thus, a mutation arising in the TP53 gene may reverse the potential from benign epithelial tumour cell into invasive epithelial cell.

If not affecting the p53-encoding gene, mutations may instead target a different protein playing a protective role, i.e., the BAX12 but also ARDI A, CTNNB I, SOX9, FAM123B and ATM.

On the other hand, hypermutated tumours progress through specific genetic events and display MSH3, MSH6, TGFBR2, ACVR2A, SLC9A9, BRAF and TCF71.2 mutated forms.

Whichever the tumour type, all these genes are involved in the Wnt and TGF-β signalling pathways, leading to higher MYC activity, as major CRC factor [13]. Role of "field defects"/"field cancerisation", the concept first emerged in the early 1950s to refer to an area of the epithelium featuring a preconditioning responsible for cancer predisposition of the area in question [14]. Despite unclear origins at the time of their introduction, the terms define premalignant tissue as potential sites for new cancer.

In time, research has progressively emphasized the importance of "field defects" in advance to CRC, and the assumption was confirmed by studies showing almost the exclusive use of discrete neoplastic foci for in vitro research and well-defined tumours for in vivo studies [15] in all cancer research.

In addition, as research further indicated, the majority of somatic mutations occurring at tumour level emerged during development of apparently normal cells [16], at the site of "field defects" (and therefore in preneoplastic stage).

A further addition to terminology refers to the term "aetiologic field effect", based on the "field defect" concept and referring to molecular and pathologic changes in preneoplastic cells at molecular level. The term also covers the extent to and manner in which exogenous environmental factors as well as molecular changes in the local microenvironment influence neoplastic progression throughout [17].

3. Epigenetic factors in tumour growth

However important mutation-induced genetic alterations, epigenetic alterations are significantly more common in CRC and involve hundreds of genes. As revealed by research, (Vogelstein and colleagues) oncogene mutations and suppressor mutations (both known as "driver mutations") are rather limited in average CRC forms (1–2 and 1–5, respectively), although accompanied by an estimated 60 additional so-called "passenger" mutations [18].

Common types of epigenetic cancer-related alterations modifying gene expression levels by action on the different types of RNA (miRNAs) may involve abnormal methylation of DNA in tumour suppressor promoters [19], such as reduced expression of miR-137 because of methylation of the miR-137-encoding DNA sequence in the CpG island [20]. Altered miR-137 expression triggers drastic (2- to 20-fold) alteration of mRNA expression of the target genes and related slighter changes in expression of proteins produced by the genes.

There are further microRNAs, of comparable numbers of target genes, which undergo even more frequent epigenetic alterations of field defects in the colon, resulting in specific CRC forms [21].

As common is direct hyper-/hypo-methylation of CpG islands of protein-encoding genes as well as histone alterations or modification of chromosomal architecture, with influence on gene expression [22]. Research has recently outlined the potential of early epigenetic decline in expression of DNA repair enzyme as cause of cancer characteristic genomic and epigenomic instability [18].

4. Colorectal cancer (CRC)

4.1. CRC clinical manifestations

Although CRC clinical signs vary with tumour location in the intestine as well as with the presence of metastases, medical practice has outlined certain warning signs and symptoms now considered typical, such as loss of appetite, weight loss, vomiting and/or nausea, rectal bleeding and anaemia in the over 50 age group [23], severe and persistent constipation and modified stools (accompanied by blood elimination and/or diminished thickness) [24]; weight loss and changed bowel habit may be considered a warning only if accompanied by bleeding [22].

4.2. CRC diagnosis

4.2.1. Diagnostic steps

Typically, CRC may be diagnosed by the sampling of colon areas suspected of tumour development during procedures suitable for the lesion site, i.e. colonoscopy or sigmoidoscopy.

Once the tumour is confirmed, the level of the disease needs to be determined, which is generally done by a CT scan involving the chest, abdomen and pelvis, but also by position imaging tomography and MRI, for certain cases.

The next diagnostic step is to determine the stage of the tumour, based on the TNM cancer staging system (where T stands for primary tumour stage, N for the presence of regional lymph nodes and M for remote metastasis). Staging criteria include the extent of initial tumour spreading, the presence and site of lymph nodes and the metastasis level [25].

4.2.2. Microscopic examination

Adenocarcinoma is a malignant tumour of the epithelium, whose source lies in the superficial glandular epithelial cells of the colon and cecum lining. This tumour invades the colon/cecum wall and further progressively permeates the respective layers (first the muscularis mucosae, then the submucosa and lastly the muscularis propria). Tumour cells in question are organized as irregular tubular, multistratified structures, featuring multiple lumens and decreased stroma (in a back-to-back growth pattern). In addition, in some cases, tumour cell lacks of cohesion may be observed, as well as a secretion of mucus pervading the interstitium and resulting in extensive mucus/colloid (optically "empty" spaces) pools (forming the so called "mucinous (colloid)"), poorly differentiated adenocarcinoma. Mucus remaining within the walls of the tumour cell drives the nucleus towards the cell membrane, and the "signet-ring cell" emerges.

In fact, differentiation may vary in adenocarcinoma, contingent on cellular pleomorphism, glandular architecture and muco-secretion of the predominant pattern; thus, three variants of adenocarcinoma may be observed as regards the degree of cell differentiation: well differentiated, moderately differentiated and poorly differentiated [26].

CRC cell characteristics may be determined by analysis of tissue samples harvested by biopsy or during surgery. The pathology report provides data on cell type and grade. In CRC, the most common cell (98% of cases) is adenocarcinoma, but other types may also occur in rare cases (squamous cell carcinoma and lymphoma) [27].

4.2.3. Immunochemistry

It is generally considered that more than half of CR adenomas and up to 90% of CRC tumours present overexpression of the COX (cyclooxygenase)-2, normally absent from healthy colon tissue but acting as fuel for abnormal cell growth [28].

The cancer variant may be determined by histologic examination.

4.2.4. Macroscopic examination

In order to predict the likely course of tumour progression and adequate management, macroscopic examination looks closely at the site of the tumour in the intestine; thus, tumour development on the ascending colon and cecum (the right side of the large intestine) is most often exophytic (growing outwards from the bowel wall), which may in infrequent cases result in faecal obstruction, accompanied by anaemia.

Tumours growing on the left bowel side are largely peripheral and may result in obstruction of the bowel lumen and thinner stools [27].

4.3. CRC prevention

One key approach to CRC (as for other cancers, in fact) and unanimously recognized as such is prevention; closer surveillance and healthier lifestyle can essentially contribute to CRC prevention.

Therefore, research has greatly been focused on effective means in that respect, in all areas of intervention.

As regards lifestyle, diets are currently recommended to include more significant amounts of vegetables, fruits and whole grains and decrease consumption of white flour products, sugars and red meat.

As in other areas of healthcare, physical exercise has been proved to be beneficial, though less significant for preventing or reducing colon cancer risk [29, 30]. However, avoiding prolonged sitting as a daily routine is important [31].

Medication has also been the target of research, which has shown the potential of aspirin and celecoxib to reduce CRC danger in high-risk groups as determined by assessment of family medical history and other personal risk factors, though not in average risk ones [32–35].

Calcium supplementation is currently under study as well, not with sufficient evidence yet.

As for protection factors, in vitro studies have shown that intake and blood levels of vitamin D act as one, as have lactic acid bacteria, due to their antioxidant activity, immunomodulation as well as promotion of programmed cell death, proliferative effects and epigenetic alteration of cancer cells [36].

Screening is an important and effective means for prevention and early detection of cancer in general and CRC in particular, the more so as most CRC cases (>80%) originate in adenomatous polyps [37].

As mentioned above, screening is also a very important means for cancer diagnosis before the emergency of actual symptoms (by 2–3 years) [25].

Close relatives of HNPCC patients need accurate and structured screening, according to a well-designed programme and schedule [38], as in certain countries such as Canada, the United Kingdom, Australia and the Netherlands [39–41].

Therefore, these should undergo a first routine colonoscopy at the age of 25, which, as a routine, should be repeated every 3 years, in the case of negative results, and every year should an adenoma be found. In cases where routine colonoscopy reveals the presence of cancer, subtotal colectomy needs to be performed.

In addition, for women, ovarian ultrasound and endometrial biopsy need to be performed as early as 25 years old.

Screening tests have been devised and researched, current practice now relying mostly on colonoscopy (both standard and virtual via CT scan), faecal occult blood testing, multitarget stool DNA screening and flexible sigmoidoscopy [25].

Although with proven efficacy in other respects, sigmoidoscopy is the only procedure able to provide screening of the right side of the colon, the site for almost half (42%) of malignancies [42].

Equally effective, standard colonoscopy is less costly than virtual colonoscopy via CT scan and avoids the additional risk of exposure to radiation and also able to eliminate any potential abnormal growth found [25].

In the 50–75 age group with standard risk factors, screening should include faecal occult blood testing or immunochemical testing every 2 years; an alternative is performance of sigmoidoscopy every 10 years, to the detriment of colonoscopy [43].

For patients with familial adenomatous polyposis, the high-malignancy risk may be offset by total proctocolectomy, ensuring elimination of the risk of both colon and rectal cancers [44].

4.4. CRC management

Given CRC's incurable character, therapeutic decisions in that respect can only be directed to either cure or as a palliative, largely depending on tumour stage [45] but also on other factors as well, such as the patient's health status and even preferences.

4.4.1. Therapy

Surgery can be a means leading to cure but in early stages only, whereas at later stages, when the metastatic disease has also been initiated, the curative potential of surgery decreases, and palliation (alleviation of tumour-related symptoms and patient's comfort and quality of life) becomes prevalent [25].

For the very first stage, one colonoscopy intervention can suffice to eliminate cancer [46], while the curative potential of surgery decreases with the tumour stage.

Therefore, one stage further, in localized cancers, cure may still be attempted through ample removal associated with ensuring adequate margins, which can be achieved laparoscopically or more often by open laparotomy [25], with colon reconnection, or by colostomy [46].

In the stage of a few emerging metastases, those in the lungs or liver may be eliminated.

In certain cases at this stage, surgery may be preceded by chemotherapy, in an attempt to minimize the tumour before removal.

If recurrence occurs, this mainly involves the lungs and liver [25].

4.4.2. Chemotherapy

This is administered in cases beyond stage 1 CRC, given the curing potential of surgery. No chemotherapy is also customary in CRC stage II; on condition no such risk factors as threats from negative lymph node sampling or the presence of a T4 tumour are present.

Chemotherapy is also not feasible in patients with identified abnormal mismatched repair genes.

On the contrary, chemotherapy is a must and an integral therapy component in stage II and stage IV CRC25, characterized by cancer spreading to remote organs or the lymph nodes; the use of the chemotherapeutic agents oxaliplatin, fluorouracil or capecitabine is instrumental in increasing life expectancy, with the disadvantage of debatable chemotherapy benefits in the case of cancer-free lymph nodes.

Turn to palliative care becomes necessary where CRC has become extensively metastatic or may not be resected, opening the alternative for several different chemotherapy medications [25], including, oxaliplatin, fluorouracil, capecitabine, irinotecan and tegafur/uracil [47, 48].

4.4.3. Radiotherapy

Given bowel sensitivity to radiation, patient with colon cancer treatment cannot benefit from addition of radiation to chemotherapy, although this may be effective for rectal cancer [25]. The same was for chemotherapy; radiotherapy may be used as neoadjuvant and adjuvant in certain rectal cancer stages only [49].

4.4.4. Palliation

For patients with incurable CRC forms, palliative care, though not a promising cure, may bring the benefit of better quality of the patient's life both directly and indirectly, via the life of their families, lessening symptoms and anxiety and also reducing the need of hospital admission [50].

Palliation is typically symptom directed and consists of procedures designed to improve symptoms or minimize the possibility of complications such as abdominal pain, tumour bleeding and/or bowel obstruction [51], thus contributing to improved quality of life.

Such procedures may include surgery, for elimination of cancer tissue to some extent, without attempting to cure, placement of a stent or performing a bypass of part of the bowel.

Non-surgical palliative care approaches include pain medication and/or radiotherapy aiming to reduce the tumour size [52].

4.4.5. Follow-up

The main purpose of follow-up is to obtain the earliest identification of later metachronous lesions, i.e., metastases or tumours not originating from the initial cancer [53].

As an underlying measure for cancer survivors, exercise as a mainstay of lifestyle may be useful as secondary therapy, as shown by results indicating important reduction in 8-oxo-dG in the urine of patients after taking moderate exercise for 2 weeks of following primary therapy [54].

4.5. CRC prognosis

The most commonly used prognosis criterion is the 5-year survival rate, which is under 60% for CRC in Europe, whereas this is the cause of death for one third of CRC patients [25] in most developed countries. The reason for these unexpectedly low outcomes despite evident progress in new therapeutic means and their improved availability worldwide is mainly CRC late identification (stage IV already present in 20% of patients seeking medical attention), with potentially resectable isolated liver metastasis in ca. 25% of these patients. Of these 25%, one third of patients undergoing resection achieve 5-year survival [55, 56].

5. Liquid biopsy

Despite the major advances in cancer therapies, the morbidity and mortality associated with this disease are still enormous. Tumour heterogeneity holds the main responsibility underlying inefficient treatment and failure of current therapeutic strategies, including the targeted therapies. For efficiency reasons, the molecular targeted therapies require constant monitoring of the tumour genome, but harvesting consecutive tissue biopsies is very difficult and inconvenient for medical and economic reasons. Therefore, the lack of real-time information regarding tumour heterogeneity during the disease evolution most commonly results in the treatment failure and requires the development of novel approaches. In this view, liquid biopsies offer a tool for real-time screening of disease particularities, stratify patients for the best treatment and also monitor the response of the treatment. Due to their non-invasive nature, liquid biopsies can be used for repeated sampling to monitor tumour genetic alterations over time, avoiding this way consecutive tissue biopsies. Liquid biopsies analyse circulating tumour cells, cell-free tumour DNA and/or exosomes, known as tumour-circulating markers.

5.1. Circulating tumour cells (CTCs)

Circulating tumour cells (CTCs) have been identified during the 1800s and presumed responsible for the metastatic process [57]. These cells are of epithelial origin and shed from the tumours in the peripheral blood of patients where they can be enriched, detected and analysed.

The detection of CTCs in the peripheral blood of patients with cancer holds a great promise for the future development of efficient anticancer therapies. However, due to the very low concentrations of CTCs in the peripheral blood (one tumour cell for millions of normal blood cells), their detection and identification still remain challenging and require high analytical sensitivity and specificity methods, which usually consist in a combination of enrichment and detection [58].

CTC enrichment strategies include a wide range of technologies based on those CTC particularities that can discriminate them out of the normal haematopoietic cells. Concrete CTCs can be detected based on physical properties such as size, density, electric charges, deformability or biological properties such as cell surface marker expression and viability. CTC separation based on their physical properties holds the great advantage of being done without labelling the cells. Some of these methods include density gradient centrifugation, filtration, photo-acoustic flow cytometry, microfluidics, etc. [59, 60].

Nevertheless, the biological properties of the CTCs hold a major role in their identification, mainly based on immunobead assays. These assays use antibodies targeting tumour-associated antigens (positive selection) or leukocyte-specific antigens such as CD45 (negative selection) in order to detect and separate CTCs from the blood cells. The positive selection usually targets the epithelial cell adhesion molecule (EpCAM). Subsequently, CTCs are confirmed with antibodies against cytokeratins (CKs) [59]. Among the current EpCAM-based technologies, the US Food and Drug Administration approved CellSearch® system (Veridex) which is the current "gold standard" for all new CTC-detection methods. According to this standard, CTCs are nucleated cells that express the epithelial cell adhesion molecule and cytokeratins but lack the expression of the common leukocyte CD45 marker ($EpCam^+\_CK18/19^+\_DAPI^+\_CD45^-$ cells).

Interestingly, some CTCs undergo the epithelial to mesenchymal transition (EMT) and loose critical epithelial markers. Capturing CTCs' lacking EpCAM expression requires the use of antibody cocktails against a panel of epithelial cell surface antigens such as HER2, MUC-1, EGFR and folate-binding protein receptor and against mesenchymal or stem cell antigens such as c-MET, N-cadherin and CD318 [61].

Regardless of the enrichment method, the isolated CTCs still contain a significant number of normal blood cells, and therefore CTCs should be next identified by a method that can discriminate between malignant cells and normal blood cells. The CellSearch® system as well as other assays is based on the fluorescent staining of the cells for the following markers: CKs (positive marker), the common leukocyte antigen CD45 (negative marker) and a nuclear dye (4,6-diamidino-2-phenylindole, DAPI).

Functional EPISPOT (for EPithelial ImmunoSPOT) assay has been introduced for CTC analysis in order to detect only the viable CTCs, able to produce metastases [62].

Other alternatives to immunologic assays of viable CTC-detection target specific mRNAs. A commercially available RNA-based CTC assay is the AdnaTest™ (AdnaGen), which uses nonquantitative RT-PCR to identify cells that express the transcripts of tumour-specific genes after immunomagnetic capture of MUC-1, HER2 and EpCAM cells [63].

5.2. Circulating tumour DNA (ctDNA)

Cell-free DNA (cfDNA) is a powerful tool for its potential use in a wide range of clinical fields such as cancer research [64, 65], non-invasive prenatal testing [66] and transplant rejection diagnostics [67]. Most cfDNA in plasma is highly fragmented (150–180 bp) [68] with a higher prevalence of tumour-associated mutations in the shorter fragments [69]. In patients suffering from cancer, a fraction of the cfDNA is tumour-derived and is known as circulating tumour DNA (ctDNA).

cfDNA reaches the systemic circulation by various pathologic or normal physiologic mechanisms [70]. However, with respect to solid tumours, the ctDNA is usually released as a result of necrosis or autophagy [71]. Notably, unlike apoptosis, necrosis generates larger DNA fragments [72]. Cancer patients generally have much higher levels of cfDNA than healthy individuals [73, 74]. ctDNA carries genomic and epigenomic alterations according to the tumour genomic alterations (copy number variation, point mutations, microsatellite instability, degree of integrity, loss of heterozygosity, rearranged genomic sequences, DNA methylation, etc.) [75]. Only on the basis of these biological characteristics, ctDNA can be discriminated from normal cfDNA. Consequently, after its validation ctDNA could be used as a specific biomarker that provides personalized information to detect residual disease or monitor tumour progression during therapy.

Due to the high degree of fragmentation as well as the small fraction of ctDNA within the cfDNA, the analysis of ctDNA is challenging and requires highly sensitive techniques. Classical methods of analysis include qRT-PCR, fluorescence and spectrophotometric approaches [76–78]. Digital droplet PCR has been developed as a high sensitive tool to detect ctDNA [79]. This technique consists in a droplet-based system [80, 81], a microfluidic platform [82, 83] and the so-called BEAMing strategy [84, 85]. Additionally, next-generation sequencing technology is currently used in plasma DNA analysis in order to identify ctDNA alterations [86–88].

6. Conclusions

There is increasing evidence that circulating tumour markers such as CTCs and ctDNA offer real-time information regarding cancer progression and tumour genotype in the view of a better systemic therapy management with direct impact on patient's disease prognosis. Additionally, future characterization of these circulating markers could contribute to approach-specific-targeted therapies to a certain population of cancer patients.

Acknowledgements

This work was done under the project PN-IIIP2-2.1-PTE-2016-0149/19PTE - TUMFLOW, financed by UEFISCDI.

Author details

Octav Ginghina[1,2]* and Cornelia Nitipir[3]

*Address all correspondence to: sciencecontactemail@gmail.com

1 Department of Surgery, "Sf. Ioan" Emergency Clinical Hospital, Bucharest, Romania

2 Department II, Faculty of Dental Medicine, "Carol Davila" University of Medicine and Pharmacy Bucharest, Bucharest, Romania

3 Department of Clinical Oncology, Elias Emergency Clinical Hospital, "Carol Davila" University of Medicine and Pharmacy, Bucharest, Romania

References

[1] Watson AJ, Collins PD. Colon cancer: A civilization disorder. Digestive Diseases. 2011;**29**(2):222-228

[2] Lynch HT, Lynch J. Clinical implications of advances in the molecular genetics of colorectal cancer. Tumori. 1995;**81**(Suppl):19-29

[3] Stein U, Walther W, Artlt F, et al. MACCI, a newly identified key regulator of HGF-MET signaling predicts colon cancer metastasis. Nature Medicine. 2008;**15**(1):59-67

[4] Stein J. MACCI-a novel target for solid cancers. Expert Opinion on Therapeutic Targets. 2013;**17**(9):1039-1052

[5] Yang K, Kurihara N, Fan K, Newmark H, Rigas B, Bancroft L, Corner G, Livote E, Lesser M, Edelmann W, et al. Dietary induction of colonic tumors in a mouse model of sporadic colon cancer. Cancer Research. 2008;**68**:7803-7810

[6] Rustgi AK. The genetics of hereditary colon cancer. Genes & Development. 2007;**21**: 2525-2538

[7] Triantafillidis JK, Nasioulas G, Kosimidis PA. Colorectal cancer and inflammatory bowel disease: Epidemiology, risk factors, mechanisms of carcinogenegis and prevention strategies. Anticancer Research. 2009;**29**(7):2727-2737

[8] Jawad N, Direkze N, Leedham SJ. Inflammatory bowel disease and colon cancer. Recent Results in Cancer Research. 2011;**185**:00115

[9] Xie J, Itzkowitz SH. Cancer in inflammatory bowel disease. World Journal of Gastroenterology. 2008;**14**(3):378-389

[10] Muzny DM, Bainbridge MN, Chang K, et al. Comprehensive molecular characterization of human colon and rectal cancer. Nature. 2012;**487**(7407):330-337

[11] Ionov Y, Peinado MA, Malkhosyan S, et al. Ubiquitous somatic mutations in simple repeated sequence reveal a new mechanism for colonic carcinogenesis. Nature. 1993;**363** (6429):558-561

[12] Markowitz SD, Betagnolli MM. Molecular origin of cancer: Molecular basis of colorectal cancer. The New England Journal of Medicine. 2009;**361**(25):2449-2460

[13] Saughter DP, Southwick HW, Smejkal W. Field cancerization in oral stratified squamous epithelium;clinical implication of multicentric origin. Cancer. 1953;**6**(5):963-968

[14] Rubin H. Fields and field cancerization: The preneoplastic origins of cancer: Asymptomatic hyperplastic fields are precursors of neoplasia, and their progression to tumors can be tracked by saturation density in culture. BioEssays. 2011;**33**(3):224-231

[15] Vogelstein B, Papadopoulos N, Velculescu VF, et al. Cancer genome landscapes. Science. 2013;**339**(6127):1546-1558

[16] Lochhead P, Chan AT, Nishihara R, et al. Etiologic field effect: Reappraisal of field effect in cancer predisposition and progression. Modern Pathology. 2014;**28**:14-29

[17] Bernstein C, Prasad AR, Nfonsam V, et al. DNA damage, DNA repair and cancer. In: Chen C, editor. New Research Directions in DNA Repair. In-Tech. 2013. ISBN: 978-51-114-6

[18] Schuebel KE, Chen W, Cope L, et al. Comparing the DNA hypermethylome with gene mutations in human colorectal cancer. PLoS Genetics. 2007;**3**(9):e157

[19] Balaguer F, Link A, Lozano JJ, et al. Epigenetic silencing of miR-137 is an early event colorectal carcinogenesis. Cancer Research. 2010;**70**(16):6608-6618

[20] Deng G, Kakar S, Kim YS. MicroRNA-124a and microRNA-34b/c are frequently methyl-ated in all histological types of colorectal cancer and polys, and in the adjacent normal mucosa. Oncology Letters. 2011;**2**(1):175-180

[21] Schnekenburger M, Diederich M. Epigenetic offer new horizons for colorectal cancer prevention. Current Colorectal CancerReports. 2012;**8**:66-81

[22] Astin M, Griffin T, Neal RD, et al. The diagnostic value of symptoms for colorectal cancer in primary care: A systematic review. British Journal of General Practitioners. 2011;**61**(586):231-243

[23] Alpers DH, Kallo AN, Kaplowtz N, et al. In: Yamada T, editor. Principles of Clinical Gastroenterology. Chichester: Wiley Blackwell; 2008. p. 381. ISBN: 978-1-4051-6910-3

[24] Terzic J, Grivennikov S, Karin E, Karin M. Inflammation and colon cancer. Gastroenterology. 2010;**138**:2101-2114.e5

[25] Kopetz S, Chang GJ, Overman MJ, Eng C, Sargent, DJ, Larson DW, Grothey A, Vauthey JN, Nagorney DM, McWilliams RR. Improved survival in metastatic colorectal cancer is associated with adoption of hepatic resection and improved chemotherapy. Journal of Clinical Oncology. 2009;**27**:3677-3683

[26] Triantafillidis JK, Nasioulas G, Kosmidids PA. Colorectal cancer and inflammatory bowel disease: epidemiology, risk factors, mechanisms of carcinogenesis and prevention strategies. Anticancer Research. 2009;**29**(7):2727-2737

[27] Sostres C, Gargallo CJ, Lanas A. Aspirin, cyclooxygenase inhibition and colorectal cancer. World Journal of Gastrointestinal Pharmacology and Therapeutics. 2014;**5**(1):40-49

[28] Campos FG, Logullo Waitzberg AG, Kiss DR, et al. Diet and colorectal cancer evidence for etiology and prevention. Nutrición Hospitalaria. 2005;**20**(1):18-25

[29] Harriss DJ, Atkinson G, Batterham A, et al. Colorectal Cancer, Lifestyle, Exercise and Research Group. Lifestyle factors and colorectal cancer risk (2): A systematic review and meta-analysis of associations with leisure – time physical activity. Colorectal Disease. 2009;**11**(7):689-701

[30] Biswas A, PI O, Faulkner GE, et al. Sedentary time and its association with risk for disease incidence, mortality, and hospitalization in adults: A systematic review and meta-analysis. Annals of Internal Medicine. 2015;**162**(2):123-132

[31] Cooper K, Squires H, Carrol C, et al. Chemoprevention of colorectal cancer: Systematic review and economic evaluation. Health Technology Assessment. 2010;**14**(32):1-206

[32] Agency for Healthcare Research and Quality. Aspirin or Anti Inflammatory Drugs for the Primary Prevention of Colorectal Cancer. United States Department of Health & Human Services; 2010/2011

[33] Weingarten MA, Zalmanovici A, Yaphe J, et al. Dietary calcium supplementation for preventing colorectal cancer and adenomatous polyps. Cochrane Database of Systematic Reviews. 2008;**1**:CD003548

[34] Ma Y, Zhang P, Wang F, et al. Association between vitamin D and risk of colorectal cancer: A systematic review of prospective studies. Journal of Clinical Oncology. 2011;**29**(28):3775-3782

[35] Zhong L, Zhang X, Covasa M. Emerging role of lactic acid bacteria in protection against colorectal cancer. World Journal of Gastroenterology. 2014;**20**(24):7878-7886

[36] What I Do to Reduce My Risk of Colorectal Cancer. Centers for Disease Control and Prevention; April 2, 2014. Retrieved March 5, 2015. https://www.cdc.gov/cancer/colorectal/basic_info/prevention.htm

[37] Westergaard H. Colorectal cancer the role of screening and surveillance. Journal of Investigative Medicine. 1996;**44**:216-227

[38] NHS Bowel Cancer Screening Programme. Available from: www.cancerscreening.nhs.uk

[39] Home-Bowel Cancer Australia. Available from: www.bowelcanceraustralia.org

[40] Bevolkingsonderzoek darmkanker. Available from: www.rivm.nl

[41] Siegel RL, Ward EM, Jemal A. Trends in colorectal cancer incidence rates in the United States by tumor location and stage, 1992-2008. Cancer Epidemiology Biomarker and Prevention. 2012;**21**(3):411-416

[42] Bacchus CM, Dunfield L, Connor GS, et al. Task Force on Prevention Health Care. Recommendations on screening for colorectal cancer in primary care. CMAJ: Canadian Medical Association Journal de1'Association medicale canadienne. 2016;**188**(5):340-348

[43] Moslein G, Pistorius S, Saeger H, et al. Preventive surgery for colon cancer in familial adenomatous polyposis and hereditary nonpolyposis colorectal cancer syndrome. Langerbecks. Archives of Surgery. 2003;**388**(1):9-11

[44] Stein A, Atanackovic D, Bokemeyer C. Current standards and new trends in the primary treatment of colorectal cancer. European Journal of Cancer. 2011;**47**(Suppl 3):S312-S314

[45] Colon Cancer Treatment (PDQ®). National Cancer Institute (NCI). May 12, 2014. Retrieved June 29, 2014. https://www.cancer.gov/types/colorectal/hp/colon-treatment-pdq

[46] Bruera G, Ricevuto E. Intensive chemotherapy of metastatic colorectal cancer: weighing between safety and clinical efficacy. Evaluation of Masi G, Loupakis F, Salvatore L, et al. Bevacizumab with FOLFOXIRI (irinotecan, oxaliplatin, fluorouracil, and folinate) as first-line treatment for metastatic colorectal cancer: a phase 2 trial. The Lancet Oncology. 2010;**1111**:845-852

[47] Devita Jr VT, Theodore SL, et al. Devita, Hellmanand Rosenberg's Cancer: Principles & Practice of Onocology. 8th ed. Philadelphia: Wolters Kluwer/Lippincott William's Wilkins; 2008. p. 1258

[48] Higginson IJ, Evans CJ. What is the evidence that palliative care teams improve outcomes for cancer patients and their families. Cancer Journal. 2010;**16**(5):423-435

[49] Wasserberg N, Kauffan HS. Palliation of colorectal cancer. Surgical Oncology. 2007;**16**(4):299-310

[50] Amersi F, Stamos MJ, Ko CY. Palliative care for colorectal cancer. Surgical Oncology Clinics of North America. 2004;**13**(3):467-477

[51] National Comprehensive Cancer Network (PDF). Available from: www.ncc.org

[52] Betof AS, Dewhist MW, Jones LW. Effects and potential mechanisms of exercise training on cancer progression. A translational perspective. Brain, Behavior, and Immunity. 2013;**30**:S75-S87

[53] Figueredo A, Rumble BR, Maroun J, et al. Follow-up of patients with curatively resected colorectal cancer: A practice guideline. BMC Cancer. 2003;**3**(26):1-23

[54] Qaseem A, Denberg TD, Hopkins RH, et al. Screening for colorectal cancer: A guidance statement from the American College of Physicians. Annals of Internal Medicine. 2012;**156**(5):378-386

[55] Available from: https://web.archive.org/web/200660925051637/ http:// www.cancer.org/ docroot/PRO/content/PRO_1_1_Cancer_Statistics_2006_Presentation. asp

[56] Simmonds PC, Primrose JN, Colquitt JL, et al. Surgical resection of hepatic metastases from colorectal cancer: A systematic review of published studies. British Journal of Cancer. 2006;**94**(7):982-999

[57] Recamier JCA. L'histoire de le meme maladie. Gabor. 1956;**1829**:110

[58] Alix-Panabieres C, Pantel K. Circulating tumor cells: Liquid biopsy of cancer. Clinical Chemistry. 2013;**59**(1):110-118

[59] Alix-Panabières C, Schwarzenbach H, Pantel K. Circulating tumor cells and circulating tumor DNA. Annual Review of Medicine. 2012;**63**:199-215

[60] Parkinson DR, Dracopoli N, Gumbs Petty B, Compton C, Cristofanilli M, Deisseroth A, et al. Considerations in the development of circulating tumor cell technology for clinical use. Journal of Translational Medicine. 2012;**10**:138

[61] Pecot CV, Bischoff FZ, Mayer JA, Wong KL, Pham T, Bottsford-Miller J, et al. A novel platform for detection of CKand CKCTCs. Cancer Discovery. 2011;**1**:580-586

[62] Alix-Panabières C. EPISPOT assay: Detection of viable DTCs/CTCs in solid tumor patients. Recent Results in Cancer Research. 2012;**195**:69-76

[63] Andreopoulou E, Yang LY, Rangel KM, Reuben JM, Hsu L, Krishnamurthy S, et al. Comparison of assay methods for detection of circulating tumor cells (CTCs) in metastatic breast cancer (MBC): AdnaGen AdnaTest BreastCancer select/detect™ versus Veridex CellSearch™ system. International Journal of Cancer. 2012;**130**:1590-1597

[64] Luo J, Shen L, Zheng D. Diagnostic value of circulating free DNA for the detection of EGFR mutation status in NSCLC: A systematic review and meta-analysis. Scientific Reports. 2014;**4**:6269

[65] Bettegowda C, Sausen M, Leary RJ, et al. Detection of circulating tumor DNA in early- and late-stage human malignancies. Science Translational Medicine. 2014;**6**:224ra24

[66] Song K, Musci TJ, Caughey AB. Clinical utility and cost of non-invasive prenatal testing with cfDNA analysis in high-risk women based on a US population. The Journal of Maternal-Fetal & Neonatal Medicine. 2013;**26**:1180-1185

[67] Macher HC, Suárez-Artacho G, Guerrero JM, et al. Monitoring of transplanted liver health by quantification of organ-specific genomic marker in circulating DNA from receptor. PLoS One. 2014;**9**:e113987

[68] Jiang P, Chan CW, Chan KC, et al. Lengthening and shortening of plasma DNA in hepatocellular carcinoma patients. Proceedings of the National Academy of Sciences of the United States of America. 2015;**112**:E1317-E1325

[69] Diehl F, Li M, Dressman D, et al. Detection and quantification of mutations in the plasma of patients with colorectal tumors. Proceedings of the National Academy of Sciences of the United States of America. 2005;**102**:16368-16373

[70] Jahr S, Hentze H, Englisch S, Hardt D, Fackelmayer FO, Hesch RD, et al. DNA fragments in the blood plasma of cancer patients: Quantitations and evidence for their origin from apoptotic and necrotic cells. Cancer Research. 2001;**61**(4):1659-1665

[71] Roninson IB, Broude EV, Chang BD. If not apoptosis, then what? Treatment-induced senescence and mitotic catastrophe in tumor cells. Drug Resistance Updates. 2001;**4**(5):303-313. DOI: 10.1054/drup.2001.0213

[72] Wang BG, Huang HY, Chen YC, Bristow RE, Kassauei K, Cheng CC, et al. Increased plasma DNA integrity in cancer patients. Cancer Research. 2003;**63**(14):3966-3968

[73] Diehl F, Schmidt K, Choti MA, Romans K, Goodman S, Li M, et al. Circulating mutant DNA to assess tumor dynamics. Nature Medicine. 2008;**14**(9):985-990. DOI: 10.1038/nm.1789

[74] Kohler C, Barekati Z, Radpour R, Zhong XY. Cell-free DNA in the circulation as a potential cancer biomarker. Anticancer Research. 2011;**31**(8):2623-2628

[75] Marzese DM, Hirose H, Hoon DS. Diagnostic and prognostic value of circulating tumor-related DNA in cancer patients. Expert Review of Molecular Diagnostics. 2013;**13**(8):827-844. DOI: 10.1586/14737159.2013.845088

[76] Bjorkman L, Reich CF, Pisetsky DS. The use of fluorometric assays to assess the immune response to DNA in murine systemic lupus erythematosus. Scandinavian Journal of Immunology. 2003;**57**(6):525-533

[77] Tuaeva NO, Abramova ZI, Sofronov VV. The origin of elevated levels of circulating DNA in blood plasma of premature neonates. Annals of the New York Academy of Sciences. 2008;**1137**:27-30. DOI: 10.1196/annals.1448.043

[78] Chen Z, Feng J, Buzin CH, Liu Q, Weiss L, Kernstine K, et al. Analysis of cancer mutation signatures in blood by a novel ultra-sensitive assay: Monitoring of therapy or recurrence in non-metastatic breast cancer. PLoS One. 2009;**4**(9):e7220. DOI: 10.1371/journal.pone.0007220

[79] Vogelstein B, Kinzler KW. Digital PCR. Proceedings of the National Academy of Sciences of the United States of America. 1999;**96**(16):9236-9241

[80] Hindson BJ, Ness KD, Masquelier DA, Belgrader P, Heredia NJ, Makarewicz AJ, et al. High-throughput droplet digital PCR system for absolute quantitation of DNA copy number. Analytical Chemistry. 2011;**83**(22):8604-8610. DOI: 10.1021/ac202028g

[81] Pekin D, Skhiri Y, Baret JC, Le Corre D, Mazutis L, Salem CB, et al. Quantitative and sensitive detection of rare mutations using droplet-based microfluidics. Lab on a Chip. 2011;**11**(13):2156-2166. DOI: 10.1039/c1lc20128j

[82] Forshew T, Murtaza M, Parkinson C, Gale D, Tsui DW, Kaper F, et al. Noninvasive identification and monitoring of cancer mutations by targeted deep sequencing of plasma DNA. Science Translational Medicine. 2012;**4**(136):136ra68. DOI: 10.1126/scitranslmed. 3003726

[83] Wang J, Ramakrishnan R, Tang Z, Fan W, Kluge A, Dowlati A, et al. Quantifying EGFR alterations in the lung cancer genome with nanofluidic digital PCR arrays. Clinical Chemistry. 2010;**56**(4):623-632. DOI: 10.1373/clinchem.2009.134973

[84] Dressman D, Yan H, Traverso G, Kinzler KW, Vogelstein B. Transforming single DNA molecules into fluorescent magnetic particles for detection and enumeration of genetic variations. Proceedings of the National Academy of Sciences of the United States of America. 2003;**100**(15):8817-8822. DOI: 10.1073/pnas.1133470100

[85] Higgins MJ, Jelovac D, Barnathan E, Blair B, Slater S, Powers P, et al. Detection of tumor PIK3CA status in metastatic breast cancer using peripheral blood. Clinical Cancer Research. 2012;**18**(12):3462-3469. DOI: 10.1158/1078-0432.CCR-11-2696

[86] Ignatiadis M, Dawson SJ. Circulating tumor cells and circulating tumor DNA for precision medicine: Dream or reality? Annals of Oncology. 2014;**25**(12):2304-2313. DOI: 10.1093/annonc/mdu480

[87] Haber DA, Velculescu VE. Blood-based analyses of cancer: Circulating tumor cells and circulating tumor DNA. Cancer Discovery. 2014;**4**(6):650-661. DOI: 10.1158/2159-8290.CD-13-1014

[88] Lanman RB, Mortimer SA, Zill OA, Sebisanovic D, Lopez R, Blau S, et al. Analytical and clinical validation of a digital sequencing panel for quantitative, highly accurate evaluation of cell-free circulating tumor DNA. PLoS One. 2015;**10**(10):e0140712. DOI: 10.1371/journal.pone.0140712

7

Epidemiology of Colorectal Cancer — Incidence, Lifetime Risk Factors Statistics and Temporal Trends

Camille Thélin and Sanjay Sikka

Abstract

Colorectal cancer is a major cause of morbidity and mortality in the entire world. Among cancers that affect both men and women, it accounts for >8% of all cancer incidence, making it the third most common cancer worldwide (behind lung and breast cancer). There were an estimated 14.1 million cancer cases around the world in 2012-last data available; 7.4 million were in men and 6.7 million in women. Of that, nearly 1.4 million new cases were from colorectal cancer. And, it has consistently been shown that the developed world carries the majority of the burden (Australia, New Zealand, Canada, the United States and parts of Western Europe), likely due to similarity in lifestyles and diets.

Keywords: Colon cancer epidemiology, colorectal cancer, SEER

1. Introduction

Colorectal cancer is a major cause of morbidity and mortality in the entire world. It has consistently been shown that the developed world carries the majority of the burden — this includes Australia, New Zealand, Canada, the United States and parts of Western Europe — likely due to similarity in lifestyles and diets. [9, 12]

Among cancers that affect both men and women, colorectal cancer accounts for >8% of all cancer incidence, making it the third most common cancer worldwide, behind lung and breast cancer (Table 1). [1]

	Cancer	New cases diagnosed in 2012 (1,000s)	Percent of all cancers*
Worldwide			
1	Lung	1,825	13.0
2	Breast	1,677	11.9
3	**Colorectal**	**1,361**	**9.7**
Men			
1	Lung	1,242	16.7
2	Prostate	1,112	15.0
3	**Colorectal**	**746**	**10.0**
Women			
1	Breast	1,677	25.2
2	**Colorectal**	**614**	**9.2**
3	**Lung**	**583**	**8.8**

*Excludes basal cell and squamous cell skin cancers and *in situ* carcinoma except urinary bladder. Source: GLOBOCAN 2012 v1.1, "Cancer Incidence and Mortality Worldwide"

Table 1. Cancer Incidence Worldwide

There were an estimated 14.1 million cancer cases around the world in 2012. [1] Of those cancers, 7.4 million were in men, while 6.7 million were in women. [1] Nearly, 1.4 million of those new cancer cases were from colorectal cancer. [1]

In the United States, the breakdown between genders is similar. Colorectal cancer is the third most common cancer in both women and men (after breast and prostate cancer, respectively, and lung cancer). Among both gender groups, it is the second leading cause of cancer deaths (behind lung cancer), with peak incidence being in the seventh decade of life. [24] In 2015, it is estimated that there will be 848,200 new cases of cancer among men and 810,000 among women in 2015 (Table 2). [2] Of those new cancer cases, 8% will comprise of colon and rectal cancer, with an estimated 69,090 in men and 63,610 in females. [2]

Men 848,200	Male	Female	Women 810,000
Prostate	26%	29%	Breast
Lung & bronchus	14%	13%	Lung & bronchus
Colon & rectum	**8% (69,090)**	**8% (63,610)**	**Colon & rectum**
Urinary bladder	7%	7%	Uterine corpus

Men 848,200	Male	Female	Women 810,000
Melanoma of skin	5%	6%	Thyroid
Non-Hodgkin lymphoma	5%	4%	Non-Hodgkin lymphoma
Kidney & renal pelvis	5%	4%	Melanoma of skin
Oral cavity & pharynx	4%	4%	Pancreas
Leukemia	4%	3%	Leukemia
Liver & intrahepatic bile duct	3%	3%	Kidney & renal pelvis
All other sites	21%	21%	All other sites

*Excludes basal cell and squamous cell skin cancers and *in situ* carcinoma except urinary bladder.

Source: American Cancer Society, —Cancer Facts and Figures 2015.‖ Projected cases are based on incidence data during 1995-2011 from 49 states and the District of Columbia, as reported by the North American Association of

Central Cancer Registries (NAACCR).

Note: Estimates should not be compared with those from previous years.

Table 2. Estimated New Cancer Cases* in the U.S. in 2015

2. Clinical presentation of colorectal cancer

The importance of screening is crucial as most early-stage colorectal cancer does not typically have symptoms. In fact, colorectal cancer may be quiescently growing for as long as 5 years before symptoms appear.

2.1. Signs and symptoms

Symptoms can be specific, such as abdominal discomfort and alarming changes in bowel movements (i.e., hematochezia, diarrhea, or obstruction). More often than not, however, symptoms are usually nonspecific, such as fatigue, weight loss, and/or changes in digestion. As such, even those with some type of symptoms have been misdiagnosed with other benign conditions. These benign conditions include examples such as diverticular disease, inflammatory bowel syndrome, or hemorrhoids. [4]

The major biochemical sign is that of new onset anemia. In fact, in those older than 40 years old, a new onset anemia — specifically hypochromic and microcytic — should prompt evaluation for colorectal cancer.

2.2. Right-sided colon cancers

Symptoms depend somewhat on the site of the tumor. In general, **right-sided colon cancers** are usually detected at an advanced stage with severe symptoms. In general, the right-sided colon cancers are commonly larger, producing vague abdominal discomfort and sometimes a palpable mass. [4, 5] Obstruction is rarely a presenting symptom, as the diameter of the right colon is larger than the left colon. [4] If the tumor involves the cecum, however, it could block the ileocecal valve causing small bowel obstruction.

Those with right-sided colon cancers are significantly older and are predominantly women (46% women versus 38% men). [6] Because of higher rates of comorbidities, survival is worse in those with right-sided carcinomas.

2.3. Left-sided colon cancers and rectal cancers

In comparison, **left-sided colon cancers and rectal cancers** tend to arise in younger, male populations with high-incidence risk. [7, 8] Cancers involving this portion of the bowel produce symptoms that range from obstruction to tenesmus, to alternating constipation and diarrhea with pencil-thin stools. [4] Often, there is blood witnessed either in the stool or coating the stool, in comparison to the right-sided colon cancers. Similarly, rectal cancers can cause obstruction and similar types of bowel movement changes as the left-sided carcinomas.

3. Risk factors of colorectal cancer

There are both modifiable and nonmodifiable risk factors associated with the incidence of colorectal cancer (Table 3).

Modifiable Risk Factors	Nonmodifiable Risk Factors
Diet	Age (≥50 years old)
Physical activity	Personal history of adenomatous colonic polyps
Body weight	Family history of colorectal cancer
Social behaviors (i.e., alcohol and cigarette smoking)	Hereditary polyposis conditions
	Personal history of inflammatory bowel disease (IBD)

Table 3. Factors Associated with Higher Risk of Colon and Rectal Cancer

Modifiable risk factors include diet, physical activity, weight, cigarette-smoking, and alcohol intake. [9] Other modifiable risk factors include low calcium content, low selenium content, and very low salt intake. [10] Occupational hazards, such as asbestos-exposure, have been linked to increased risk of colorectal cancer when compared to the rest of the general population. [10]

Socioeconomic factors, along with access to (and use of) health care services, are also important contributing risk factors. In fact, there is a disproportionately high incidence of colorectal cancers in low socioeconomic status populations. [11]

Nonmodifiable risk factors associated with higher risk of colorectal cancer include increasing age, personal history of adenomatous polyps, personal history of inflammatory bowel disease, genetic inheritance, race/ethnicity, and gender. [9] Unlike modifiable risk factors that could theoretically have been avoided, these risk factors are not considered part of the "environmental nature" of this disease. Thus, they are not controllable. They do, however, play an important role in screening and identifying susceptible patients.

3.1. Modifiable risk factors: Diet

Diets associated with high incidence of colorectal cancer include diets with high consumption of red or processed meat, diets high in fat, beer-drinking, diets low in calcium intake, and diets low in whole-grain fiber, fruits and vegetables. [9] This represents a typical "Western diet."

On average, 40–45% of Western diets have total caloric intake made up from fatty foods (including meat products), while fat only accounts for about 10–15% of dietary makeup in lower-risk populations — China, India, and parts of Africa and South America. Consequently, it has been shown that the developed world carries the majority of the burden (Australia, New Zealand, Canada, the United States and parts of Western Europe), [9, 12] likely due to similarity in lifestyles and diets.

The hypothesis behind dietary fat as a risk factor is that the fat enhances hepatic cholesterol and bile acid synthesis resulting in increased sterols in the colon. [4] Those sterols are then converted into secondary bile acids, cholesterol metabolites, and potentially toxic metabolic compounds. [4, 13]

While the exact pathogenesis remains unknown, what is known is that these sterols and bile acid metabolites cause damage to colonic mucosa, thus enhancing proliferative activity which could lead to dysplasia. [4, 13] This has been demonstrated in animal models, where animals fed polyunsaturated and saturated fats have higher numbers of adenocarcinoma than those on a low-fat diet. [4] This has also been shown in human population studies where those with colorectal cancer tend to have higher fecal bile acid levels, [4] while a recent meta-analysis has shown that consumption of red meat and processed meat is positively associated with risk of both colon — particularly the descending and sigmoid colon — and rectal cancer. [14]

The "Western diet" also comprises of lower amounts of fiber intake. Multiple epidemiology studies have shown a geographical difference of lower colorectal cancer incidence rates in places with higher fiber intake. [9] It is even postulated that due to the ability of fiber to change the colonic pH, carcinogenesis may be impeded. [4, 9]

Dietary fiber also increases fecal bulk, thus diluting the aforementioned carcinogenic compounds and reducing transit time and mucosal contact. In fact, fiber has been found to decrease the concentration of sterol and bile acid metabolites that could be implicated in creating carcinogenic compounds. [4] Again, this has been demonstrated in animal models, where increased fiber intake led to decreased concentration of specific bacterial metabolic enzymes that could be implicated in creating carcinogenic compounds. [4] Unfortunately, for all its experimentally demonstrative protective roles, increased fiber supplementation has been unable to prevent adenoma recurrence in several randomized-controlled trials.

3.2. Modifiable risk factors: Physical activity and body weight

Other modifiable risk factors are physical inactivity and excess body weight. Decreased gut motility, increased insulin resistance, lower metabolic rates, and increased circulating estrogens are all mechanisms implicated in the higher risk of colorectal cancer associated with this modifiable risk factor. [9, 10]

3.3. Modifiable risk factors: Social behaviors

Associated with a higher risk is regular consumption of cigarettes and alcohol. [10] Carcinogenic metabolites found in both tobacco and alcohol are considered promoters of tumor growth, based on experimental studies in animals. [15]

Cigarette-smoking has been attributed to 12% of colorectal cancer deaths, while alcohol consumption has been linked with early onset colorectal cancers, specifically tumors in the distal colon. [9, 16, 17] There is information showing that there is higher risk in active smokers for development of rectal cancer.[9, 18]

3.4. Nonmodifiable risk factors: Age

Increasing age carries a higher likelihood of colorectal cancer, specifically after the age of 40. [2]

Cancer incidence rises progressively after the age of 40 in the general population, with 90% of colorectal cancers occurring in those aged 50 years and older. [2] In fact, a 50-year old has 5% chance of developing cancer and 2.5% chance of dying from this cancer after the age of 80 years. [2, 9]

As such, the US Preventative Task Force (USPSTF) has defined "average risk" as those aged 50 years or more with no personal history of colorectal cancer or adenomas, no inflammatory bowel disease, and with negative family history. [19] Put in other terms, the incidence rate is more than 50 times higher in those 60–79 years old than in those less than 40 years old.

In contrast, those with "increased risk" include those with a personal history of colorectal cancer, personal history of colonic adenomas, family history of sporadic colorectal cancer, as well as family history of sporadic adenoma. [4, 9]

Finally, those with "high risk" include those with hereditary nonpolyposis colorectal cancer (Lynch syndrome), polyposis syndromes, and inflammatory bowel diseases (IBD). [4] *See below for a discussion on hereditary polyposis conditions and IBD.*

3.5. Nonmodifiable risk factors: Personal history of colonic adenomatous polyps

Carrying a personal history of adenomatous polyps has an increased risk of developing colorectal cancer, in comparison to those with no history of adenomas. In recent literature, it was reported that 95% of sporadic colorectal cancers developed from such adenomas, usually after a protracted period, which has been estimated anywhere from 5 to 10 years. [4, 9] However, while nearly all colorectal cancer arise from adenomas, only a small minority of these dysplastic polyps actually progress to cancer (5% or less). [4]

3.6. Nonmodifiable risk factors: Family history of colonic adenomatous polyps or colorectal cancer

The majority of cases occur in those with family history of either colorectal cancer or adenomatous cancer. In fact, there is a two- to three-fold increased risk of sporadic cancer in those with first-degree relatives. This means that up to 20% of those with colorectal cancer have family members affected by this disease. [4, 9] This risk becomes even higher when there are two or more relatives involved and when those family members are affected by the disease at an age younger than 60.

3.7. Nonmodifiable risk factors: Hereditary polyposis conditions

Those with recognized inherited polyposis syndromes carry an even higher risk. Recent literature estimates that about 5–10% of sporadic colorectal cancers are the outcome of inherited conditions, such as the familial adenomatous polyposis (FAP) and hereditary nonpolyposis colorectal cancer (HPNCC). [4, 9]

HPNCC (also called Lynch syndrome) is thought to comprise of about 1–6% of all colorectal cancers. It carries a lifetime risk of cancer as high as 70–80%. [4, 9] FAP and its variants account for less than 1% of all colorectal cancer cases, but almost all those diagnosed with this disorder will develop cancer if the colon is not removed by the age of 40. [4]

Other hereditary conditions that are associated with sporadic colorectal cancers include Gardner's syndrome (high-risk), Turcot's syndrome (high-risk), and Peutz-Jeghers syndrome (low-to-moderate risk). [4] Appropriate screening recommendations are made for this population subtype, which will not be discussed here.

3.8. Nonmodifiable risk factors: Personal history of Inflammatory Bowel Disease (IBD)

Those with IBD — ulcerative colitis and Crohn's disease — also carry an increased risk of developing colorectal cancer. It has been estimated that the relative risk of colorectal cancer in patients with IBD ranges from 4- to 20-fold. [4, 9] Thus, appropriate screening recommendations are made for this population subtype, which will not be discussed here.

4. Statistics

4.1. Methods

The following statistical data were obtained from the Surveillance, Epidemiology and End Results (SEER) Program of the National Cancer Institute (NCI), specifically from the data previously published in the *SEER Cancer Statistic Review (CSR) 1975–2012*, which was released in April 23, 2015. The NCI funds for the program through Centers for Disease Control and Presentation (CDC), National Program of Cancer Registries, and involved states' contributions.

The SEER program was conceptualized in 1973, with a mission to report the "most recent cancer incidence, mortality, survival, prevalence, and lifetime risks statistics. It originally only represented about 10% of the US population.

Since then, it has expanded to include the following population-based cancer registries: Alaska Native Tumor Registry, Arizona Indians, Cherokee Nation, Connecticut, Detroit, Georgia Center for Cancer Statistics (Atlanta, Greater Georgia, Rural Georgia), Greater Bay Area Cancer Registry (San Francisco-Oakland, San Jose-Monterey), Greater California, Hawaii, Iowa, Kentucky, Los Angeles, Louisiana, New Jersey, New Mexico, Seattle-Puget Sound, and Utah. This translates to approximately 26% of African Americans, 41% of Hispanics, 43% of American Indians and Alaska Natives, 54% of Asians, and 71% of Hawaiian/Pacific Islanders. It is published annually, with 2012 being the most recent year for which data are available.

4.2. Temporal trends in the united states

How common is this cancer? It is estimated that there will be 132,700 new colorectal cancer cases in 2015. [21] This comprises 8% of all new cancer cases (Figure 1). [21] Of those new cancer cases, there will be an estimated 49,700 deaths. [21] This comprises 8.4% of all cancer deaths (Table 4).

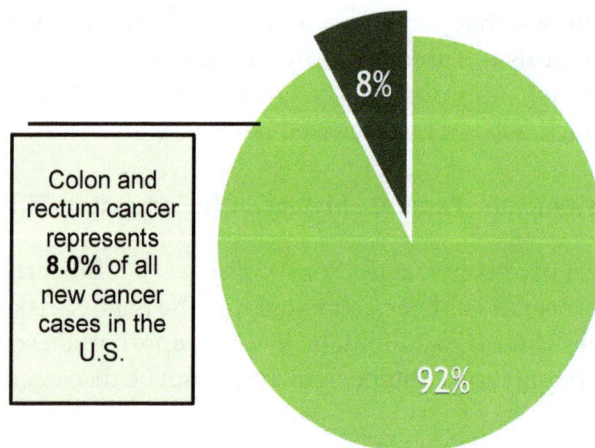

Colon and rectum cancer represents **8.0%** of all new cancer cases in the U.S.

8%

92%

Figure 1. Colon and rectum cancer in the U.S.

Who gets this cancer? Colorectal cancer is more common in men than in women. In 2014, there were a total of 135,260 people diagnosed with colorectal cancer: 70,099 men versus 65,161 women. [22] Based on SEER 18, this means that 48.9 per 100,000 persons new cases were male, while 37.1 per 100,000 persons were female. [20]

Common Type of Cancer	Estimated New Cases 2015	Estimated Deaths 2015
Breast cancer (female)	231,840	40,290
Lung and bronchus cancer	221,200	158,040
Prostate cancer	220,800	27,540
Colon & rectal cancer	**132,700**	**49,700**
Bladder cancer	74,000	16,000
Melanoma of the skin	73,870	9,940
Non-Hodgkin Lymphoma	71,850	19,790
Thyroid cancer	62,450	1,950
Kidney & renal pelvis cancer	61,560	14,080
Endometrial cancer	54,870	10,170

Source: SEER 2015

Table 4. Comparison of Common Cancers

While colorectal cancer is more common in men than in women, the gender bias is smaller when all races are included. However, the gender bias remains wide when race and ethnicity are factored in. The greatest divide was found in African American males versus females, with 61.2 per 100,000 new cases in black men versus 46.0 per 100,000 new cases in black women. [20]

Other race/ethnicities also showed a divide, but not as wide. Hispanic male new cases were 30/100,000 while female new cases were 43.3/100,000. American Indian/Alaska Native male new cases were 35.7/100,000 while female new cases were 46.3/100,000. Asian/Pacific Islander male new cases were 31.3/100,000 while female new cases were 42.2/100,000. White male new cases were 36.3/100,000 while female new cases were 47.8/100,000 (Table 5). [20]

At what age is this cancer most frequently diagnosed? Colorectal cancer is most frequently diagnosed among those aged 65–74 years old. [20] This age group comprises 23.9% of new cases. [20] The median age is 68 years old (Table 6; Figure 2).

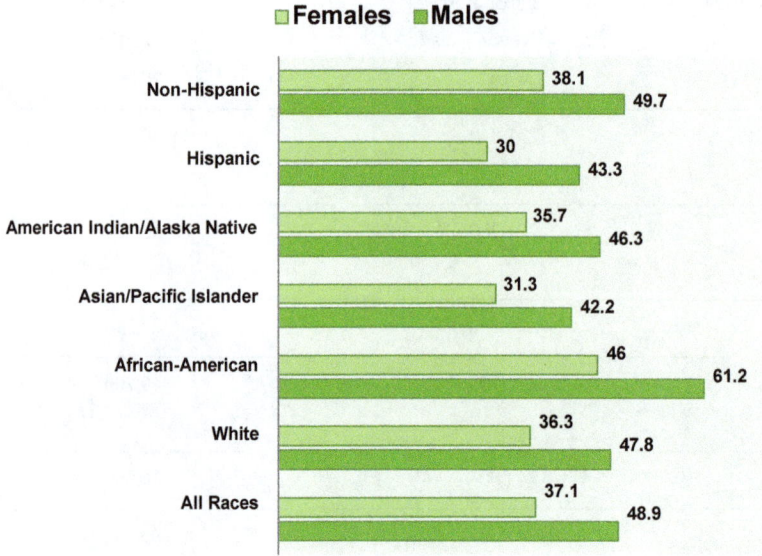

□Females ■Males

Source: SEER 18 2008-2012, Age Adjusted

Table 5. Number of New Colon and Rectal Cancer Cases/100,000 Persons by Race/Ethnicity & Sex

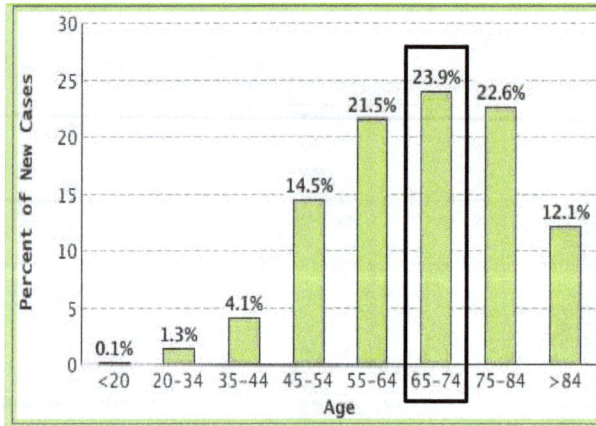

Source: SEER 2015

Table 6. Percent of Deaths by Age Group

There is different distribution based on age at diagnosis in different gender groups. In women, colon cancer tends to arise in an older population (mean age being 73 years old; Figure 2; in comparison, colon cancer tends to arise in a younger population in men (mean age being 69 years old; Figure 2). [9]

In the younger age groups (all races, both sexes), those <20 years old comprised of 0.1% of new cases; 20–34 years old comprised of 1.3%; 45–54 years old comprised of 14.5%; 55–64 years old comprised of 21.5%.

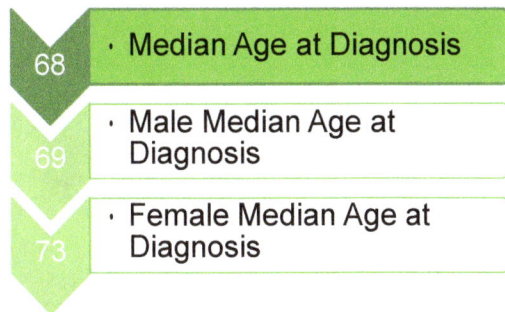

Figure 2. Median age at which colorectal cancer is most frequently diagnosed.

In the older age groups (all races, both sexes), 75–84 years old comprised of 22.6% (75–84 years old) and those >84 years old comprised of 12.1%. [20]

What are the survival rates? Based on the data from SEER 18 2005–2011, relative survival statistics show that 64.9% of people survive 5 years or more after being diagnosed with colon or rectal cancer (all races/sexes, Figure 3). [20, 22]

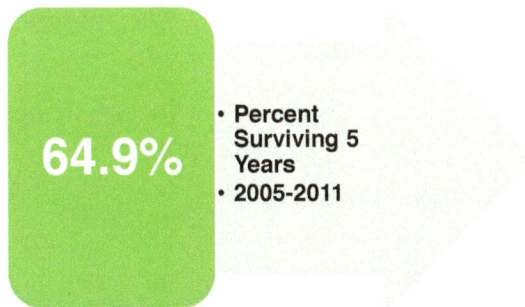

Figure 3. Relative survival rate of colon or rectal cancer.

Does staging influence survival rates? Cancer stage at diagnosis will determine both treatment options and has a strong influence on the length of survival. Obviously, the earlier the cancer is caught, the better the chance of survival.

Current statistics show that 39.5% of colon and rectal cancers are diagnosed at the local stage (confined to primary site), with a 5-year survival for localized colon and rectal cancer being very high at 90.1% [20] (Table 7).

Thirty-six percent of cancers in the regional stage (those spread to regional lymph nodes) have a 70.8% 5-year relative survival rate. [20] Twenty percent of cancers in the distant stage (those that metastasized) carry a 13.1% 5-year relative survival rate. [20] Lastly, those that are unstaged (5%) have a 34.5% 5-year survival rate [20] (Table 7).

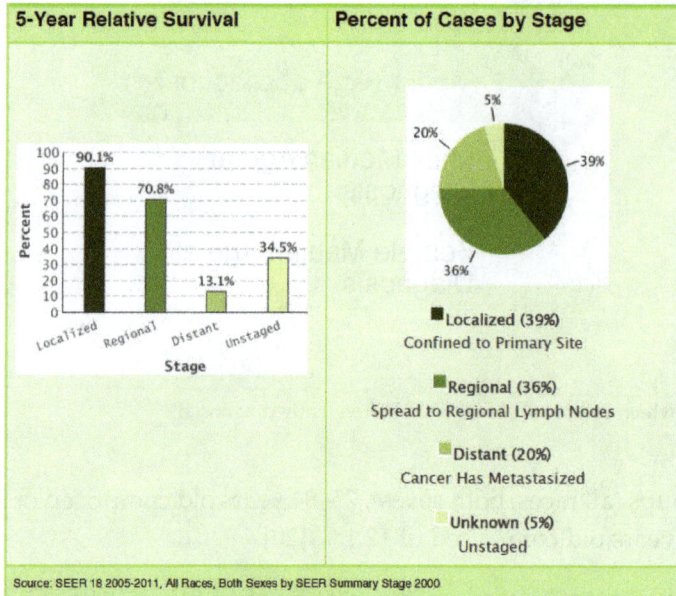

Table 7. 5-Year Relative Survival and Percent of Colon and Rectal Cancer Cases by Stage at Diagnosis [20]

Does the site of cancer change the incidence? Distribution of colon cancers also vary. This suggests that there are different pathogenic etiologies and carcinogenic mechanisms involved in different sites of the colon (and rectum).

The most common tumor locations in decreasing order are the descending colon (40–42%), rectosigmoid and rectum (30–33%), cecum and ascending colon (25–30%), and transverse colon (10–13%). [22, 23] In other words, 50% of colon cancers are within reach of a flexible sigmoidoscope [24] (Table 8).

Who dies from this cancer? As with all cancers, the death rates increase with age. Among both gender groups, it is the second leading cause of cancer deaths — behind lung cancer — with peak incidence being in the seventh decade of life. [2, 20]

In the United States, colorectal cancer is the second leading cause of death. [2] Unfortunately, each year there are >55,000 deaths (26,804 men; 24,979 women). [20]

The percent of deaths is highest among those aged 75–84 at 26.6%. [20] The median age at death is 73 years old (Figure 4). [20] This age group comprises 26.6% of all colorectal cancer deaths [20] (Table 9).

In the younger age groups (all races, both sexes), percent of deaths in those <20 years old comprised of 0% of new cases; 20–34 years old comprised of 0.7%; 35–44 years old comprised of 2.5%; 45–54 years old comprised of 9.3%; 55–64 years old comprised of 17.9%.

In the older age groups (all races, both sexes), percent of deaths in those 65–74 years old comprised of 22.1% and those >84 years old comprised of 21.0%. [20]

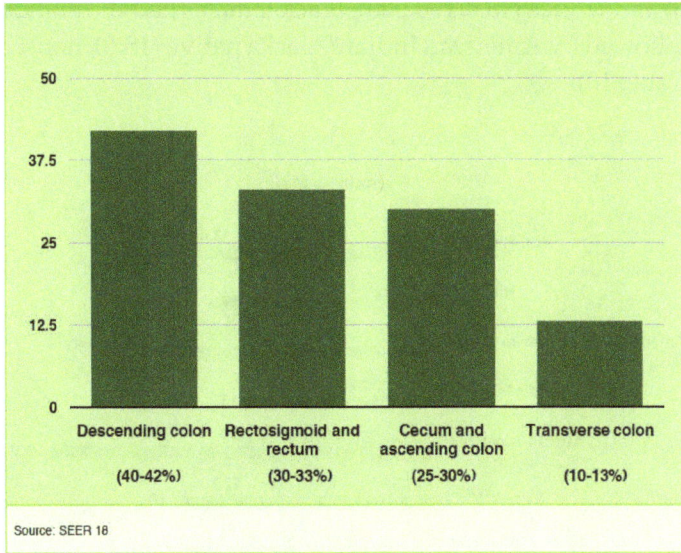

Source: SEER 18

Table 8. Incidence Rates of Colon and Rectal Cancer by Location [20]

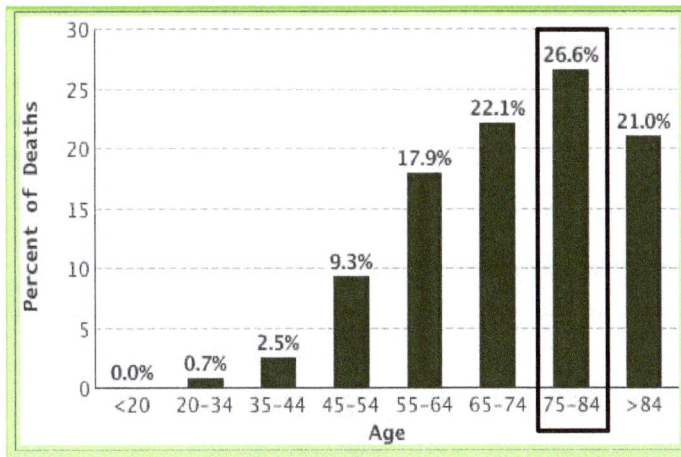

Source: SEER 18 2008-2012, All Races/Both Sexes

Table 9. Percent of Deaths by Age Group

As more males are diagnosed each year than females, there are more male number of deaths than females. In all races, there were 18.6 number of deaths per 100,000 males versus 13.1 number of deaths per 100,000 females.

The divide between the genders was even greater when race and ethnicity were factored in. African American males had the highest number of deaths per 100,000: 26.9 (versus 17.8/100,000 females). [25] Males who were identified as non-Hispanic (but not white or black) had the second highest number of deaths (18.9/100,000), followed by American Indian/Alaska native (18.8/100,000) and whites (18.0/100,000). Black females had the higher number of deaths per 100,000 (17.8), followed by American Indian/Alaska native (15.6), non-Hispanic (13.4), and whites (12.7) [20] (Table 10).

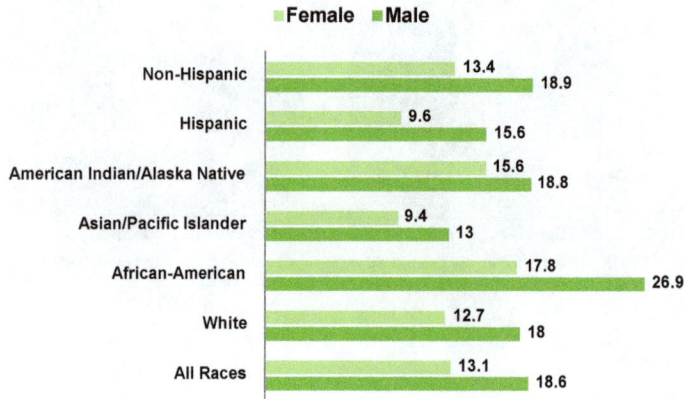

Source: U.S. 2008-2012, Age-Adjusted

Table 10. Number of Colon and Rectal Cancer Deaths per 100,000 Persons by Race/Ethnicity & Sex

What are the projection rates of colorectal cancer? Rates of new colon and rectal cancer diagnosis have been falling each year, over the past 10 years. [26] This is true not only for the United States but also for New Zealand, Australia, and Western Europe.[9] Despite these numbers, the death rate has not changed significantly, however (Table 11).

Year	1975	1980	1985	1990	1995	1999	2003	2007
5-Year Relative Survival	48.6%	51.1%	58.0%	60.8%	59.7%	64.5%	65.3%	66.5%

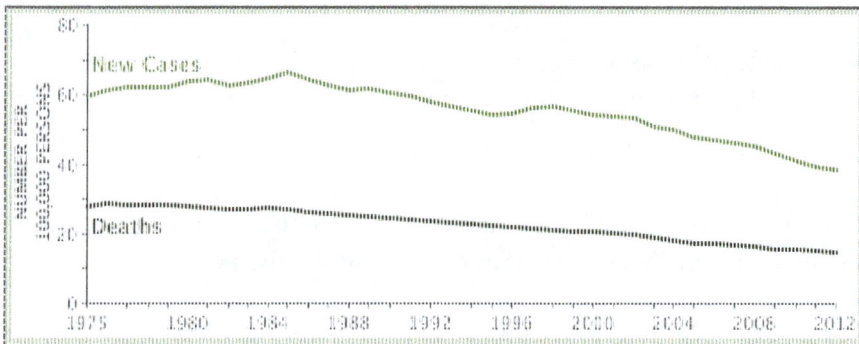

Source: SEER 9 Incidence & U.S. Mortality 1975-2012, all races/both sexes/rates are age-adjusted

Table 11. Incidence & U.S Mortality 1975-2012

5. Conclusion

Although new diagnosis rates of colorectal cancer have lowered significantly in both women and men since 1975, more can be done in terms of screening. The drama in these numbers is that colorectal cancer is a preventative cancer, both in screening and in identification of modifiable (i.e., theoretically preventable) risk factors. In fact, if everyone aged 50 years or older had regular screening tests, at least 60% of deaths from this cancer could have been avoided. [3, 19] And with the knowledge that the 5-year survival is close to 90% when colorectal cancer is diagnosed at an early stage, the statistics becomes even more dramatic. **Bottom-line:** colorectal cancer is susceptible to screening and aggressive campaigns toward educating the public dictate the future of its incidence and survival.

Author details

Camille Thélin* and Sanjay Sikka

*Address all correspondence to: cthelin1@tulane.edu

Department of Internal Medicine, Division of Gastroenterology and Hepatology, Tulane University, New Orleans, LA, United States

References

[1] Ferlay J, Soerjomataram I, Ervik M, Dikshit R, Eser S, Mathers C, Rebelo M, Parkin DM, Forman D, Bray, F. GLOBOCAN 2012 v1.1, Cancer Incidence and Mortality Worldwide: IARC CancerBase No. 11 [Internet]. Lyon, France: International Agency for Research on Cancer; 2014. Available from: http://www.wcrf.org/int/cancer-facts-figures/worldwide-data, accessed January 16, 2015.

[2] American Cancer Society, "Cancer Facts and Figures 2015." Reported by the North American Association of Central Cancer Registries (NAACCR). Available at http://www.cancer.org/acs/groups/content/@editorial/documents/document/acspc-044552.pdf.

[3] Centers for Disease Control and Prevention, Division of Cancer Prevention and Control. Colorectal Cancer Control Program (CRCCP) Fact Sheet. Available at cdc.gov/cancer/crccp/pdf/CRCCP_FactSheet.pdf, accessed December 2, 2013.

[4] Feldman M, Friedman LS, Brandt LJ. *Sleisenger and Fordtran's Gastrointestinal and Liver Disease: Pathophysiology, Diagnosis, Management, 10th Edition*. Philadelphia: Saunders/Elsevier, February 2010.

[5]   Nawa T, Kato J, Kawamoto H, Okada H, Yamamoto H, Kohno H, Endo H, Shiratori Y. Differences between right- and left-sided colon cancer in patient characteristics, cancer morphology and histology. J Gastroenterol Hepatol 2008;23:418–23.

[6]   American Cancer Society. Colorectal Cancer Facts and Figures 2014-2016. Atlanta: American Cancer Soceity, 2014. Available at http://www.cancer.org/acs/groups/content/documents/document/acspc-042280.pdf.

[7]   Iacopetta B. Are there two sides to colorectal cancer? Int J Cancer 2002;101:403–8.

[8]   Siegel RL, Jemal A, Ward EM. Increase in incidence of colorectal cancer among young men and women in the United States. Cancer Epidemiol Biomarkers Prev 2009;18:1695–8.

[9]   Haggar FA, Boushey RP. Colorectal Cancer Epidemiology: Incidence, Mortality, Survival, and Risk Factors. Clinics in Colon and Rectal Surgery. 2009;22(4):191–7. doi: 10.1055/s-0029/1242458.

[10] Tárraga L, Pedro J, Albero JS, Rodríguez-Montes JA. "Primary and Secondary Prevention of Colorectal Cancer." Clinical Medicine Insights. Gastroenterology 2014;7:33–46. PMC. Web. 16 May 2015

[11] Doubeni CA, Laiyema AO, Major JM, et al. Socioeconomic status and the risk of colorectal cancer an analysis of more than a half million adults in the national Insittuaes of Health-AARP Diet and Health Study. Cancer 2012;118:3636–44.

[12] Boyle P, Langman JS. ABC of colorectal cancer: Epidemiology. BMJ 2000 Sept 30;321(7264):805–8.

[13] Santarelli R L, Pierre F, Corpet D E. Processed meat and colorectal cancer: a review of epidemiologic and experimental evidence. Nutr Cancer 2008;60(2):131–44

[14] Larsson S C, Wolk A. Meat consumption and risk of colorectal cancer: a meta-analysis of prospective studies. Int J Cancer 2006;119(11):2657–64

[15] Pöschl G, Seitz HK. Alcohol and cancer. Alcohol Alcohol 2004 May–Jun;39(3):155–65.

[16] Zisman AL, Nickolov A, Brand RE, Gorchow A, Roy HK. Associations between the age at diagnosis and location of colorectal cancer and the use of alcohol and tobacco: implications for screening. Arch Intern Med 2006;166(6):629–34.

[17] Botteri E, Iodice S, Raimondi S, Maisonneuve P, Lowenfels AB. Cigarette smoking and adenomatous polyps; a meta-analysis. Gastroenterology 2008;134(2);388–96; e3.

[18] Hooker CM, Gallicchio L, Genkinger JM, Comstock GW, Alberg AJ. A prospective cohort study of rectal cancer risk in relation to active cigarette smoking and passive smoke exposure. Ann Epidemiol 2008;18:28–35.

[19] US Preventative Task Force. Evaluating Test Strategies for Colorectal Cancer Screening: A Decision Analysis for the U.S. Preventive Services Task Force: Colorectal Cancer: Screening. November 2014. Available at http://

www.uspreventiveservicestaskforce.org/Page/SupportingDoc/colorectal-cancer-screening/evaluating-test-strategies-for-colorectal-cancer-screening-a-decision-analysis-for-the-us-preventive-services-task-force

[20] Howlader N, Noone AM, Krapcho M, Garshell J, Miller D, Altekruse SF, Kosary CL, Yu M, Ruhl J, Tatalovich Z,Mariotto A, Lewis DR, Chen HS, Feuer EJ, Cronin KA (eds). SEER Cancer Statistics Review, 1975-2012, National Cancer Institute. Bethesda, MD, http://seer.cancer.gov/csr/1975_2012/, based on November 2014 SEER data submission, posted to the SEER web site, April 2015

[21] U.S. Cancer Statistics Working Group. United States Cancer Statistics: 1999–2011 Incidence and Mortality Web-based Report. Atlanta: U.S. Department of Health and Human Services, Centers for Disease Control and Prevention and National Cancer Institute; 2014. www.cdc.gov/uscs.

[22] Siegel RL, Ward EM, Jemal A. Trends in colorectal cancer incidence rates in the United States by tumor location and stage, 1992-2008. Cancer Epidemiol Biomarkers Prev 2012;21:411–6.

[23] Seigel RL, DeSantis C, Jemal A. Colorectal cancer statistics, 2014. CA: Cancer J Clinicians 2014;64:104–17.

[24] Ferri F. *Ferri's Clinical Advisor 2015*, 1st ed. St. Louis, MO: Elsevier Mosby. 2014.

[25] American Cancer Society. Cancer facts & figures for African Americans 2005–2006. American Cancer Society, 2005. Available at http://www.cancer.org/docroot/STT/stt_0.asp, accessed November 8, 2005

[26] Chu KC, Tarone RE, Chow WH, Hankey BF, Ries LAG. Temporal patterns in colorectal cancer incidence, survival, and mortality from 1950 through 1990. J Natl Cancer Inst 1994;86:997–100.

8

Treatment Strategies in Colorectal Cancer

Hamid Elia Daaboul and Mirvat El-Sibai

Abstract

Colorectal cancer is known to be one of the most commonly diagnosed cancers worldwide. It maintains a high mortality rate despite the newest methodological therapeutic approaches adopted in various academic establishments. The treatment modalities in colorectal cancer follow the degree of disease progression based on staging information. Earliest the cancer is diagnosed, the highest the possibility to be cured. Different strategies are being involved in treating colorectal cancer, starting from simple endoscopic polypectomy to remove a potential malignant polyp, to wider surgical intervention to get rid of a primary unmetastasized tumor, to other concomitant radio-chemotherapy combinations to reduce a bulky tumor rendering it operable, ending in more sophisticated chemotherapeutical regimens combined with targeted drugs to shrink the metastatic lesions and prolong survival rate. Different new treatments are being investigated with a sole aim to preserve the patient's quality of life and extend life span.

Keywords: colorectal cancer, colorectal polyps, chemotherapy, targeted therapy, immunotherapy, Lynch syndrome, familial adenomatous polyposis syndrome

1. Introduction

Colorectal cancers (CRC) are considered the third most commonly diagnosed cancers in the world. The incidence and mortality rates vary worldwide from lowest in Africa and Asia to highest in Australia, North America, and Europe. The etiology is mainly due to changes in dietary habits, from low-fiber ingestion to high-fat diet, increased body mass index (BMI), low physical activity, cigarette smoking, alcohol consumption, diabetes mellitus, ulcerative colitis, Crohn's disease, some inherited syndromes (familial adenomatous polyposis syndrome and nonpolyposis colorectal cancer or Lynch syndrome (LS), MUTYH-associated and Turcot-associated polyposis syndromes, Peutz-Jeghers syndrome, Juvenile polyposis syndrome, and Cowden syndrome), in addition to radiation therapy for another abdominal cancer [1–3]. Early diagnosis is necessary to get full remission, and screening has proved to be fundamental in decreasing the mortality rate. The treatment of CRC is multidisciplinary and implies a collaboration of many therapeutic teams including surgical, chemotherapy, as well as radiotherapy experts. In the following chapter, we will be studying the different treatment modalities and strategies approved and administered worldwide, according to CRC stages.

The staging classification of CRC has been conceived according to collaboration between the Union for International Cancer Control (UICC) and the seventh edition of the American Joint Committee on Cancer (AJCC-7), taking into consideration the Dukes' staging with its modifications by Astler-Coller (MAC) and Kirklin system (**Table 1**).

Stage	UICC/AJCC			Dukes	MAC
0	Tis	N0	M0	—	—
I	T1	N0	M0	A	A
	T2	N0	M0	A	B1
II A	T3	N0	M0	B	B2
B	T4a	N0	M0	B	B2
C	T4b	N0	M0	B	B3
III A	T1–T2	N1–N1c	M0	C	C1
	T1	N2a	M0	C	C1
B	T3–T4a	N1–N1c	M0	C	C2
	T2–T3	N2a	M0	C	C1–C2
	T1–T2	N2b	M0	C	C1
C	T4a	N2a	M0	C	C2
	T3–T4a	N2b	M0	C	C2
	T4b	N1–N2	M0	C	C3
IV A	Any T	Any N	M1a	D	D
B	Any T	Any N	M1b	D	D

Tis, Tumor confined to the mucosa; T1, tumor invades the submucosa; T2, tumor invades the muscularis propria; T3, tumor invades subserosa or beyond, without invading other organs; T4, tumor invades nearby organs (T4a, without perforation of visceral peritoneum; T4b, with perforation of visceral peritoneum); N1, metastasis to one to three regional lymph nodes (RLNs) (N1a, metastasis to one RLN; N1b, metastasis to two to three RLNs; N1c, metastasis into areas of fat near lymph nodes but not the nodes themselves); N2, metastasis to four or more RLNs (N2a, metastasis to four to six RLNs; N2b, metastasis to seven or more RLNs); M1, distant metastases present (M1a, metastasis to distant organ, as the liver or lung, or distant set of lymph nodes; M1b, metastasis to distant organs, to distant set of lymph nodes, or to distant parts of the peritoneum as the lining of the abdominal cavity).

Table 1. Anatomic AJCC-7 staging for CRC.

2. Treatment of CRC by stage

2.1. Treatment of stage 0 CRC

In stage 0 colorectal cancer, the tumor is still confined to the inner lining of the colon (T in situ). A surgical removal of the cancer is all that is needed. A polypectomy or a colonoscopic local excision is usually sufficient. Partial colectomy is required in case of bigger tumors.

2.2. Treatment of malignant polyps

2.2.1. Definition, classification, and staging

Malignant polyps are adenomas that have been identified histologically, after endoscopic excision, to be adenocarcinomas which have invaded through the muscularis mucosa into the basic submucosa (pT1) [4]. They can occur sporadically or as part of a polyposis syndrome. They can be classified endoscopically by their size and morphology and histologically as favorable (low risk) and unfavorable (high risk). In 1985, Haggitt reconceived the Japanese society classification and the Paris endoscopic classification into a new one taking into consideration the level of invasion depth (**Table 2**).

Despite the big advantage and wide use of Haggitt's classification in assessing the quality of resection of endoscopic polypectomies, the sessile, flat, or depressed lesions yet were not successfully evaluated using this classification. In the early 1990s, Kikuchi succeeded in quantifying the grade of vertical and horizontal submucosal invasion, dividing the invasion into three levels (**Table 3**).

Morphologically, polyps are known to be either pedunculated or sessile. Pedunculated polyps are usually attached to the colonic mucosa via a stalk of variable length, while sessile polyps are devoid of stalk, are flattened in shape, and overlay the mucosa with less separation of the adenomatous epithelium part from the underlying layers of the colon [5].

Histologically, polyps can be divided into low-risk versus high-risk features (**Table 4**) [4].

Level	Location of carcinoma
0	Carcinoma in situ or confined to the mucosa. Not invasive
I	Carcinoma invading through the muscularis mucosa into the submucosa but limited to the head of the polyp
II	Carcinoma invading the level of the neck of the polyp
III	Carcinoma invading in any part of the stalk of the polyp
IV	Carcinoma invading into the submucosa of the bowel wall below the stalk of the polyp but above the muscularis propria

Table 2. Haggitt's classification according to the level of invasion.

Submucosal level	Submucosal invasion
Sm1*	Characterizes lesions that are limited to the upper third of the submucosal layer
Sm1a	Submucosal invasion under one fourth of tumoral width
Sm1b	Submucosal invasion between one fourth and a half of the tumoral width
Sm1c	Horizontal affection of the superior third of the submucosa over half of the tumoral width
Sm2	Characterizes lesions that are limited to the middle third of the submucosal layer
Sm3	Characterizes lesions that are limited to the lower third of the submucosal layer

*Sm1 lesions are further subdivided into three categories (a, b, and c) with regard to the degree of horizontal involvement of the upper submucosal layer (B), to the horizontal involvement of the total lesion (A). B/A ratios of 0.25, 0.25–0.5, and >0.5 correspond to a, b, and c, respectively.

Table 3. Kikuchi's classification according to submucosal invasion level.

Low-risk features (favorable)	High-risk features (unfavorable)
• Pedunculated (levels 1–3 according to Haggitt classification)	• Tumor budding
• Well-differentiated adenocarcinoma	• Poorly differentiated adenocarcinoma (grade 3)
• Free resection margin (2 mm)	• Positive, indeterminate, or <1 mm resection margin
• En bloc resection	• Piecemeal removal
• Neither lymphatic nor vascular invasion	• Presence of either lymphatic or vascular invasion
• Submucosal invasion Sm < 1 mm	• Submucosal invasion Sm* >1 mm

*While Sm1a + b lesions have a very low risk for metastasis, the malignant potential increases with depth of submucosal invasion [6].

Table 4. Polyp classification according to histological criteria.

2.2.2. Treatment

All of the aforementioned classifications are mandatory for accurate assessment of the degree of malignancy and aggressiveness of the resected polyp for rational clinical decision. Studies have shown polyps smaller than 5 mm in diameter, have negligible risk of malignancy, and are easily managed by standard techniques of endoscopic snare removal. Protruding polyps (Haggitt levels I, II, or III) with favorable histological features should be subjected to local excision or endoscopic polypectomy. Haggitt level IV lesions with favorable histology are considered low risk and can be favorably managed with endoscopic polypectomy provided margins are safe (>2 mm). Haggitt level IV protruding polyps and/or polyps exhibiting unfavorable features should be surgically excised due to the high incidence of lymph node metastasis. Excision can be performed either through traditional open approach or via more conservative laparoscopic techniques [7]. For sessile non-protruding polyps, a wider excision should be reconsidered requiring endoscopic mucosal resection (EMR) or endoscopic submucosal dissection

(ESD) [4]. Endoscopic mucosal resection is more specific for removal of sessile polyps limited to the mucosa and submucosa (Sm1a + b) and is typically used for complete excision of lesions up to 2 cm [8]. Endoscopic submucosal dissection is usually adopted for larger gastrointestinal lesions, where it more easily promotes the en bloc resection, yet it carries greater risk of perforation (31%) and late bleeding (15%) [9]. Lesions with a deep level of invasion (Sm1c, Sm2, or Sm3) or rectal lesions (specifically those of the distal third) showed higher incidence of lymph node metastasis 12–25% and should be treated by a definitive oncologic segmental resection due to the high risk of regional lymph node involvement.

2.2.3. Surveillance

Local recurrence is basically common in managed malignant polyps. Regular endoscopic follow-up is recommended to detect any disease recurrence; however, the duration of subsequent surveillance varies [10, 11]. In favorable histological criteria, protruding (levels I, II, or III), and noninvasive Sm1a + b polyps, it is recommended that a colonoscopy be carried out 3 months after the polypectomy [12, 13]. Further regular checkup is advised within 1, 3, and 5 years [14]. In malignant pedunculated polyps with unfavorable histological criteria, the risk of relapse or residual lesions reached 39% in treated patients. These patients are also found to have distant metastasis on follow-up, even 5 years after surgery [15]. Accordingly, in addition to the regular endoscopic surveillance, monitoring the serum level of carcinoembryonic antigen (CEA) and imaging techniques as computerized tomography or magnetic resonance imaging would enable early detection of disease recurrence. According to the American Cancer Society and the US Multi-Society Task Force on Colorectal Cancer's guidelines, shorter follow-up intervals are recommended in case of senility, positive family history, or hereditary nonpolyposis colorectal cancer (HNPCC). Furthermore, endoscopic ultrasound or flexible sigmoidoscopy at 3- to 6-month intervals for the first 2 years after polypectomy can be considered for detecting early curable recurrences.

2.3. Treatment of stage I CRC

Stage I CRC includes T1 and T2, where cancer is still limited to and has not yet invaded the layers of the colon into other nearby organs. T1 cancers are usually parts of polyps that were discussed hereinabove. For T2 cancers, the standard of care consists of partial colectomy with regional lymph node dissection. A laparoscopic-assisted colectomy can be an acceptable choice for patients who are not candidates for open colectomy.

Stage I adenocarcinoma of the rectum is relatively rare, and a surgical removal of the cancer is usually curable. For the low-risk stage I rectal cancer, both endoscopic resection and transanal excision can be used. Transanal endoscopic microsurgery (TEM) is a transanal operation suitable for small tumors and not too far from the anus. It involves wide excision of all layers of the invaded rectum with the surrounding tissue to secure negative margins. If the cancer is located in the upper part of the rectum, a low anterior resection (LAR) is recommended, where the incision takes part across the abdomen to remove the affected rectum along with some surrounding tissue and lymph nodes, and followed by anorectal anastomosis. If the cancer occupies the lower part of the rectum (alongside the anus), an abdominoperineal resection

(APR) with permanent colostomy is advised, when the distance between tumor and anus is too short to allow safe anastomosis. No additional therapy is needed after these operations, unless the surgeon finds the cancer with high-risk features. Then, an adjuvant concomitant chemoradiotherapy is appropriate with 5-fluorouracil (5-FU) or capecitabine [16].

2.3.1. Surveillance

Regular follow-up testing after the end of treatment aims at seizing any early disease recurrence. Colonoscopy should be repeated 1 year after therapy completion. In case of normal results, the next checkup should be after 3 years and then after 5 years. In case of finding any advanced adenoma (polyps with ruffled structure, larger than 1 cm, or with high-grade dysplasia), colonoscopy should be repeated within 1 year [17].

2.4. Treatment of stage II CRC

2.4.1. Assessing risk factors

The role of adjuvant chemotherapy remains undetermined in stage II CRC. Surgical intervention should aim at a wide resection of the tumor with the involved bowel segment, all together with cutting out of the lymphatic system draining that part. The resection should include at least 5 cm colon segment of either side of the resected tumor. For adequate tumor staging (II or III), and to determine and eliminate any possible lymph node metastases (pN), at least 12 lymph nodes should be excised and subjected to histological analysis. Partial colectomy may be the only needed treatment for low- and medium-risk stage II CRC patients. High-risk patients should be subjected to chemotherapy if one of the following risk factors was identified:

- High pT4 stage (T4 or tumor invading into adherent organs)
- Suboptimal lymph node resection (less than 12)
- Presence of lymphovascular or perineural invasion
- Bowel obstruction or perforation
- Poorly differentiated histology
- High carcinoembryonic antigen (CEA) marker level
- Positive margins

Various additional risk factors are being implied in assessing the additive benefit to the high-risk factors in stage II colorectal cancer using adjuvant chemotherapy.

One of the most promising risk factors is the microsatellite instability (MSI)/mismatch repair (MMR), which is regarded as a good prognostic factor. Microsatellites are short, tandemly repeated DNA sequences in the genome that are susceptible to errors of DNA replication in the presence of a defective mismatch repair (MMR) system. They are detected in about 15% of all colorectal cancers and can be used to determine stage II patients who are at very low risk of recurrence and with low benefit of adjuvant chemotherapy [18, 19]. Moreover, it has been established in a multivariate analysis that microsatellite instability was significantly associated with survival advantage independently of any other prognostic factors (hazard ratio (HR) 0.42; 95% confidence interval 0.27–0.67; p < 0.001) [20].

Another potential predictive colorectal marker is the allelic deletion of chromosome 18q, or the loss of heterozygosity (LOH) of chromosome 18, which is considered as a bad prognostic factor. The 18q loci hold several genes that are highly related to apoptosis and carcinogenesis. Patients (stage II or III) presenting 18qLOH were found to have less disease-free survival and overall survival than those with retained chromosome 18 (DFS 44% versus 64%, p = 0.002; OS 50% versus 69%, p = 0.005) [21].

Another prognostic marker in CRC is the expression of guanylyl cyclase C (GCC) in resected lymph nodes. GCC is a protein that is usually expressed by intestinal cells but universally overexpressed in colorectal cancer. GCC is an intestinal tumor-suppressing receptor which regulates epithelial homeostasis. Silencing of GCC contributes to tumorigenesis by reflecting dysregulation of the cell cycle and DNA repair [22]. The presence of GCC in resected lymph nodes reflects the detection of prognostically important occult metastases [23].

The Kirsten rat sarcoma (*KRAS*) oncogene is a proto-oncogene involved in the normal tissue signaling pathways. *KRAS* mutation can occur via a single amino acid substitution or a single nucleotide substitution. The resulting protein is implicated in various malignancies, including colorectal cancer [24]. Even though the British QUASAR trial in 2007 did not succeed to show any significant difference in overall survival between fluorouracil-treated and folinic acid–treated observation groups in stage II CRC [25], the risk of disease recurrence was found significantly higher for *KRAS*-mutant than *KRAS* wild-type tumors (28% versus 21%), and the risk of recurrence appeared larger in *KRAS*-mutant rectal than colon tumors [26].

The tumor suppressor TP53, or genome guardian, is another important predictive prognostic factor in CRC. TP53 is the most commonly mutated gene in human cancers, and its prevalence in CRC comprises 34% of the proximal colon tumors where it is mostly related to lymphatic invasion and 45% of the distal colorectal tumors where it is majorly correlated with lymphovascular invasion [27]. Clinical studies have shown that CRC patients with mutant p53 are more 5-fluorouracil-based chemotherapy resistant and have poorer prognosis than those with wild-type p53 [28].

The transforming growth factor beta (TGF-β) signaling pathway plays a central but paradoxical role in the predisposition and progression of colorectal cancer. TGF-β acts as a potent tumor suppressor in normal intestinal epithelial cells by inhibiting cell proliferation and inducing apoptosis. However, mutations in the genes encoding for TGFB receptor 2 (TGFBR2), with high levels of microsatellite instability, promote colon tumorigenesis by perturbing the function of TGF-β signaling pathways and stimulating the proliferation and invasion of poorly differentiated and metastatic colon cancer cells [29, 30].

Thymidylate synthase (TS) is an enzyme implicated in the formation of thymidine, one of DNA nucleotides. It catalyzes the methylation of deoxyuridine monophosphate (dUMP) to deoxythymidine monophosphate (dTMP). This role in nucleotide metabolism has made TS an important target of many chemotherapeutic agents such as 5-FU and the new folate-based TS inhibitors (raltitrexed and pemetrexed). Elevated intracellular TS levels have been implicated in emerging resistance to fluoropyrimidines and other TS inhibitors due to the increase in transcription and translation roles of TS. Therefore, high TS expression in early-stage CRC patients is correlated to a poorer overall survival in both chemotherapy-treated and chemotherapy-untreated patients following surgery [31].

2.4.2. Choice of chemotherapy

5-Fluorouracil remains the backbone chemotherapy in treating CRC. In MOSAIC study, patients with stage II or III disease were randomly assigned to receive adjuvant FOLFOX4 or 5-FU/leucovorin (LV). In stage II disease, no improvement in DFS or OS was noted in 899 patients upon adding oxaliplatin to 5-FU (DFS HR = 0.84, p = 0.258; OS HR = 1.00, p = 0.986). Moreover, in patients with high-risk stage II disease, the estimated 10-year overall survival was 75.4% in FOLFOX arm versus 71.7% in 5-FU/leucovorin arm (p = .058) [19]. Similar results were obtained with the NSABP C-07 trial, where patients were randomized to receive either bolus 5-FU/LV alone or with oxaliplatin. While the addition of oxaliplatin to 5-FU/LV improved DFS, no benefit in OS was observed at all [32]. Furthermore, the QUASAR study investigated the role of adjuvant 5-FU in disease recurrence in "average-risk" patients (patients without any high-risk feature). As a result, 5-FU decreased the risk of recurrence compared to observation alone (relative risk (RR) for colon cancer = 0.78, p = 0.004; RR for rectal cancer =0.68, p = 0.004). And, the risk of death was improved in treated patients (RR = 0.84; p = 0.046), with an absolute survival benefit of 3.6% [25]. A major predictive prognostic factor in stage II CRC is microsatellite instability. As known, microsatellites are repeated DNA sequences in the genome. They are very susceptible to errors in DNA replication and especially in case of a defective mismatch repair (MMR) system, where they really can substitute it [19]. In colon cancer, the high level of MSI is associated with mutations in the MMR system. Based on findings from over 7000 patients classified as MSI-high (MSI-H), MSI-low (MSI-L), or MSI-stable (MSS) colon cancers, those with MSI-H had a better prognosis compared to those with MSI-L or MSS tumors by 15% [33]. Another important predictive factor in stage II CRC is 18qLOH. Loss of heterozygosity of chromosome 18 is highly associated with decreased overall survival [21, 34, 35]. The ECOG 5202 trial aimed at stratifying patients according to the molecular prognostic factors, MSI and 18qLOH. The recommendations were for stage II patients with low-risk (MSI-H or with either MSS or MSI-L together with 18qLOH retention) observation without any treatment. However, for those with high-risk observation (either MSS or MSI-L with 18qLOH), chemotherapy with FOLFOX is suggested [19].

As a conclusion for stage II CRC adjuvant treatment, the following algorithm is reasonable (**Table 5**).

2.4.3. Access to radiotherapy

According to Johns Hopkins colorectal health team, radiotherapy can be used adjuvantly in case of pT4, where the lesion is fixed and adherent to the abdominal wall or bladder, as it provides a lower chance of recurrence. Similarly, in case of rectal cancer, neoadjuvant chemoradiotherapy is indicated in order to shrink the tumor size prior to surgery and to avoid colostomy if

Low risk (with MSI-H or with either MSS or MSI-L and retention of 18qLOH)	Observation
Average risk (with MSS)	Observation or fluoropyrimidine* as single agent (optional)
High risk**: • (with MSI-H and 18qLOH retention) • (with MSS or MSS-L and 18qLOH)	• Fluoropyrimidine as single agent • FOLFOX or CAPOX***

*Fluoropyrimidines are a class of antimetabolites that are converted in the body to 5-fluorouracil. These include 5-fluorouracil, capecitabine, doxifluridine, tegafur, and carmofur.
**The high-risk factors are mentioned hereinabove in the text.
***FOLFOX denotes folinic acid/5-FU/oxaliplatin; CAPOX denotes capecitabine/oxaliplatin.

Table 5. Stage II CRC adjuvant treatment algorithm.

possible. Radiotherapy is indicated when the rectal tumor has invaded the wall of the bowel or has spread into adjacent lymph nodes. 5-Fluorouracil or capecitabine are being used concomitantly with radiotherapy to sensitize tumor cells to radiation. In addition, concomitant chemoradiotherapy is indicated when the margins of resection are positive. However, no significant differences in overall survival were reported till now. EORTC 22921 was one randomized trial of 1011 patients that assessed the role of adjuvant 5-FU after preoperative chemoradiation for patients with T3 or T4 resectable tumor. Patients were divided in four arms including preoperative radiotherapy with or without chemotherapy and preoperative radiotherapy with or without chemotherapy followed by adjuvant chemotherapy. The OS for a median follow-up of 10.4 years was similar in the four groups (48.4–52.9%). There were no differences either in DFS rates or in the cumulative incidence of distant metastases [36]. A number of treatment strategies have been recently studied by various clinical trials, yet still no conclusive decisions have been taken. The major aim remains the patient's benefit from a better tumor resection with less side effects, longer survival, and minor recurrence rates.

2.4.4. Surveillance

Survivorship care is a follow-up that takes place after the end of treatment to provide a better disease control and a less recurrence morbidity. A thorough physical examination with a tumor marker CEA should be performed systematically every 3–6 months for 2 years. In case of normal results, the frequency can be reduced to 6 months for an additional 3 years. Radiological imaging including CT scans or MRIs is indicated once a year for a total of 5 years. Colonoscopy is also suggested at an interval of 1 year after treatment and then after 3 and 5 years if results are normal.

2.5. Treatment of stage III CRC

Stage III colon cancer is characterized by tumor of any size (T1–T4) with metastasis to regional lymph nodes. A partial colectomy to remove the involved part of the colon along with adjacent lymph nodes, followed by adjuvant chemotherapy (not beyond 8 weeks of surgery), is considered the standard of care for this stage. However, in rectal cancer, tumor size (T3–T4, with invasion through intestinal muscular layer) with clinical positive lymph nodes is suggestive for neoadjuvant chemoradiotherapy and followed by adjuvant chemotherapy for a lower risk of recurrence rate. The European Society for Medical Oncology (ESMO) guidelines recommended in 2013 a stratification of the risk factors for disease recurrence of rectal cancer according to the following items identified by pretreatment MRI. These included the tumor invasion depth (T staging), the number of metastatic lymph nodes (N staging), the distance to anus, invasion of mesorectal fascia (MRF), and extramural vascular invasion (EMVI). Four risk groups were stratified (ultralow-, low-, medium-, and high-risk groups). Surgery alone was the choice for the ultralow-risk group, while neoadjuvant chemoradiotherapy with adjuvant chemotherapy was the best choice for the medium- and high-risk groups; the low-risk group showed a beneficial effect of adding chemoradiotherapy or chemotherapy [37]. These findings are compatible with the NCCN guidelines which recommended neoadjuvant chemoradiotherapy and adjuvant chemotherapy for those patients with high risk of local recurrence, including stage II (T3–T4, with tumor invading through the intestinal muscle layer) and stage III (positive lymph nodes) [17].

2.5.1. Choice of chemotherapy

After a wide surgical resection with anastomosis, the standard chemotherapy protocol is approved to be oxaliplatin and 5-FU/folinic acid (FOLFOX4 or FLOX). In the MOSAIC study, the addition of oxaliplatin to 5-FU/LV (FOLFOX) showed a significantly increased DFS at 6 years, with a reduction in the risk of recurrence of 23% compared with the control arm (5-FU/LV), with an OS absolute gain of 4.2%. Similar results were obtained in the NSABP C-07 study, either in DFS at 3 years or in terms of reduction in the risk of recurrence. As a result of these studies, FOLFOX has been adopted adjuvantly on a biweekly basis, for a period of 12 cycles. In case of contradiction to oxaliplatin, 5-FU/LV administered intravenously according to de Gramont, AIO, or Mayo Clinic regimen, or oral fluoropyrimidines (capecitabine) are comparable in benefit. Other drugs such as topoisomerase I inhibitor (irinotecan) or anti-VEGFR agent (bevacizumab) or *KRAS* wild-type drug (cetuximab) did not succeed in adding any advantage either in DFS or in OS in stage III colon cancer [38].

In neoadjuvant rectal treatment, 5-fluorouracil remains the standard chemotherapeutic agent to be administered concomitantly with radiation. In ASCO 2011, NASBP R-04 firstly randomly compared the effect of capecitabine (an oral fluoropyrimidine) and 5-FU in preoperative concurrent chemoradiotherapy of rectal cancer. The results showed neither significant difference in pathological complete response (pCR) rate nor in third and fourth degree of adverse reaction rate [39]. Recently, in Germany, a randomized clinical phase III multicenter non-inferiority study showed no statistical difference of 3 years of DFS and local recurrence rate between capecitabine and 5-FU, concluding that capecitabine can substitute 5-FU as adjuvant or neoadjuvant chemotherapy for locally advanced rectal cancer [40]. The role of oxaliplatin in radiotherapy has been thoroughly examined as in many randomized studies as STAR-01, ACCORD 12/0405, NSABP R-04, and PETACC 6. Unfortunately, neither study succeeded in showing any significant increase of the pCR rate or downstage rate comparing to single drug (5-FU or capecitabine). In addition, ACCORD 12/0405 reported same OS (88%) in both combined two drugs (capecitabine with oxaliplatin) and single drug (capecitabine) [39, 41]. As a conclusion, single-agent fluoropyrimidine (5-FU or capecitabine) used concomitantly with pelvic radio-therapy remains the standard of care in stage III CRC.

2.5.2. Surveillance

Regular follow-up is highly advised in stage III CRC due to the high rate of recurrence. Detecting early relapse can be performed through a meticulous regular physical checkup with tumor marker CEA every 3 months for the first 2 years. A thoraco-abdomino-pelvic CT scan is required every 6 months for the first 2 years. A colonoscopy is advised in a 6-month period for the first year after treatment. The period of physical examination with CEA can be elongated for a 6-month period for the following 3 years in case of normal results. The CT scan period can be lengthened to 1 year for the following 5 years, and the colonoscopic evaluation can be further extended to once every 3 years in case of normal previous results.

2.6. Treatment of stage IV CRC

Almost 20–30% of the newly diagnosed CRC patients present with distant metastatic dis-ease at the time of initial presentation. And, up to 50% of the early-stage CRC patients will eventually relapse with metastatic disease. Metastasis can occur in different organs and most commonly to the liver (50–60% of the cases). The lungs are less frequent (10–20%) and are more common in rectal than in colon cancer. Other less often places are the peritoneum, ovaries, adrenal glands, bones, and brain. In case of locally recurrent disease or with resectable metastases, the standard of care remains curative surgical interven-tion. Chemoradiotherapy or chemotherapy alone can also be considered an acceptable approach in case of rendering a tumor resectable. For non-resectable tumors and/or dis-seminated metastatic disease, systemic chemotherapy stays the main therapeutic approach. Fluoropyrimidines (5-FU and capecitabine) are the mainstay in all protocols used in meta-static colorectal cancer (mCRC). For nearly 40 years (mid-1950 to 1996), 5-FU was the only agent approved for mCRC treatment. Later on, different cytotoxic agents appeared, as the topoisomerase I inhibitor (irinotecan) and the third-generation platinum analog (oxalipla-tin), which both led to considerable advances in mCRC treatment along with fluoropyrimi-dines. Targeted monoclonal antibodies, such as VEGF inhibitor (bevacizumab) and EGFR inhibitor wild-type *KRAS* (cetuximab and panitumumab), opened a new era in the manage-ment of mCRC. Many other promising targeted therapies include the anti-VEGF recom-binant fusion protein (ziv-aflibercept), the dual targeting VEGFR2-TIE2 tyrosine kinase inhibitor (regorafenib), the human monoclonal antibody (IgG1) anti-VEGFR2 (ramuci-rumab), the anti-immune checkpoint programmed cell death protein 1 (PD-1)/programmed death-ligand 1 (PD-L1) (nivolumab and pembrolizumab), and the combination of trifluri-dine, a nucleoside analog, with tipiracil, an inhibitor of the enzyme thymidine phosphory-lase (trifluridine/tipiracil) which have been approved for combination treatment of mCRC, in addition to many other new drugs under investigations.

2.6.1. Choice of chemotherapy

Various randomized clinical trials have been designed to determine the efficacy of oxaliplatin versus irinotecan together with 5-FU/LV or capecitabine. The most well-known trial was the GERCOR C97-3 study conducted by Tournigand and coworkers [42] in France which investigated 5-FU/LV (46-hour infusion) and oxaliplatin (FOLFOX6) compared with 5-FU/LV and irinotecan (FOLFIRI) in mCRC. A similar efficacy was observed in both arms with respect to overall response rate (ORR, 56% versus 54%, respectively), median time to tumor progression (8.5 versus 8.1 months), and median OS (20.6 versus 21.5 months). Similar results were obtained by CALGB Cooperative Group (CALGB 80203) and the Hellenic Cooperative Oncology Group in Greece. Based on these results, both FOLFOX and FOLFIRI have been approved for first-line treatment in mCRC. A meta-analysis of six clinical studies was conducted by Guo et al. [43] to investigate the clinical efficacy of the oral capecitabine (Xeloda) plus irinotecan (XELIRI) versus FOLFIRI regimen in the first-line treatment of mCRC. The results showed no significant differences in terms of ORR, PFS, or OS between the two arms. Another important randomized study to compare XELOX non-inferiority with respect to FOLFOX6 in the first-line treatment of mCRC was conducted by Ducreux and coworkers [44]. No differences were observed between both arms in terms of the clinical efficacy endpoints of ORR (42% versus 46%, respectively), PFS (8.8 versus 9.3 months, respectively), and OS (19.9 versus 20.5 months, respectively). Based on these and many other studies, it has been established that both protocols FOLFOX and FOLFIRI can be safely substituted by oral XELOX and XELIRI in terms of clinical efficacy (PFS and OS).

It is has been proven that doublet chemotherapy has superior clinical efficacy over single-agent fluoropyrimidine chemotherapy. However, a new question emerged: is triplet chemotherapy with 5-FU, oxaliplatin, and irinotecan can provide improved clinical efficacy over doublet chemotherapy? To answer this question, the Gruppo Oncologico Nord Ovest (GONO) of Italy conducted the first randomized phase III study to compare 5-FU/LV, oxaliplatin, and irinotecan (FOLFOXIRI) with FOLFIRI in the front-line setting [45]. After a median follow-up of 5 years, the final analysis confirmed the superiority of the FOLFOXIRI regimen over FOLFIRI, in terms of improved ORR, PFS, and median OS [46]. However, there was significantly higher grade 2/grade 3 neurotoxicity (19% versus 0%) and grade 3/grade 4 neutropenia (50% versus 28%) compared with FOLFIRI, the matter that limits the use of this regimen to relatively more fit patient population (ECOG performance status 0–1).

2.6.2. Chemotherapy in association with targeted therapy

In order to understand the role of targeted therapy in treating mCRC, we should first perceive their mode of action on a molecular level. Bevacizumab (Avastin®) is a recombinant humanized monoclonal antibody that blocks angiogenesis by inhibiting vascular endothelial growth factor A (VEGF-A), which stimulates angiogenesis in a variety of diseases, including cancer [47]. In 2004, bevacizumab has been approved in the United States for use in combination with standard chemotherapy for metastatic colon cancer. The CALGB/SWOG 80405 phase III randomized study compared the potential benefit of cetuximab and bevacizumab added to conventional chemotherapy (FOLFOX or FOLFIRI) [48]. In contrast to the FIRE study that showed identical ORR and PFS, but a 3.7-month improvement in OS toward the cetuximab arm, CALGB/SWOG 80405 study showed no significant difference at all either in PFS (10.4 versus 10.8 months) or in OS (29.9 versus 29.0 months) in patients treated with cetuximab compared with bevacizumab. Recently, Venook and coworkers investigated the potential effect of primary tumor location on the clinical efficacy of patients treated on CALGB/SWOG 80405 study. It was strange to report that there was a significant improvement in OS (p < .0001) for patients with left-sided tumors compared with right-sided tumors (33.3 versus 19.4 months). For the bevacizumab arms, the OS was maintained high in both groups (left-sided tumors versus right-sided tumors) and significantly higher for left-sided primary tumors (31.4 versus 24.2 months). However, in the cetuximab arms, the OS in left-sided tumors was 19.3 months (which was 36.0 months) and only 16.7 months for right-sided tumors. These findings highlighted the importance of sidedness as an important predictive marker and in determining response to anti-EGFR antibody in mCRC [49].

Cetuximab (Erbitux®) and panitumumab (Vectibix®) are both monoclonal antibodies that inhibit the epidermal growth factor receptor (EGFR). Both drugs were approved by the FDA to treat mCRC that exhibit *KRAS* wild-type genes in 2009. However, due to high rate of cetuximab resistance (45%), further studies identified the role of *NRAS* and *BRAF V600E* in treatment response [50]. The *KRAS*, *NRAS*, and *BRAF* are oncogenes that encode proteins involved in the mitogen-activated protein kinase (MAPK) signaling pathway, which regulates cell proliferation and survival. Mutations in these genes are found in about 45%, 4%, and 8% of mCRC, respectively [51], and this is responsible for activating excess proteins, whose activation does not require EGFR upstream signaling, leading to negative feedback loops that limit EGFR activation, the fact that limits the role of anti-EGFR drugs. Therefore, only the wild type of *KRAS* and *NRAS* is indicated for the treatment of EGFR inhibitors. Mutation in *BRAF V600E* was also considered as bad indicator in response to EGFR inhibitors and a strong negative prognostic marker in mCRC. Data from the randomized phase III Medical Research Council COIN trial in mCRC showed an OS of 8.8 versus 14.4 versus 20.1 months, respectively, for patients with *BRAF*-mutant, *KRAS* exon 2-mutant, and *KRAS* exon 2 wild type [52]. Moreover, the presence of *BRAF* mutation in mCRC has been associated with big primary tumors (T4), poor histologic differentiation, and peritoneal carcinomatosis [53–55].

Due to the poor prognosis factor of the BRAF V600E-mutated gene, many trials tried to establish a standard treatment for BRAF-mutated mCRC. Vemurafenib is a BRAF enzyme inhibitor, which interrupts the B-Raf/MEK step on the B-Raf/MEK/ERK pathway, in case where BRAF possesses V600E mutation. In 2017, it has been approved by the FDA for the treatment of late-stage melanoma with BRAF V600E-mutated gene. In 2010, a phase I trial for solid tumors including colorectal cancer was launched to study the effect of vemurafenib (PLX4032) on mCRC patients with mutant BRAF. Unfortunately, the results were not as promising as they were in malignant melanoma, with median PFS of 3.7 months [56]. Loupakis and coworkers studied in a retrospective exploratory analysis of a phase II trial the effect of FOLFOXIRI regimen with bevacizumab on BRAF-mutated mCRC patients. Data found PFS and OS of 11.8 and 24.1 months, respectively [57]. Two limitations were reported in the study: the first was that only patients older than 70 were included, or those who fit (ECOG PS 0) 71–75 old patients, and the second was the rarity of BRAF-mutant patients (8% of the population). In TRIBE phase III study, FOLFOXIRI regimen was studied either with bevacizumab or alone as first-line treatment mCRC, and the median OS was 31 versus 25.8 months in favor of the combination.

However, in the mutant BRAF subgroup, the median OS was 13.4 months [58, 59]. According to ASCO recommendations in 2017, FOLFOXIRI with or without bevacizumab should be considered in patients with a BRAF mutation and good performance status.

The programmed death-ligand 1 (PD-L1) with its receptor programmed cell death protein 1 (PD-1) is T-cell surface checkpoint protein that plays a major role in suppressing the immune system, promoting self-tolerance by downregulating T-cell inflammatory activity, and leading to carcinogenesis [60]. In the recently updated 2017 NCCN guideline, two novel anti-PD-1 antibodies, nivolumab (Opdivo®) and pembrolizumab (Keytruda®), have been indicated as treatment options for patients with unresectable MSI-H- or MMR-deficient CRC, although not yet FDA approved for mCRC [17]. This was based on the interim results of two ongoing studies: KEYNOTE-016, a phase II study of pembrolizumab as monotherapy in MSI-H-/MMR-deficient tumors, and CheckMate 142, a study of nivolumab versus nivolumab combination with ipilimumab, another monoclonal antibody, in recurrent or mCRC. This decision has been taken into account due to the impressive durable response in both studies [61, 62].

Ziv-aflibercept (Zaltrap®), a novel anti-VEGF, is a recombinant fusion protein that consists of vascular endothelial growth factor (VEGF)-binding portions from the extracellular domains of human VEGF receptors 1 and 2 fused to the Fc portion of the human immunoglobulin (IgG) 1 [63]. In 2012, it has been approved by the FDA for use in combination with FOLFIRI for the treatment of patients with mCRC that is resistant to or has progressed following an oxaliplatin-containing regimen treatment. A randomized double-blind placebo-controlled global multicenter phase III VELOUR trial randomized two groups: one to receive FOLFIRI with ziv-aflibercept and the other FOLFIRI with placebo. A statistically significant improvement in OS was observed in patients in the FOLFIRI plus ziv-aflibercept group compared with the FOLFIRI plus placebo group [HR 0.82 (95% CI, 0.71–0.94), p = 0.0032, stratified log-rank test]. The median OS was 13.5 versus 12.06 months, and the median PFS was 6.9 versus 4.7 months, respectively, in the ziv-aflibercept group compared with the placebo group [64].

Regorafenib (Stivarga®), a new oral anti-angiogenic drug, is an oral multi-kinase inhibitor which targets angiogenic, stromal, and oncogenic receptor tyrosine kinase (RTK). It inhibits many membrane-bound and intracellular kinases that are involved in normal cellular functions and pathologic processes, mainly the VEGFR2-TIE2 tyrosine kinase receptors. In 2012, it has been approved by FDA for the treatment of mCRC patients which have been previously treated with fluoropyrimidine-, oxaliplatin-, and irinotecan-based chemotherapy and with the anti-VEGF therapy bevacizumab and, if KRAS wild type, with an anti-EGFR therapy. The approval was based on the results of an international randomized (2:1), double-blind, placebo-controlled CORRECT trial. The patients were randomized to get either oral regorafenib or placebo. A statistically significant prolongation in overall survival was observed in regorafenib arm [hazard ratio (HR) 0.77 (95% CI 0.64–0.94), p = 0.0102]. The median survival time was 6.4 versus 5 months in favor of the regorafenib group (phase III, 2011; FDA, 2012) [65].

Ramucirumab (Cyramza®) is a fully human monoclonal antibody (IgG1), which works by blocking the binding of VEGF to its receptor VEGFR2, hence preventing the downstream effect of VEGF in angiogenesis. Recently, it has been approved by FDA for use in combination with

FOLFIRI for the treatment of patients with mCRC whose disease has progressed on a first-line regimen containing bevacizumab, oxaliplatin, and fluoropyrimidine [66]. A randomized double-blind multinational trial divided patients into FOLFIRI plus ramucirumab-receiving group and FOLFIRI plus placebo. A statistically significant improvement in OS was observed in patients who received FOLFIRI plus ramucirumab compared with those who received FOLFIRI plus placebo [median overall survival 13.3 versus 11.7 months; HR 0.85 (95% CI 0.73–0.98), p = 0.023, stratified log-rank test]. The DFS was also in favor of ramucirumab arm (5.7 versus 4.5 months) [67].

Trifluridine/tipiracil (TFD/TPI) (Lonsurf®) is a new combination drug approved in 2015 for the treatment of mCRC. It is a combination of two active components: trifluridine, a nucleoside analog, and tipiracil, a thymidine phosphorylase inhibitor, which prevents trifluridine rapid metabolism, hence increasing its bioavailability. In 2015, it has been approved by the FDA for use in patients with mCRC who have been treated with fluoropyrimidine-, oxaliplatin-, and irinotecan-based chemotherapy, an anti-vascular endothelial growth factor (VEGF) biological therapy and an anti-epidermal growth factor receptor (EGFR) therapy, if RAS wild type [68]. Based on a pivotal phase III study (RECOURSE) to assess the efficacy and safety of TFD/TPI compared with that of placebo in a large international population, the outcomes were in favor of TFD/TPI arm, in terms of median OS (7.1 versus 5.3 months) and median PFS (2.0 versus 1.7 months) [69].

2.6.3. Disease recurrence

In case of recurrence, surgical option for liver or lung metastases should be considered in the first place followed by adjuvant chemotherapy, albeit others prefer to administer neoadjuvant chemotherapy for 2–3 months before any metastasectomy. In non-resectable tumors and disseminated metastasis, chemotherapy remains the mainstay in treating disease recurrence. It should be based on non-previously used protocols, i.e., if FOLFOX was used in previous treatment modalities, FOLFIRI should be the right option, and if both FOLFOX and FOLFIRI have been used, the choice shifts toward XELOX or XELIRI. Another alternative is to use infusional 5-FU or oral capecitabine as monotherapies. Other possibilities are the use of newly approved drugs as ziv-aflibercept with FOLOIRI, ramucirumab plus FOLFIRI, oral regorafenib, trifluridine/tipiracil, and nivolumab or pembrolizumab in case of MSI-H or dMMR. According to the last NCCN guideline in 2017, adjuvant Stereotactic Body Radiation Therapy (SBRT) should be considered in some localized lung or liver lesions. Moreover, the hepatic arterial infusion (HAI) pump therapy can be used as a substitute to systemic chemotherapy in unresectable CRC liver metastases, where it demonstrated significant tumor response rates [70]. Chemoembolization or embolization via radioactive beads is another way to treat liver metastases through the hepatic artery in chemorefractory colorectal tumors [71]. In case of peritoneal carcinomatosis, a novel strategy has emerged combining cytoreductive peritonectomy with hyperthermic intraperitoneal chemoperfusion (HIPEC), with a median survival of 3 years [72]. Many other options are being studied to be used as palliative treatment in advanced metastatic disease, such as external-beam radiotherapy, photodynamic therapy, cryotherapy, and radiofrequency ablation, in addition to oncothermia and many others under trials to palliate and manage the disease burden (**Table 6**).

Locally recurrent disease, with resectable metastases	Colectomy + metastasectomy	
Locally recurrent disease (T4)	Chemoradiotherapy or chemotherapy alone followed by colectomy	
Non-resectable tumors and/or disseminated metastatic disease	Chemotherapy	FOLFOX or FOLFIRI (substitutable by XELOX or XELIRI)
		FOLFOXIRI (ECOG good performance status and BRAF V600E mutation)
	Targeted therapy[*]	Bevacizumab (for right-sided tumors)
		bevacizumab or cetuximab, or panitumumab (for left-sided tumors and wild-type *KRAS* and *NRAS* genes)
		Bevacizumab (for left-sided tumors and mutant-type KRAS and NRAS genes)
Disease recurrence		Nivolumab or pembrolizumab as monotherapy (for MSI-H or dMMR)
		FOLFIRI + ziv-aflibercept
		FOLFIRI + ramucirumab
		Regorafenib as monotherapy
		Trifluridine/tipiracil as monotherapy
		Clinical trials

[*]Targeted therapy should be added to chemotherapy, unless otherwise mentioned.

Table 6. Metastatic CRC treatment algorithm.

2.7. Miscellaneous

2.7.1. Lynch syndrome and familial adenomatous polyposis syndrome

Lynch syndrome, or hereditary nonpolyposis colorectal cancer (HNPCC), is an autosomal dominant disorder that increases the risk of many types of cancer, including endometrial, ovary, stomach, small intestine, hepatobiliary tract, upper urinary tract, brain, skin, and particularly colon cancer [73]. It is considered the most common hereditary colorectal diseases and accounts for 1–3% of all CRC. It is associated with inherited mutation in the mismatch repair (MMR) genes MLH1, MSH2, MSH6, and PMS2. This defect in MMR genes leads to tumor DNA microsatellite instability (MSI) and promotes carcinogenesis [74]. For this reason MSI profiling with immunohistochemistry testing for DNA mismatch repair has been considered essential in diagnosing Lynch syndrome (LS). The revised Bethesda guidelines have endorsed the testing for MSI, for families at high risk, in any of the following situations in CRC diagnosed in patients <50 years of age, the presence of Lynch-associated tumors, and MSI-H identified in patients <60 years old, identifying Lynch-related tumors in one or more first-degree relative and in patients <50 years of age and identifying Lynch-related tumors in two or more second-degree relatives regardless of age [75, 76]. The mainstay in the treatment of Lynch syndrome is colectomy. However, due to the risk of developing synchronous or metachronous secondary tumors, subtotal colectomy with ileorectal anastomosis should be considered in young patients [76]. Recently, three kinds of chemotherapy have been investigated for the treatment of LS: 5-FU with leucovorin, oxaliplatin, and irinotecan. Most studies showed no benefit of chemotherapy in such patients, just one small study on stage IV CRC reported one complete response and three partial responses with MSI-H tumors compared to MSI-L/MSS tumors [77]. The use of acetylsalicylic acid (aspirin) as chemo-prevention by patients with LS is highly supported to reduce the risk of CRC [78]. The Colorectal Adenoma/Carcinoma Prevention Programme 2 (CAPP2) trial was conducted to study aspirin chemoprevention that has colorectal cancer as the primary endpoint. The initial findings did not show any significant difference in colorectal adenoma or cancer formation up to 4 years. In 2010, after a longer follow-up (56 months), the results showed a significant decrease in the incidence of CRC and LS-related cancers between the aspirin (600 mg) and placebo groups. Prescription of aspirin for people at high risk was recommended, but the optimum dose and duration of treatment remain to be established, hopefully in CAPP3 [79]. The colonoscopic surveillance in Lynch syndrome is recommended from the age of 20–25 years and repeated at 1–2 years of interval.

Familial adenomatous polyposis (FAP) is an autosomal dominant disorder caused by a germline mutation in the adenomatous polyposis coli (APC) gene, on chromosome 5q21, and characterized by the presence of numerous adenomatous polyps in the colon and rectum. It is responsible for about 1% of all CRC cases, and, often, extracolonic manifestations can take place as in Gardner syndrome (sebaceous cysts, epidermoid cysts, fibromas, desmoid tumors, osteomas, dental anomalies and congenital hypertrophy of the retinal pigment epithelium (CHRPE)), Turcot syndrome (brain tumors), gastric and duodenum polyps, soft tissue tumors, and thyroid cancers. FAP can be subdivided into classical FAP, attenuated FAP (AFAP), and gastric adenocarcinoma and proximal polyposis of the stomach (GAPPS) [80]. Clinical diagnosis can be based on the number of polyposis, where more than 100 adenomas can be counted in case of FAP, from 10 to 99 in case of AFAP, and gastric polyps restricted to the body and fundus of the stomach (gastric fundic gland polyposis) in case of GAPPS [81]. Identification of a heterozygous germline pathogenic variant in APC should be confirmed by a molecular genetic testing for a definitive diagnosis. Proctocolectomy with ileal pouch-anal anastomosis (IPAA) is recommended in case of diffuse spreading out of the polyps with severe familial phenotype presence. Total colectomy with ileorectal anastomosis (IRA) is advised in case of scarce adenomas with a mild familial phenotype presence. In AFAP, endoscopic polypectomy can be considered in case of reduced polyposis number. In GAPPS, gastrectomy is recommended since gastric carcinoma is detected in 13% of GAPPS. Regular yearly endoscopic surveillance should be taken into account to detect any disease recurrence. In families with classic FAP, endoscopic evaluation should begin at age of 12–14 years and be continued lifelong in mutation carriers. Regular physical examination and screening via CT scans or MRI for extracolonic manifestations should also start early in life or as soon as colorectal polyposis is diagnosed [82].

MUTYH-associated polyposis (MAP) is another inheritable form of FAP that is caused by autosomal recessive mutations of the MUTYH gene [83]. It accounts for about 10–20% of all polyposis patients [2]. Clinically, in MAP patients, between 20 and 99 adenomas should be present upon endoscopy [84]; however, a molecular genetic testing is necessary to differentiate between APC and MUTYH mutations [85]. In case of reduce polyposis number, endoscopic polypectomy can be sufficient. In case of polyp dissemination all around the colic frame, IPAA is the treatment of choice, and if the rectum is intact, IRA can be used to conserve it [85, 86]. Regular annual checkup by endoscopy should be maintained in all families presenting MAP disorder [87].

Author details

Hamid Elia Daaboul and Mirvat El-Sibai*

*Address all correspondence to: mirvat.elsibai@lau.edu.lb

Department of Natural Sciences, School of Arts and Sciences, Lebanese American University, Byblos, Lebanon

References

[1] Haggar FA, Boushey RP. Colorectal cancer epidemiology: Incidence, mortality, survival, and risk factors. Clinics in Colon and Rectal Surgery. 2009;**22**(04):191-197

[2] Nielsen M, et al. Genotype–phenotype correlations in 19 Dutch cases with APC gene deletions and a literature review. European Journal of Human Genetics. 2007;**15**(10):1034-1042

[3] Johnson CM, et al. Meta-analyses of colorectal cancer risk factors. Cancer Causes & Control. 2013;**24**(6):1207-1222

[4] Aarons CB, Shanmugan S, Bleier JI. Management of malignant colon polyps: Current status and controversies. World Journal of Gastroenterology: WJG. 2014;**20**(43):16178

[5] Gordon PH, Nivatvongs S. Principles and Practice of Surgery for the Colon, Rectum, and Anus. NW, USA: CRC Press; 2007

[6] Kashida H, Kudo S-E. Early colorectal cancer: Concept, diagnosis, and management. International Journal of Clinical Oncology. 2006;**11**(1):1-8

[7] Ramirez M, et al. Management of the malignant polyp. Clinics in Colon and Rectal Surgery. 2008;**21**(04):286-290

[8] Chandrasekhara V, Ginsberg GG. Endoscopic mucosal resection: Not your father's polypectomy anymore. Gastroenterology. 2011;**141**(1):42-49

[9] Takahashi T, et al. Borderline cases between benignancy and malignancy of the duodenum diagnosed successfully by endoscopic submucosal dissection. Scandinavian Journal of Gastroenterology. 2009;**44**(11):1377-1383

[10] Repici A, et al. Endoscopic mucosal resection for early colorectal neoplasia: Pathologic basis, procedures, and outcomes. Diseases of the Colon & Rectum. 2009;**52**(8):1502-1515

[11] Williams J, et al. Management of the malignant colorectal polyp: ACPGBI position state-
      ment. Colorectal Disease. 2013;**15**(s2):1-38

[12] Rex DK, et al. Guidelines for colonoscopy surveillance after cancer resection: A consen-
      sus update by the American Cancer Society and US Multi-Society Task Force on colorec-
      tal cancer. CA: A Cancer Journal for Clinicians. 2006;**56**(3):160-167

[13] Castells A, et al. Clinical practice guideline. Prevention of colorectal cancer. 2009 update.
      Asociación Española de Gastroenterología. Gastroenterologia y Hepatologia. 2009;**32**(10):
      717 e1

[14] Alabi AA, et al. Preoperative serum vascular endothelial growth factor-a is a marker for
      subsequent recurrence in colorectal cancer patients. Diseases of the Colon & Rectum. 2009;
      52(5):993-999

[15] Bujanda L, et al. Malignant colorectal polyps. World Journal of Gastroenterology: WJG.
      2010;**16**(25):3103

[16] Carrara A, et al. Analysis of risk factors for lymph nodal involvement in early stages
      of rectal cancer: When can local excision be considered an appropriate treatment?
      Systematic review and meta-analysis of the literature. International Journal of Surgical
      Oncology. 2012;**2012**

[17] Benson AB, et al. Colon Cancer, version 1.2017, NCCN clinical practice guidelines in
      oncology. Journal of the National Comprehensive Cancer Network. 2017;**15**(3):370-398

[18] Boland CR, Goel A. Microsatellite instability in colorectal cancer. Gastroenterology.
      2010;**138**(6):2073-2087 e3

[19] Dotan E, Cohen SJ. Challenges in the management of stage II colon cancer. Seminars in
      Oncology. 2011

[20] Gryfe R, et al. Tumor microsatellite instability and clinical outcome in young patients
      with colorectal cancer. New England Journal of Medicine. 2000;**342**(2):69-77

[21] Watanabe T, et al. Molecular predictors of survival after adjuvant chemotherapy for
      colon cancer. New England Journal of Medicine. 2001;**344**(16):1196-1206

[22] Pitari G, et al. The paracrine hormone hypothesis of colorectal cancer. Clinical Pharma-
      cology & Therapeutics. 2007;**82**(4):441-447

[23] Hyslop T, Waldman SA. Guanylyl cyclase C as a biomarker in colorectal cancer. Biomar-
      kers in Medicine. 2013;**7**(1):159-167

[24] Hartman D, et al. Mutant allele-specific imbalance modulates prognostic impact of
      KRAS mutations in colorectal adenocarcinoma and is associated with worse overall sur-
      vival. International Journal of Cancer. 2012;**131**(8):1810-1817

[25] Group QC, Adjuvant chemotherapy versus observation in patients with colorectal can-
      cer: A randomised study. The Lancet, 2007. **370**(9604): p. 2020-2029

[26] Hutchins G, et al. Value of mismatch repair, KRAS, and BRAF mutations in predicting recurrence and benefits from chemotherapy in colorectal cancer. Journal of Clinical Oncology. 2011;**29**(10):1261-1270

[27] Russo A, et al. The TP53 colorectal cancer international collaborative study on the prognostic and predictive significance of p53 mutation: Influence of tumor site, type of mutation, and adjuvant treatment. Journal of Clinical Oncology. 2005;**23**(30):7518-7528

[28] Iacopetta B. TP53 mutation in colorectal cancer. Human Mutation. 2003;**21**(3):271-276

[29] Grady WM, Markowitz SD. Genetic and epigenetic alterations in colon cancer. Annual Review of Genomics and Human Genetics. 2002;**3**(1):101-128

[30] Xu Y, Pasche B. TGF-β signaling alterations and susceptibility to colorectal cancer. Human Molecular Genetics. 2007;**16**(R1):R14-R20

[31] Calascibetta A, et al. Analysis of the thymidylate synthase gene structure in colorectal cancer patients and its possible relation with the 5-fluorouracil drug response. Journal of Nucleic Acids. 2010;**2010**

[32] Yothers G, et al. Oxaliplatin as adjuvant therapy for colon cancer: Updated results of NSABP C-07 trial, including survival and subset analyses. Journal of Clinical Oncology. 2011;**29**(28):3768-3774

[33] Popat S, Hubner R, Houlston R. Systematic review of microsatellite instability and colorectal cancer prognosis. Journal of Clinical Oncology. 2005;**23**(3):609-618

[34] Jen J, et al. Allelic loss of chromosome 18q and prognosis in colorectal cancer. New England Journal of Medicine. 1994;**331**(4):213-221

[35] Bertagnolli M, et al. Presence of 18q loss of heterozygosity (LOH) and disease-free and overall survival in stage II colon cancer: CALGB protocol 9581. Journal of Clinical Oncology. 2009;**27**(15_suppl):4012-4012

[36] Bosset J-F, et al. Fluorouracil-based adjuvant chemotherapy after preoperative chemoradiotherapy in rectal cancer: Long-term results of the EORTC 22921 randomised study. The Lancet Oncology. 2014;**15**(2):184-190

[37] Van Cutsem E, et al. Metastatic colorectal cancer: ESMO Clinical Practice Guidelines for diagnosis, treatment and follow-up. Annals of Oncology. 2014;**25**(suppl_3):iii1-iii9

[38] Labianca R, et al. Primary colon cancer: ESMO Clinical Practice Guidelines for diagnosis, adjuvant treatment and follow-up. Annals of Oncology. 2010;**21**(suppl_5):v70-v77

[39] Roh M, et al. The impact of capecitabine and oxaliplatin in the preoperative multimodality treatment in patients with carcinoma of the rectum: NSABP R-04. Journal of Clinical Oncology. 2011;**29**(15_suppl):3503-3503

[40] Hofheinz R-D, et al. Chemoradiotherapy with capecitabine versus fluorouracil for locally advanced rectal cancer: A randomised, multicentre, non-inferiority, phase 3 trial. The Lancet Oncology. 2012;**13**(6):579-588

[41] Rödel C, et al. Preoperative chemoradiotherapy and postoperative chemotherapy with flu-orouracil and oxaliplatin versus fluorouracil alone in locally advanced rectal cancer: Initial results of the German CAO/ARO/AIO-04 randomised phase 3 trial. The Lancet Oncology. 2012;**13**(7):679-687

[42] Tournigand C, et al. FOLFIRI followed by FOLFOX6 or the reverse sequence in advanced colorectal cancer: A randomized GERCOR study. Journal of Clinical Oncology. 2004;**22**(2): 229-237

[43] Guo Y, et al. Capecitabine plus irinotecan versus 5-FU/leucovorin plus irinotecan in the treatment of colorectal cancer: A meta-analysis. Clinical Colorectal Cancer. 2014;**13**(2): 110-118

[44] Ducreux M, et al. Capecitabine plus oxaliplatin (XELOX) versus 5-fluorouracil/leucovo-rin plus oxaliplatin (FOLFOX-6) as first-line treatment for metastatic colorectal cancer. International Journal of Cancer. 2011;**128**(3):682-690

[45] Falcone A, et al. Phase III trial of infusional fluorouracil, leucovorin, oxaliplatin, and irinotecan (FOLFOXIRI) compared with infusional fluorouracil, leucovorin, and iri-notecan (FOLFIRI) as first-line treatment for metastatic colorectal cancer: The Gruppo Oncologico Nord Ovest. Journal of Clinical Oncology. 2007;**25**(13):1670-1676

[46] Masi G, et al. Randomized trial of two induction chemotherapy regimens in metastatic colorectal cancer: An updated analysis. Journal of the National Cancer Institute. 2010;**103**(1): 21-30

[47] Los M, Roodhart JM, Voest EE. Target practice: Lessons from phase III trials with beva-cizumab and vatalanib in the treatment of advanced colorectal cancer. The Oncologist. 2007;**12**(4):443-450

[48] Venook AP, et al. CALGB/SWOG 80405: Phase III Trial of Irinotecan/5-FU/Leucovorin (FOLFIRI) or Oxaliplatin/5-FU/Leucovorin (mFOLFOX6) with Bevacizumab (BV) or Cetuximab (CET) for Patients (Pts) with KRAS Wild-Type (Wt) Untreated Metastatic Adenocarcinoma of the Colon or Rectum (MCRC). American Society of Clinical Oncology; 2014

[49] Venook AP, et al. Impact of Primary (1°) Tumor Location on Overall Survival (OS) and Progression-Free Survival (PFS) in Patients (Pts) with Metastatic Colorectal Cancer (mCRC): Analysis of CALGB/SWOG 80405 (Alliance). American Society of Clinical Oncology; 2016

[50] Hsu H-C, et al. Mutations of KRAS/NRAS/BRAF predict cetuximab resistance in meta-static colorectal cancer patients. Oncotarget. 2016;**7**(16):22257

[51] Douillard J-Y, et al. Panitumumab–FOLFOX4 treatment and RAS mutations in colorectal cancer. New England Journal of Medicine. 2013;**369**(11):1023-1034

[52] Maughan TS, et al. Addition of cetuximab to oxaliplatin-based first-line combination chemotherapy for treatment of advanced colorectal cancer: Results of the randomised phase 3 MRC COIN trial. The Lancet. 2011;**377**(9783):2103-2114

[53] Tran B, et al. Impact of BRAF mutation and microsatellite instability on the pattern of meta-static spread and prognosis in metastatic colorectal cancer. Cancer. 2011;**117**(20):4623-4632

[54] Yaeger R, et al. BRAF mutation predicts for poor outcomes after metastasectomy in patients with metastatic colorectal cancer. Cancer. 2014;**120**(15):2316-2324

[55] Atreya CE, et al. Differential radiographic appearance of BRAF V600E–mutant metastatic colorectal cancer in patients matched by primary tumor location. Journal of the National Comprehensive Cancer Network. 2016;**14**(12):1536-1543

[56] Kopetz S, et al. PLX4032 in metastatic colorectal cancer patients with mutant BRAF tumors. Journal of Clinical Oncology. 2010;**28**(15_suppl):3534-3534

[57] Loupakis F, et al. FOLFOXIRI plus bevacizumab as first-line treatment in BRAF mutant metastatic colorectal cancer. European Journal of Cancer. 2014;**50**(1):57-63

[58] Loupakis F, et al. FOLFOXIRI plus Bevacizumab (Bev) Versus FOLFIRI plus Bev as First-Line Treatment of Metastatic Colorectal Cancer (MCRC). Results of the phase III randomized TRIBE trial. Alexandria VA, USA: American Society of Clinical Oncology; 2013

[59] Falcone A, et al. FOLFOXIRI/Bevacizumab (Bev) Versus FOLFIRI/Bev as First-Line Treatment in Unresectable Metastatic Colorectal Cancer (mCRC) Patients (Pts). Results of the phase III TRIBE trial by GONO group. Alexandria VA, USA: American Society of Clinical Oncology; 2013

[60] Wang X, et al. PD-L1 expression in human cancers and its association with clinical outcomes. OncoTargets and Therapy. 2016;**9**:5023

[61] Le DT, et al. PD-1 blockade in tumors with mismatch-repair deficiency. New England Journal of Medicine. 2015;**372**(26):2509-2520

[62] Overman MJ, et al. Nivolumab in Patients with DNA Mismatch Repair Deficient/Microsatellite Instability High Metastatic Colorectal Cancer: Update from CheckMate 142. Alexandria VA, USA: American Society of Clinical Oncology; 2017

[63] Mullard A. 2012 FDA drug approvals. Nature Reviews. Drug Discovery. 2013;**12**(2):87

[64] Van Cutsem E, et al. Addition of aflibercept to fluorouracil, leucovorin, and irinotecan improves survival in a phase III randomized trial in patients with metastatic colorectal cancer previously treated with an oxaliplatin-based regimen. Journal of Clinical Oncology. 2012;**30**(28):3499-3506

[65] Yoshino T, et al. Randomized phase III trial of regorafenib in metastatic colorectal cancer: Analysis of the CORRECT Japanese and non-Japanese subpopulations. Investigational New Drugs. 2015;**33**(3):740-750

[66] Verdaguer H, Tabernero J, Macarulla T. Ramucirumab in metastatic colorectal cancer: Evidence to date and place in therapy. Therapeutic Advances in Medical Oncology. 2016; **8**(3):230-242

[67] Tabernero J, et al. Ramucirumab versus placebo in combination with second-line FOLFIRI in patients with metastatic colorectal carcinoma that progressed during or after first-line therapy with bevacizumab, oxaliplatin, and a fluoropyrimidine (RAISE): A randomised, double-blind, multicentre, phase 3 study. The Lancet Oncology. 2015;**16**(5):499-508

[68] Raedler LA. Lonsurf (Trifluridine plus Tipiracil): A new oral treatment approved for patients with metastatic colorectal cancer. American Health & Drug Benefits. 2016;**9**(Spec Feature):97

[69] Kish T, Uppal P. Trifluridine/tipiracil (lonsurf) for the treatment of metastatic colorectal cancer. Pharmacy and Therapeutics. 2016;**41**(5):314

[70] Ko Y, Karanicolas P. Hepatic arterial infusion pump chemotherapy for colorectal liver metastases: An old technology in a new era. Current Oncology. 2014;**21**(1):e116

[71] Fiorentini G, et al. Chemoembolization in colorectal liver metastases: The rebirth. Anticancer Research. 2014;**34**(2):575-584

[72] Ceelen W. Current management of peritoneal carcinomatosis from colorectal cancer. Minerva Chirurgica. 2013;**68**(1):77-86

[73] Kastrinos F, et al. Risk of pancreatic cancer in families with lynch syndrome. JAMA. 2009;**302**(16):1790-1795

[74] Buecher B, et al. Role of microsatellite instability in the management of colorectal cancers. Digestive and Liver Disease. 2013;**45**(6):441-449

[75] Umar A, et al. Revised Bethesda guidelines for hereditary nonpolyposis colorectal cancer (lynch syndrome) and microsatellite instability. Journal of the National Cancer Institute. 2004;**96**(4):261-268

[76] Vasen HF et al. Guidelines for the clinical management of lynch syndrome (hereditary non-polyposis cancer). Journal of Medical Genetics. 2007;**44**(6):353-362

[77] Fallik D, et al. Microsatellite instability is a predictive factor of the tumor response to irinotecan in patients with advanced colorectal cancer. Cancer Research. 2003;**63**(18):5738-5744

[78] Ait Ouakrim D, et al. Aspirin, ibuprofen, and the risk for colorectal cancer in Lynch Syndrome. JNCI: Journal of the National Cancer Institute. 2015;**107**(9)

[79] Burn J, et al. Long-term effect of aspirin on cancer risk in carriers of hereditary colorectal cancer: An analysis from the CAPP2 randomised controlled trial. The Lancet. 2012; **378**(9809):2081-2087

[80] Galiatsatos P, Foulkes WD. Familial adenomatous polyposis. The American Journal of Gastroenterology. 2006;**101**(2):385

[81] Jasperson KW, Patel SG, Ahnen DJ. APC-Associated Polyposis Conditions. In: Adam MP, Ardinger HH, Pagon RA, Wallace SE, Bean LJH, Mefford HC, Stephens K, Amemiya A, Ledbetter N, editors. SourceGeneReviews® [Internet]. Seattle (WA): University of Washington, Seattle; 1993-2017

[82] Provenzale D, et al. Genetic/familial high-risk assessment: Colorectal version 1.2016, NCCN clinical practice guidelines in oncology. Journal of the National Comprehensive Cancer Network. 2016;**14**(8):1010-1030

[83] Al-Tassan N, et al. Inherited variants of MYH associated with somatic G: C [arrow right] T: A mutations in colorectal tumors. Nature Genetics. 2002;**30**(2):227

[84] Nielsen M, et al. MUTYH-associated polyposis (MAP). Critical Reviews in Oncology/ Hematology. 2011;**79**(1):1-16

[85] Sieber OM, et al. Multiple colorectal adenomas, classic adenomatous polyposis, and germ-line mutations in MYH. New England Journal of Medicine. 2003;**348**(9):791-799

[86] Bolocan A, et al. Map syndrome (MYH associated polyposis) colorectal cancer, etio-pathological connections. Journal of Medicine and Life. 2011;**4**(1):109

[87] Syngal S, et al. ACG clinical guideline: Genetic testing and management of hereditary gastrointestinal cancer syndromes. The American Journal of Gastroenterology. 2015;**110**(2):223

9

Basic Endoscopic Findings — Normal and Pathological Findings

Parth J. Parekh and Sanjay K. Sikka

Abstract

Since its inception, colonoscopy has evolved to become the cornerstone for colorectal imaging. The increasing indications for endoscopic evaluation and potential therapeutic intervention parallels technological advances and the expanding diagnostic and therapeutic capabilities of colonoscopy. The diagnostic and therapeutic yield of colonoscopy is highly user dependent. Thus, it is essential for the clinical endoscopist to perform a thorough endoscopic evaluation and be cognizant of normal and pathologic findings. This review details normal and pathologic endoscopic findings in a variety of disease states that are often encountered by the clinical endoscopist including colon polyps, inflammatory bowel disease, and infectious and non-infectious colitides. In addition, we review the diagnostic and therapeutic role of colonoscopy in the evaluation of an acute lower gastrointestinal bleed.

Keywords: Polyp, pseudopolyp, hyperplastic polyp, adenoma, tubular adenoma, tubulovillous adenoma, sessile adenoma, sessile serrated adenoma, colitis, diverticulosis, hemorrhoids, anal fissure

1. Introduction

The advent of retrograde colonoscopy in June 1969 revolutionized the field of gastroenterology [1]. It has since evolved to become the gold standard for colorectal imaging [2, 3].

As technology continues to advance, so too does the diagnostic utility and therapeutic capabilities of colonoscopy. Thus, it becomes imperative for the clinical endoscopist to perform a thorough colonoscopic evaluation and be cognizant of normal and pathologic findings as indications for colonoscopy expand. Here, we detail normal and pathologic endoscopic findings in a variety of disease states that are often encountered by the clinical endoscopist including colon polyps, inflammatory bowel disease (IBD), and infectious and non-infectious colitides. In addition, we review the diagnostic and therapeutic role of colonoscopy in the evaluation of an acute lower gastrointestinal bleed.

2. Polyps and potential progression to colorectal cancer

Colorectal cancer is the third most common cancer among men and women, and the third leading cause of cancer-related death in the United States [4]. It is estimated that in 2014, 71,830 men and 65,000 women were diagnosed with colorectal cancer with approximately 50,000 mortalities (26,270 men and 24,040 women) as a result of the disease. Globally, colorectal cancer is the fourth leading cause of cancer-related death accounting for approximately 700,000 deaths in 2012 [5]. The vast majority of colorectal cancers stem from benign polyps arising from the mucosal layer. Winawer et al. were among the first to demonstrate that colorectal adenomas have the potential to progress to colorectal adenocarcinoma, thus stressing the importance of colonoscopic polypectomy in colorectal cancer prevention [6]. Subsequent long term data has validated the importance of colonoscopy and colonoscopic polypectomy in the prevention of colorectal cancer-related deaths [7]. To date, colonoscopy remains the cornerstone in colorectal cancer prevention. Unfortunately, the "miss rate" of colonoscopy for colorectal cancer and adenomas larger than 1 cm has been reported to be as high as 6% [8] and 17% [9, 10], respectively.

Adenomas and hamartomatous polyps, later discussed in depth, are polyps that carry malignant potential. They are indolent in nature, typically growing slowly over the span of a decade or more. There is a direct correlation between the size of the adenoma and its risk of developing future advanced adenomas or carcinoma with studies demonstrating this risk to be as high as 7.7% [11], 15.9% [11], and 19.3% [12], for adenomas <5mm, 5–20mm, and >20mm, respectively.

Chromosomal instability and common point mutations occurring in colorectal cancer-related tumor suppressor genes (e.g., APC, P53) or tumor promoter genes (e.g., K-Ras) architect the progression from benign polyps to colorectal cancer. Figure 1 depicts key point mutations and its impact on morphologic changes of a benign polyp to colorectal cancer. There is, however, considerable genetic and epigenetic heterogeneity resulting in different pathways to tumorigenesis [13]. Luo et al. sought to evaluate the effect of these alterations on the progression to colorectal cancer by conducting genome-wide array-based studies and comprehensive data analysis of aberrantly methylated loci in normal colon tissue (n=41), colon adenomas (n=42), and colorectal cancer (n=64) [14]. They identified three classes of cancers and two classes of adenomas, high-frequency methylation and low-frequency methylation based on their DNA methylation patterns. Mutant K-Ras was found in a subset of high-frequency methylated adenomas. In addition, they found the methylation signatures of high-frequency methylation adenomas to be similar to those of cancer with low or intermediate levels of methylation, and low-frequency methylation adenomas to have methylation signatures similar to that of normal colon tissue. These findings demonstrated genome-wide alterations in DNA methylation to occur during the early stages of progression of adenomas to colorectal cancer, and the presence of heterogeneity in tumorigenesis, even at the adenoma step of the process.

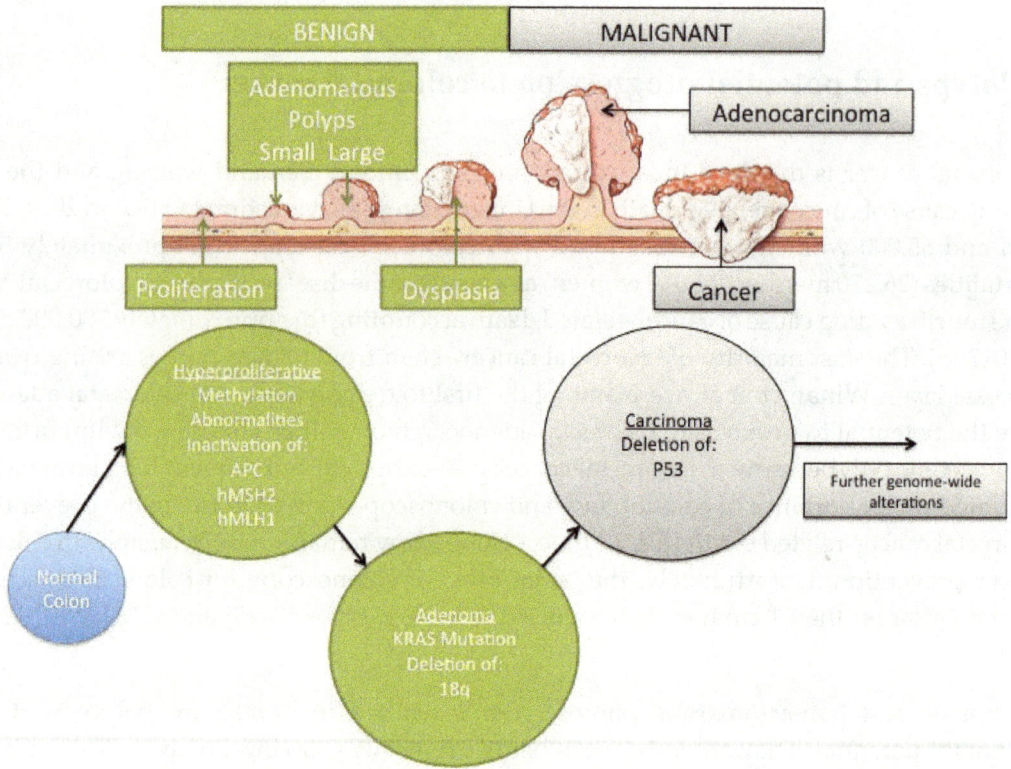

Figure 1. Key point mutations and its impact on morphologic changes of a benign polyp to colorectal cancer.

3. Polyps and pseudopolyps

In 2003, the Paris Endoscopic Classification arose to describe polyp morphology [15], which can potentially guide the endoscopist toward its malignancy potential [16–18]. Figure 2 provides a schematic overview of the Paris Endoscopic Classification and Figure 3 provides an endoscopic view of differing polyp morphology under traditional white-light colonoscopy. A recent study by van Doom et al. evaluated the interobserver agreement for the Paris Endoscopic Classification among seven expert endoscopists [19]. The seven expert endoscopists assessed 85 endoscopic video clips depicting polyps. Afterwards, they underwent a digital training module and then assessed the same 85 polyps again. A calculated Fleiss kappa of 0.42 and a mean pairwise agreement of 67% suggested moderate interobserver agreement among the seven experts. In addition, the proportion of lesions labeled as "flat" lesions ranged between 13–40% (p<0.001). The interobserver agreement did not change significantly after the digital training module, which led the investigators to conclude there to be only moderate interobserver agreement among experts for this classification system and that use of this classification system in daily practice is questionable and unsuitable for comparative endoscopist research. Thus, the need for a simplified classification system is necessary to better aid the clinical endoscopist.

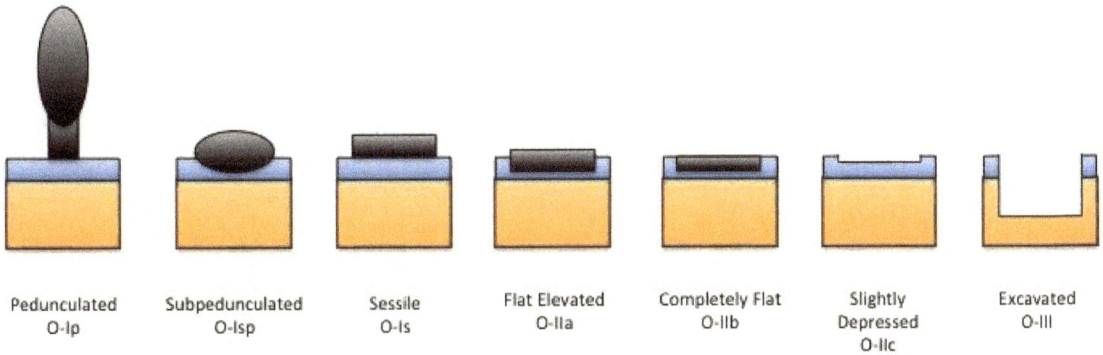

| Pedunculated O-Ip | Subpedunculated O-Isp | Sessile O-Is | Flat Elevated O-IIa | Completely Flat O-IIb | Slightly Depressed O-IIc | Excavated O-III |

Figure 2. The Paris Classification based on polyp appearance.

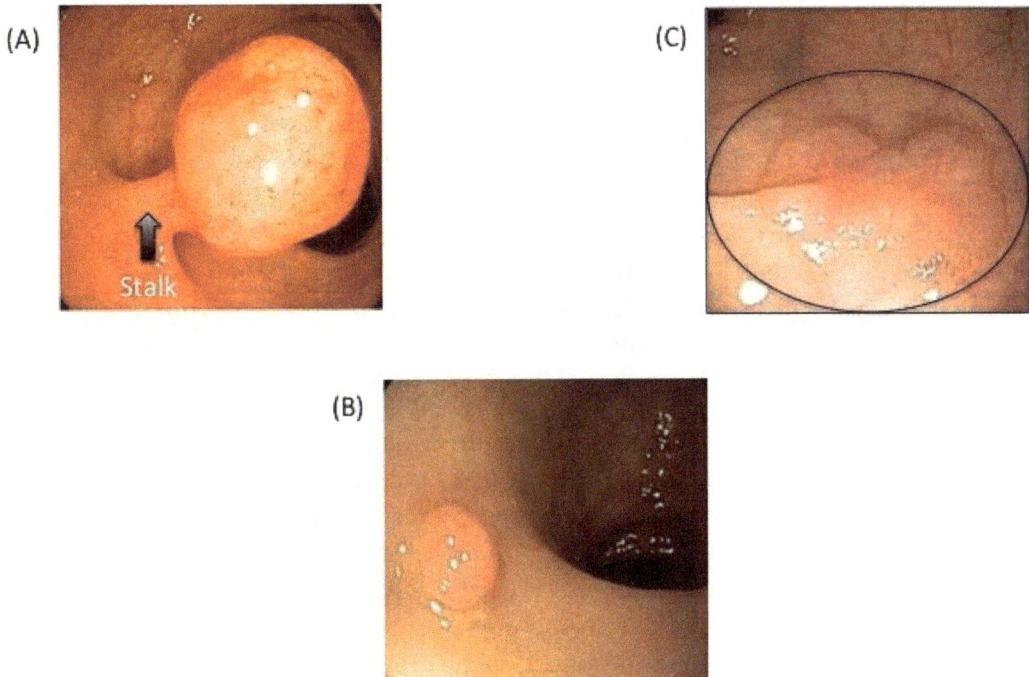

Figure 3. Endoscopic views of differing polyp morphology under traditional white-light colonoscopy: (A) Pedunculated polyp, (B) Sessile polyp, (C) Flat polyp.

In addition to traditional white-light colonoscopy, several studies have demonstrated the utility of narrow-band-imaging (NBI) to be useful in adenoma detection [20–23]. Under NBI, adenomas appear to have thicker and higher volumes of microvasculature compared to normal mucosa and hyperplastic polyps, resulting in distinct pit patterns that may increase diagnostic yield [23]. This section will review the morphology and histology, malignant potential, and provide endoscopic and pathologic depictions of different polyp subtypes.

3.1. Adenomas

Adenomatous polyps by definition are dysplastic and thus carry malignant potential. They can further be characterized as being an advanced adenoma, synchronous adenoma, or metachronous adenoma. An advanced adenoma is defined as an adenoma with high-grade dysplasia, an adenoma with a size >10 mm, an adenoma with significant villous components (>25%), or an adenoma with evidence of invasive carcinoma [24]. Synchronous adenomas are polyps that are diagnosed at the same time as an index colorectal cancer and metachranous adenomas are ones diagnosed at least six months before or after the diagnosis of an index colorectal cancer [25]. The diagnosis of synchronous and metachranous adenomas are of utmost importance as it can potentially identify individuals at risk for hereditary conditions, thus impacting therapeutic intervention and screening intervals for relatives [26].

3.1.1. Tubular, villous, and tubulovillous adenomas

Adenomas are characterized as tubular, villous, or tubulovillous (a mixture of the two) based on their glandular architecture. Tubular adenomas, which account for the vast majority of colon adenomas, are characterized by a network of branching adenomatous epithelium and a tubular component of >75% [16]. Figure 4 depicts a histologic representation of a tubular adenoma in the background of normal colon tissue. Villous adenomas, which account for up to 15% of adenomas, are characterized by long glands that extend straight down to the center of the polyp from its surface with a villous component of >75% [16]. Figure 5 depicts a histologic representation of a villous adenoma in the background of normal colon tissue. Lastly, tubulovillous adenomas, which account for up to 15% of adenomas, are a mixture of the two previous adenomas with a villous component of anywhere from 26–75%. Figure 6 depicts a histologic representation of a tubulovillous adenoma in the background of normal colon tissue.

The CpG island methylator phenotype (CIMP) pathway is composed of methylated promoter regions of multiple putative tumor suppressor genes occurring in colorectal cancer and also in adenomatous polyps [27]. Kakar et al. examined villous/tubulovillous adenomas (n=32) and tubular adenomas (n=30) for BRAF/K-Ras mutations and CIMP-status (characterized by methylation of three or more loci at hMLH1, p16, HIC1, RASSF2, MGMT, MINT1, and MINT31) [28]. They found 44% of villous/tubulovillous to be CIMP-positive compared with 27% of tubular adenomas (p=0.08). In addition, villous/tubulovillous adenomas demonstrated significantly higher methylation rates at MGMT (87% vs. 37%; p<0.01) and RASSF2 (94% vs. 70%; p=0.02) when compared to tubular adenomas. Lastly, CIMP-positive adenomas correlated with increased size, right-sided location, and increased villous component in villous/tubulovillous adenomas. This led the authors to conclude that CIMP status is indicative of size, location, and malignant potential, and that methylation of MGMT and RASSF2 increases as adenomas progress from tubular adenomas to villous/tubulovillous adenomas.

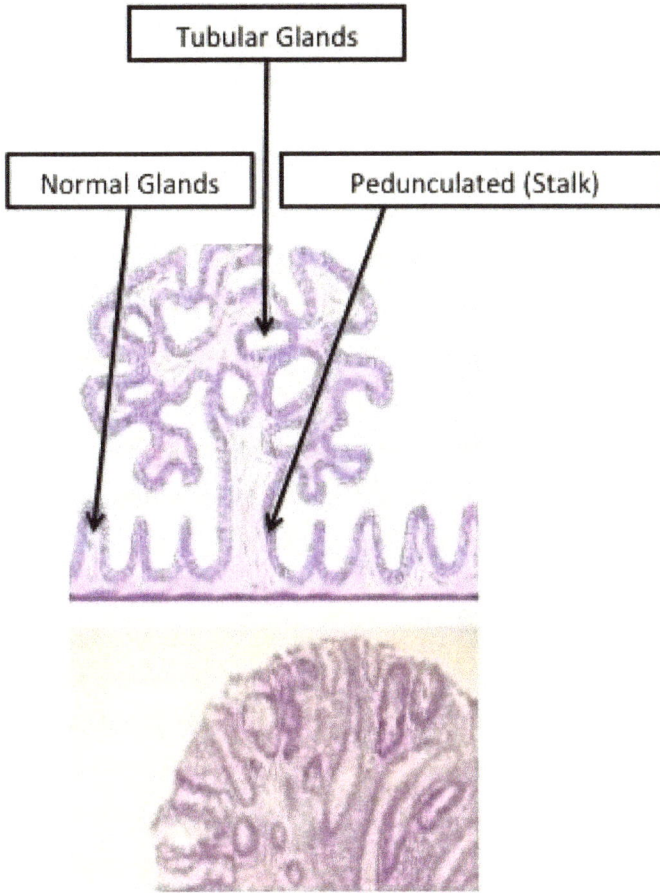

Figure 4. Histologic representation of tubular adenoma in the background of normal colon tissue.

3.1.2. Sessile serrated adenomas, traditional serrated adenomas, and hyperplastic polyps

Serrated lesions account for approximately 30% of colorectal cancers, arising via the serrated neoplasia pathway characterized by widespread DNA methylation and *BRAF* mutations [29]. They are classified histologically as sessile serrated adenomas/polyps (SSA/Ps), traditional serrated adenomas (TSAs), or hyperplastic polyps, with only SSA/Ps and TSAs carrying malignant potential [30]. SSA/Ps typically lack classic dysplasia, however, those that demonstrate foci of classic histologic dysplasia and molecular profiles exhibiting methylation of DNA repair genes (e.g., MLH-1) are thought to be precursor lesions to sporadic unstable microsatellite (MSI-H) cancers. SSA/Ps also exhibit activation of the *BRAF* oncogene, a feature seen in many sporadic MSI-H cancers [31]. Figure 7 depicts two potential molecular pathways of serrated neoplasia.

SSA/Ps tend to be more prominent in the proximal colon [32] as compared with TSAs [33] and hyperplastic polyps [34], which tend to be more prominent in the rectosigmoid. Thus, expert recommendations are to completely remove all serrated lesions proximal to the sigmoid colon and all serrated lesions in the rectosigmoid >5mm [30]. They may be more difficult to detect

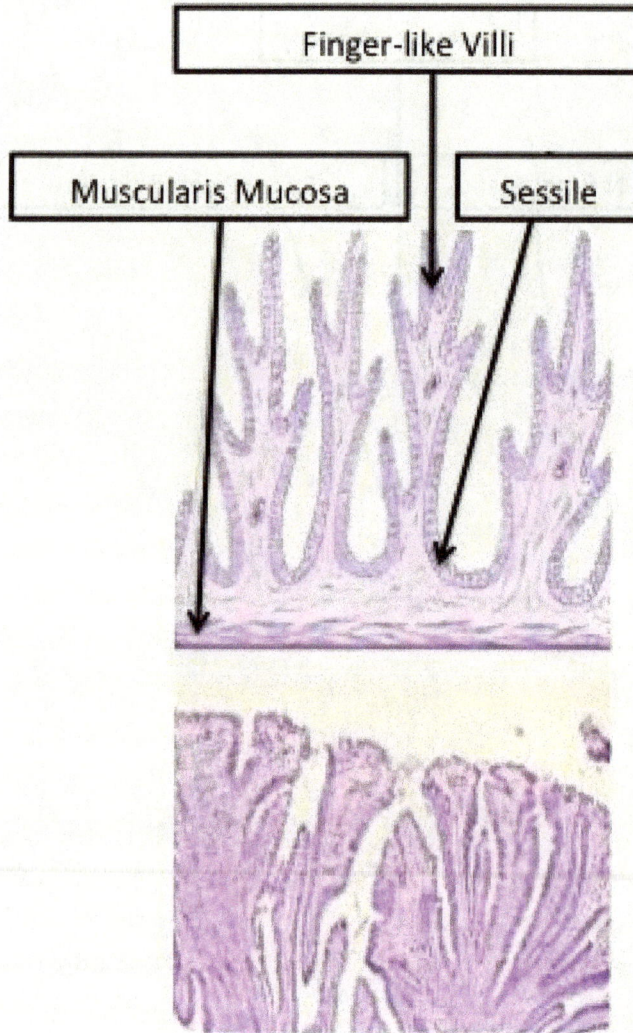

Figure 5. Histologic representation of villous adenoma in the background of normal colon tissue.

than conventional adenomatous polyps, in particular SSA/Ps, since they are more likely to be flat lesions, and so recent studies have advocated for a longer withdrawal time to increase serrated lesion detection rates [35, 36].

Serrated lesions have a distinct endoscopic appearance albeit often very subtle. A retrospective analysis of high-resolution endoscopic video clips by Tadepalli et al. analyzed the gross morphologic characteristics of 158 SSPs [37]. They found the most prevalent visual descriptors to be the presence of a mucous cap (which may be yellow or green in white light and red under NBI) (63.9%), rim of debris or bubbles (51.9%), alteration of the contour of a fold (37.3%), and interruption of underlying vascular pattern (32%). Figure 8 depicts an SSP under traditional white-light colonoscopy with a superficial mucous cap, its appearance under NBI, and a histologic representation.

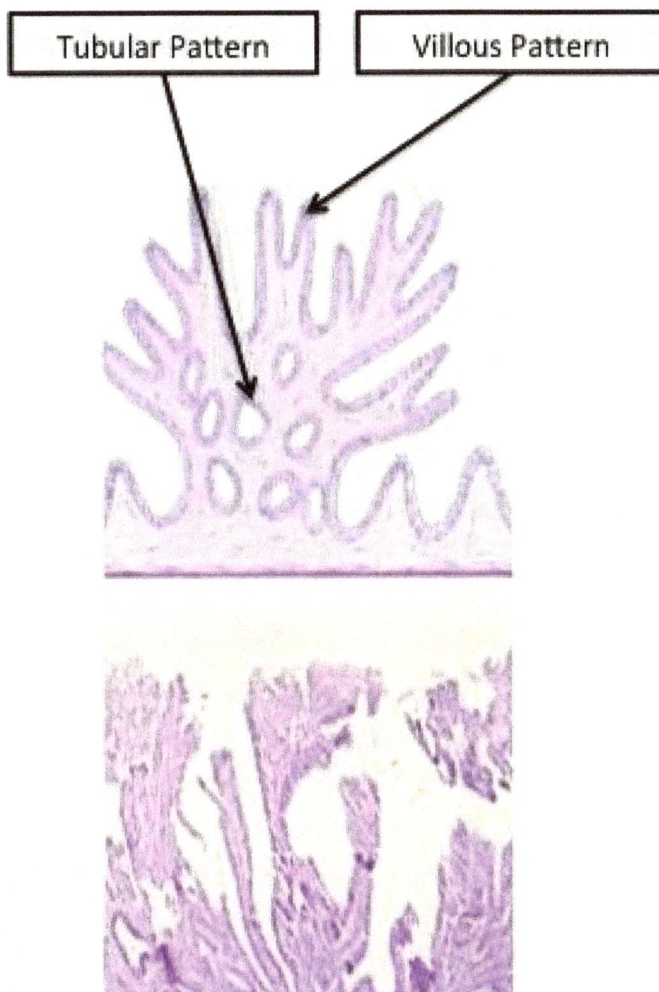

Figure 6. Histologic representation of a tubulovillous adenoma in the background of normal colon tissue.

Hyperplastic polyps are the most common non-neoplastic polyps in the colon; however, they are oftentimes grossly indistinguishable from adenomatous polyps. Histologically, hyperplastic polyps resemble normal colonic tissue with the exception of proliferation in the basal portion of the crypt and a characteristic "saw tooth" pattern along the crypt axis [38]. The relationship between diminutive hyperplastic polyps in the left colon and proximal neoplasia has long been a topic of debate with studies producing mixed results [39–42]. Hyperplastic polyps found proximal to the left colon, however, have consistently been shown to carry malignant potential and should be resected [39, 43].

3.2. Hamartomatous polyps

Hamartomatous polyps are polyps that may grossly resemble normal colonic tissue but are histologically a mixture of tissues growing in disarray. Histologically, they contain mucous-filled glands, retention cysts, abundant connective tissue, and/or chronic eosinophilic infiltra-

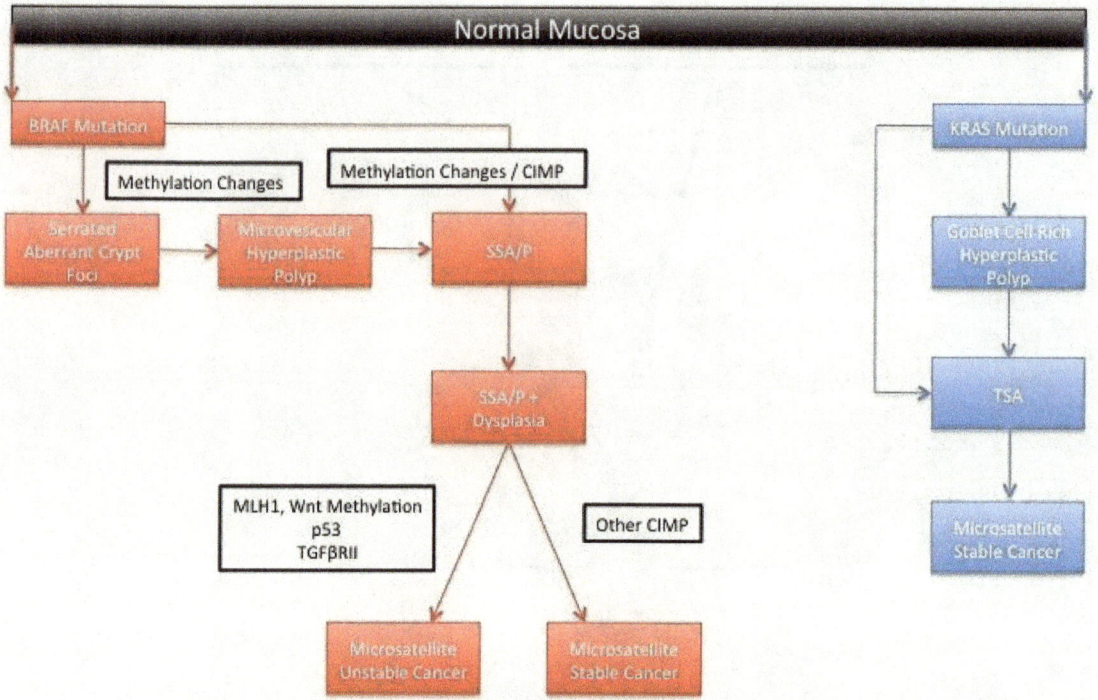

Figure 7. Potential molecular pathways of serrated neoplasia.

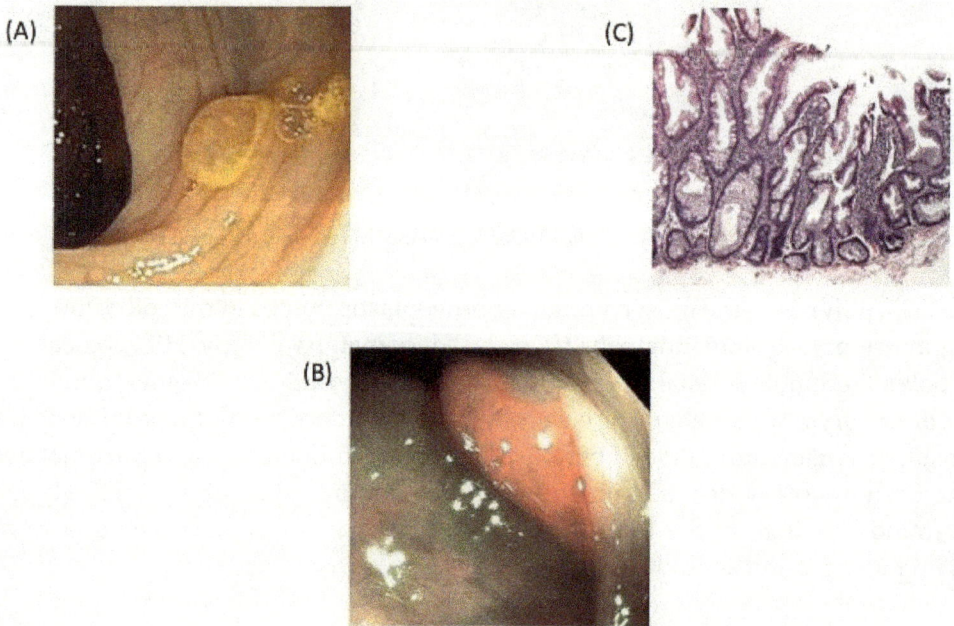

Figure 8. A) Sessile serrated polyp with mucosal cap under white-light colonoscopy. (B) Sessile serrated polyp under NBI. (C) Histology of sessile serrated polyp demonstrating expanded crypt proliferative zone, exaggerated architecture in crypt region with basilar crypt dilation, inverted crypts, and a predominance of crypts with minimal cell maturation.

tion [44]. Traditionally, they have been classified as non-neoplastic but several associated polyposis syndromes (e.g., Juvenile Polyposis Coli, Peutz-Jegher Syndrome, Cronkhite Canada Syndrome, and Cowden Syndrome) do carry a predilection towards colorectal cancer and other gastrointestinal malignancies.

Juvenile polyps are a type of hamartomatous polyp characterized by dilated cystic glands rather than an increased number of epithelial cells [44]. They can be found at any age, but as the name implies, are more commonly diagnosed during childhood. They are typically removed due to their propensity to bleed. Peutz-Jegher polyps are a type of hamartomatous polyp characterized by glandular epithelium supported by smooth muscle cells contiguous with the muscularis mucosa. Figure 9 depicts an endoscopic view of a hamartomatous polyp and histologic view of a Peutz-Jegher polyp.

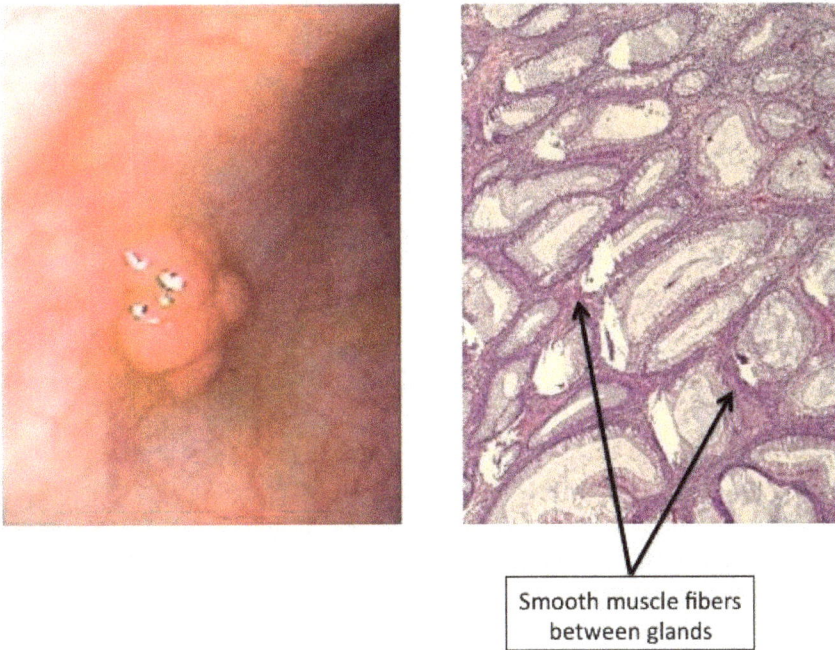

Smooth muscle fibers between glands

Figure 9. Endoscopic view of a hamartomatous polyp and histologic view of a Peutz-Jegher polyp.

3.3. Inflammatory pseudopolyps

Inflammatory polyps, typically seen in IBD, are indicative of regenerative and/or healing phases of mucosal ulceration and possess no malignant potential. They are formed from discrete islands of residual intact colonic mucosa that result from the ulceration and tissue regeration that is inherent to the disease course [45]. Scattered throughout the colitic region of the colon, they are often numerous, filiform, and can be large enough to encompass the lumen resulting in intussusception or luminal obstruction [45, 46]. The clinical endoscopist ought to be cognizant of clusters of localized giant pseudopolyposis as they may be associated with occult dysplasia [47]. Histologically, inflammatory pseudopolyps are characterized by inflamed lamina propria and distorted colonic epithelium [48]. Surface erosions, congestion, hemorrhage and/or crypt abscesses may also be present [48]. Figure 10 depicts an endoscopic and histologic view of an inflammatory pseudopolyp.

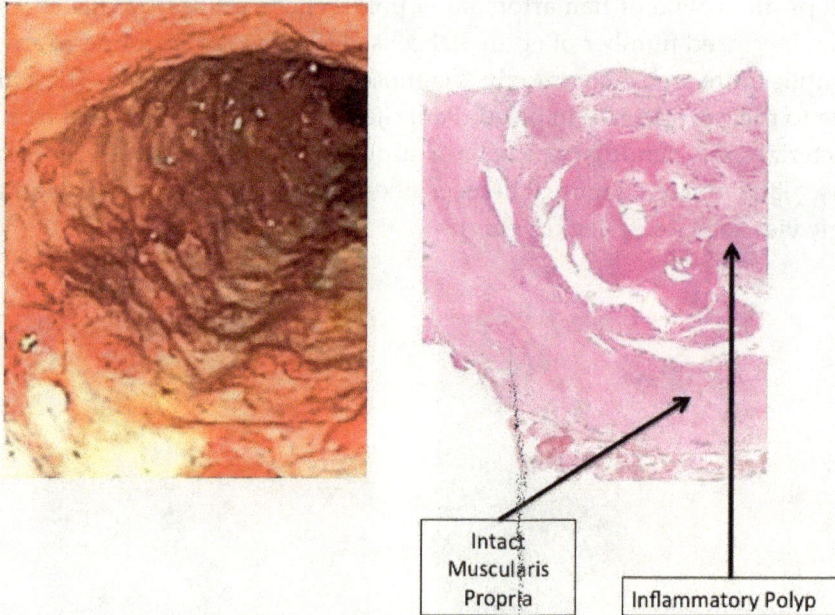

Figure 10. Endoscopic and histologic view of an inflammatory pseudopolyp.

4. Colitis

4.1. Inflammatory bowel disease

In patients with a clinical presentation suggestive of IBD, colonoscopy with ileoscopy can be used to make the initial diagnosis as it allows for direct visualization and biopsy of rectal, colonic, and terminal ileum mucosa [49]. In addition, it can assess disease activity and monitor therapeutic response, provide surveillance of dysplasia or neoplasia, and lastly provide therapeutic intervention such as stricture dilation [49] or closure of fistulae and anastomotic leakages [50].

The use of endoscopic appearance in distinguishing IBD from other non-IBD colitides is limited [51] as there are a number of 'IBD mimickers' including but not limited to colonic tuberculosis [52], Behçet's disease [53], and segmental colitis associated with diverticular disease [54]. In addition to tuberculosis, there are hosts of other infectious colitides that can also endoscopically mimic IBD [51, 55]. Table 1 provides an endoscopic description of various infectious colitides. Once these other etiologies have been excluded, colonoscopy can often shed light in distinguishing Crohn's disease (CD) from ulcerative colitis (UC), which is important for disease management. The data gathered from an index colonoscopy is of utmost importance owning to the fact that once therapy is initiated for IBD, discriminating features of CD from UC may be obscured [56, 57].

Infectious Etiology	Endoscopic Appearance
Apergillus	Hemorrhagic ulcerations
Campylobacter	Colonic erythema and ulceration
Chlamydia	Perianal abscesses, ulcerations, and fistulae
C. difficile	Pseudomembranes and moderately severe colitis, predominantly left sided
Cytomegalovirus	Colitis with ulceration (typically punched out and shallow)
Entamoeba	Acute colitis with ulceration
E. coli 0157:H7	Moderately severe colitis
Herpes	Proctitis with ulceration, there may be perianal involvement as well.
Histoplasma	Moderately severely colitis, predominantly right sided
Klebsiella	Hemorrhagic colitis
Mycobacterium	Ileal ulceration, may be transverse or circumferential
Nessieria	Proctitis with ulceration, there may be perianal involvement as well
Salmonella	Friable mucosa, ileal and colonic hemorrhages often present
Schistosoma	Extensive colitis may be segmental, polyps often times present
Shigella	Intense patchy colonic erythema that can also include the ileum
Treponema	Proctitis with ulceration, there may be perianal involvement as well
Yersinia	Patchy colitis with ileal ulceration (apthoid)

Table 1. Endoscopic description of various infectious colitides [54].

4.1.1. Endoscopic features of UC and Mayo Scoring System

Endoscopically, classic UC starts in the rectum and progresses proximally, sometimes as far as the ileo-cecal valve, in a circumferential and contiguous fashion with diffused and continuous inflammation [58]. Endoscopic features suggestive of UC include erythema, edema resulting in a loss of the usual vascular patter, granular appearing mucosa, increased friability, and small superficial erosions and ulcers surrounded by diffuse inflammation [59]. These classic visual features are used to endoscopically score the extent of the disease. The Mayo

Scoring System was derived in order provide an objective measure describing the endoscopic extent of the disease. Lemmens et al. sought to evaluate the correlation between endoscsopy and histology with use of the Mayo Scoring System [60]. This retrospective study included 236 biopsy sets from 131 patients with known UC. Endoscopy was performed by IBD specialists and graded using the Mayo Scoring System. Biopsy specimens were analyzed by expert gastrointestinal pathologists using the Geboes and Riley histologic scoring systems. They found that at both extremes, inactive and severely active disease, there was a very high concordance rate. For mild disease, however, there were important differences, as histologic examination seemed to have detected more severe disease than endoscopically suspected, thus stressing the need for a combined histologic and endoscopic scoring system when assessing disease activity. Figure 11 depicts the classic endoscopic appearance of UC in relation to the Mayo Scoring System.

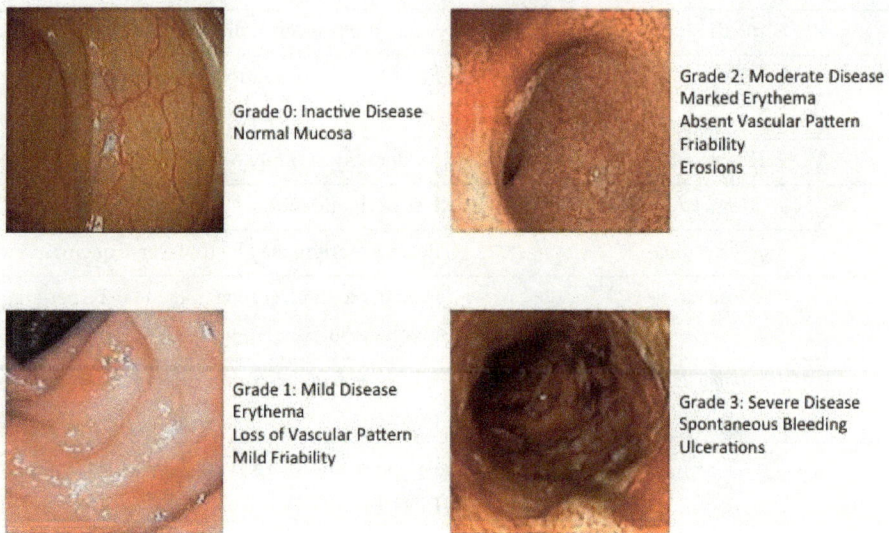

Figure 11. Classic endoscopic appearance of UC in relation to the Mayo Scoring System.

4.1.2. Endoscopic features of CD and the Simple Endoscopic Score for CD (SES-CD)

Inflammation in CD can span the entire gastrointestinal tract with nearly 55% of cases involving the terminal ileum and colon, 40% involving exclusively the ileum, and 25% involving the colon alone [61]. Rectal involvement occurs in up to 50% of patients with CD [62]. It should be noted that while terminal ileal involvement is strongly suggestive of CD, it might also occur in patients with UC, particularly pan-colitic UC, by way of "backwash" of cecal contents or "backwash ileitis" [63, 64]. The exact pathogenesis of "backwash ileitis" remains poorly understood, however it is believed that in patients with pan-colitic UC, the terminal ileum becomes inflamed stemming from chronic exposure to cecal contents.

Endoscopically, classic CD appears as "skip lesions" or areas of inflammation interposed between islands of normal mucosa, "cobblestone" appearance of the mucosal surface due to submucosal inflammation and edema, and deep, longitudinal, polycyclic ulcers [55]. In 2004, the SES-CD was derived in order to provide an objective measure describing the endoscopic extent of the disease [65]. To date, prospective data evaluating the utility of SES-CD in predicting corticosteroid-free clinical remission and long-term disease progression is lacking [66, 67]. Figure 12 depicts the classic endoscopic appearance of CD as well as the SES-CD. Table 2 illustrates the key endoscopic differences between UC and CD.

	SES-Score			
Variable	**0**	**1**	**2**	**3**
Size of ulcer (diameter in cm)	None	Aphthous ulcers (0.1-0.5)	Large ulcers (0.5-2)	Very large ulcers (>2)
Ulcerated surface (%)	None	<10	10-30	>30
Affected surface (%)	Unaffected segment	<50	50-75	>75
Presence of strictures	None	Single, can be passed	Multiple, can be passed	Cannot be passed

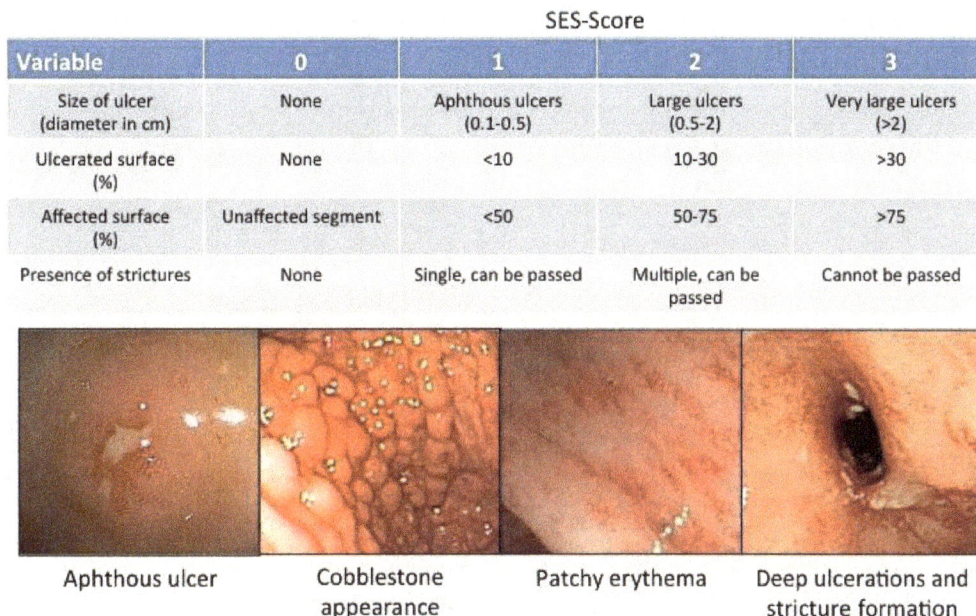

Aphthous ulcer | Cobblestone appearance | Patchy erythema | Deep ulcerations and stricture formation

Figure 12. Classic endoscopic appearance of CD as well as the SES-CD.

Endoscopic Features	Ulcerative Colitis	Crohn's Disease
Aphthous Ulcers	√	√√√
Cobblestone Appearance	x	√√
Deep Ulcers	x	√√√
Erythema	√√√	√√
Granular Mucosa	√√√	√
Ileal Ulcers	x	√√√
Loss of Vascular Pattern	√√√	√
Pseudopolyp	√√√	√√√
Patchy Inflammation	x	√√√
Rectal Involvement	√√√√	√√

Table 2. Key endoscopic differences between UC and CD [54].

4.2. Microscopic (Lymphocytic and collagenous) and eosinophilic colitis

While microscopic colitis by definition is a histologic diagnosis, emerging data suggests that it may not always present with normal endoscopic findings [68–72]. Microscopic colitis is further subdivided into lymphocytic colitis and collagenous colitis depending on the presence of lymphocytic predominant infiltration or collagen deposition, respectively [73]. There have been several macroscopic lesions associated with collagenous colitis including longitudinal ulcers [69,70], hypervascularity [71], loss of normal vascularity [72], and exudative bleeding [73]. A retrospective study by Park et al. sought to investigate macroscopic lesions seen on the endoscopy in 14 patients with diagnosed lymphocytic colitis [68]. Patients with more severe diarrhea demonstrated macroscopic lesions on colonoscopy that included hypervascularity and exudative bleeding, which led to the conclusion that lymphocytic colitis may not always present with a normal endoscopically appearing mucosa. Figure 13 depicts lymphocytic colitis associated with hypervascular mucosa and exudative bleeding.

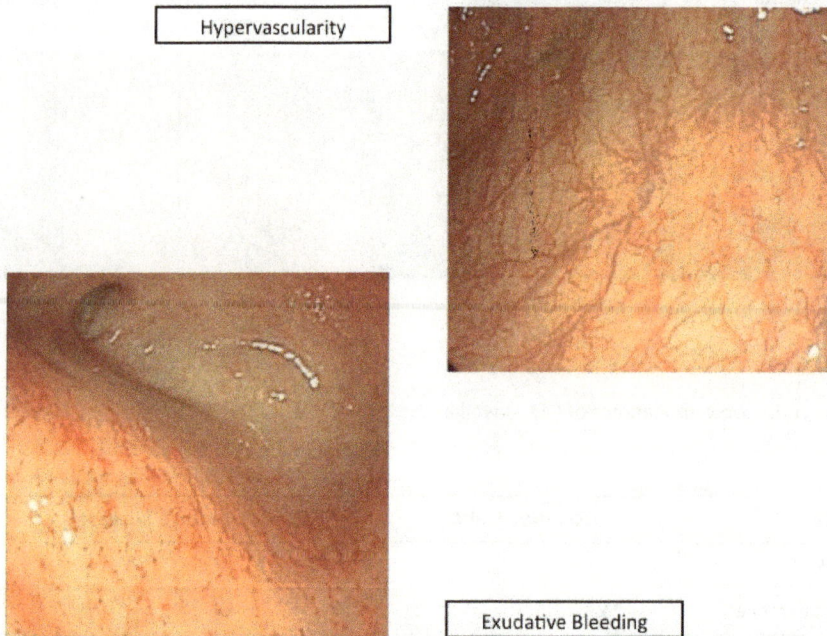

Figure 13. Hypervascular mucosa and exudative bleeding associated with lymphocytic colitis.

Eosinophilic disorders can span the entirety of the gastrointestinal tract, including the esophagus (eosinophilic esophagitis), stomach and small intestine (eosinophilic gastroenteritis), and the colon (eosinophilic colitis). Eosinophilic colitis is the least frequent manifestation of primary eosinophilic gastrointestinal disorders with only a few reports reported over the last four decades [74]. Secondary eosinophilic colitis can stem from several conditions including parasitic infections (e.g., *Strongyloides stercoralis* [75], *Enterobius vermicularis* [76], and *Trichuris trichiura* [77]), drug-induced (e.g., clozapine [78], carbamazepine [79], rifampicin [80], non-steroidal anti-inflammatory drugs [81, 82], tacrolimius [83], and gold [84]), auto-immune disorders (e.g., scleroderma [85], dermatomyositis and polymyositis [86, 87], and vasculitides (e.g., Churg-Strauss syndrome [88]). Endoscopic features suggestive of eosinophilic colitis include an edematous mucosa with loss of normal vascular pattern, patchy erythema, and superficial ulcerations [74].

4.3. Ischemic colitis

Ischemic colitis occurs as a result of inadequate blood supply to the large colon, typically affecting the critically ill and elderly population [89]. A recent retrospective study by Church et al. examined the role of urgent bedside colonoscopy in critically ill patients [90]. This study included 41 patients totaling 49 bedside colonoscopies with the most common indication being to exclude ischemic colitis (n=25). Of those 25, the diagnosis was confirmed in 19 with 14 patients subsequently undergoing surgical intervention, which led the authors to conclude that bedside colonoscopy is helpful in the diagnosis of acute lower gastrointestinal disease and can potentially guide therapeutic management in critically ill patients. There are several endoscopic findings that may assist in the diagnosis of ischemic colitis, one of which is the colon single-stripe sign. Zuckerman retrospectively studied 26 patients with endoscopic evidence of the colon single-stripe sign and compared it with 58 consecutive patients without a stripe [91]. All patients in the colon single-strip cohort had a stripe that was >5cm in length predominantly in the left colon (89%). Patients with the colon single-stripe sign were significantly more likely to have evidence of a preceding ischemic event (62%) compared to the colitis comparison group (7%). Histologically, patients with the colon single-stripe sign had microscopic evidence of ischemic injury compared to the colitis cohort (75% vs. 13%, respectively; p<0.0001). Next, the clinical course and outcome of the 26 patients with the colon single-stripe sign was compared with 22 patients with circumferentially involved ischemic colitis. None of the patients with the colon single-stripe sign required surgical intervention compared with 27% of patients with circumferential ischemic colitis. In addition, mortality rates were higher in the circumferential ischemic colitis group compared with patients with the colon single-stripe sign (41% vs. 4%, respectively; p<0.05). This led the authors to conclude that the colon-single stripe sign can manifest endoscopically, typically in a milder disease in the clinical spectrum of ischemic colitis [91]. Other endoscopic manifestations of ischemic colitis include petechial hemorrhages, edematous and fragile mucosa, segmental erythema, scattered erosions, and longitudinal ulcerations [92]. The 'watershed areas' areas (e.g., splenic flexure and transverse colon) are areas most vulnerable to ischemia due to the fact that they have the fewest collateral circulation. Figure 14 depicts various endoscopic manifestations of ischemic colitis.

4.4. Graft-Versus-Host Disease (GVHD)

Acute GVHD is associated with significant morbidity and mortality in the first 100 days following allogeneic hematopoietic progenitor stem cell transplant [93]. Acute GVHD can have GI manifestations (abdominal pain, nausea/vomiting, and diarrhea), obstructive jaundice, or skin rash. Gastroenterologists are often times consulted for endoscopic evaluation to rule out GHVD, when post-transplant patients present with GI manifestations in the absence of liver

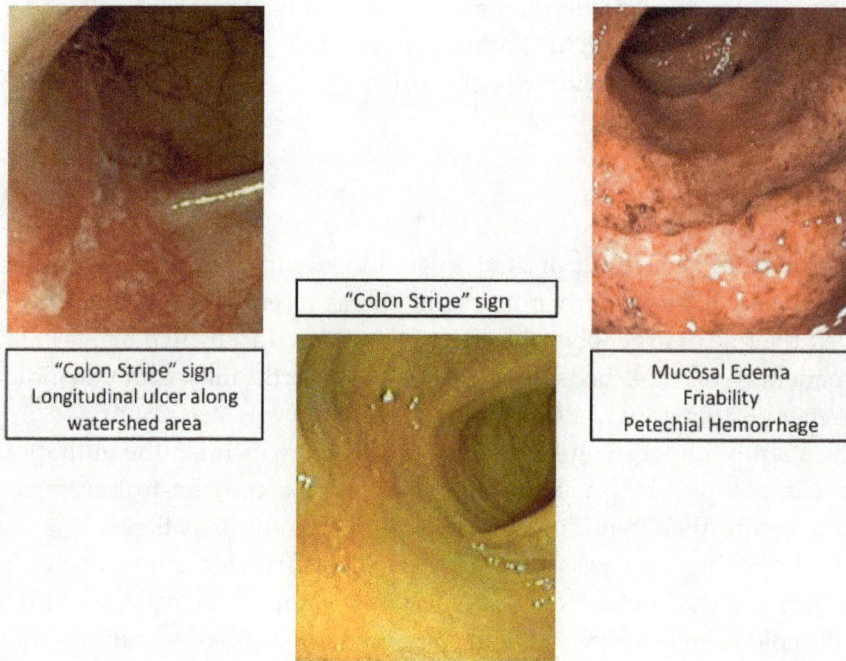

Figure 14. Various endoscopic manifestations of ischemic colitis.

or dermatologic involvement. In a majority of patients, flexible sigmoidoscopy with rectal biopsies allow for histologic diagnosis of GVHD and thus colonoscopy is not necessary [94, 95]. Endoscopic features of GVHD include diffuse edema, hyperemia, patchy erosions, scattered ulcers, sloughing, and active bleeding [96].

5. Evaluation of Lower Gastrointestinal Bleeding (LGIB)

The incidence of LGIB is approximately 20 per 100,000, with an associated all cause mortality of 3.9% [97]. The three most common causes of LGIB include angioectasias, diverticular bleeding, and hemorrhoidal bleeding [98]. Colonic ulcerations secondary to underlying IBD or chronic NSAID use, stercoral ulcer, Dieulafoy's lesion, or colorectal varices are less common etiologies of LGIB. In addition, an upper gastrointestinal source should also be included in the differential being that upwards of 15% of patients with severe hematochezia are found to have an upper gastrointestinal source [99]. In a hemodynamically stable patient, colonoscopy remains the cornerstone in the diagnosis of an LGIB. Figure 15 is a suggested algorithm by Parekh et al. for the role of colonoscopy in the evaluation of a hemodynamically stable LGIB [100].

Diverticulosis of the colon is an out-pouching of colonic mucosa through weakened layers of muscle in the colon wall. The incidence of diverticular increases after the age of 40 [101]. While in itself benign, complications of diverticular disease include diverticulitis, which is the inflammation or infection of diverticula, and painless bleeding, which may be life threatening.

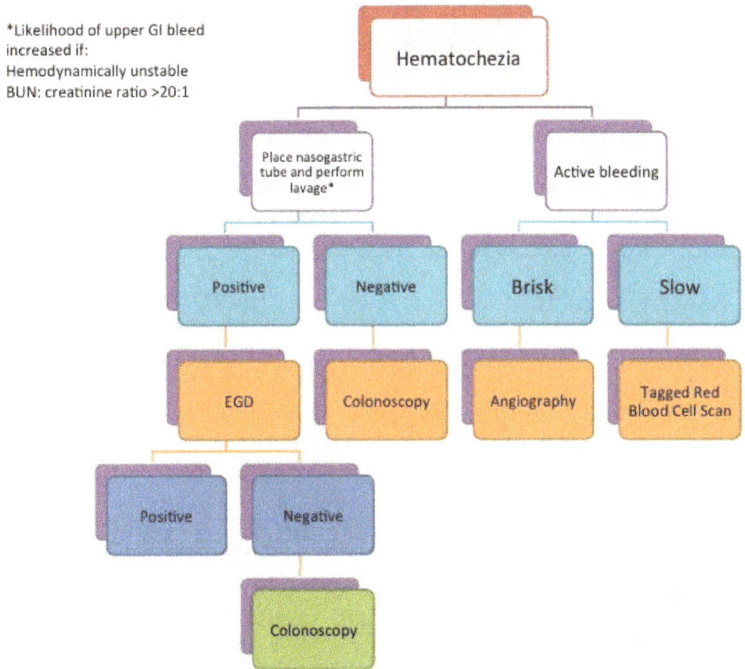

Figure 15. Suggested algorithm by Parekh et al. for the role of colonoscopy in the evaluation of a hemodynamically stable LGIB [100].

Therefore, it is important for the endoscopist to inform the patient of symptoms of potential complications of diverticular disease.

Colonic angioectasias, previously referred to as arteriovenous malformations or angiodysplasias, are a common source of lower gastrointestinal bleeding [102]. They can often times be difficult to identify if not actively bleeding. Figure 16 is an example of colonic diverticula and an angioectasia seen endoscopically.

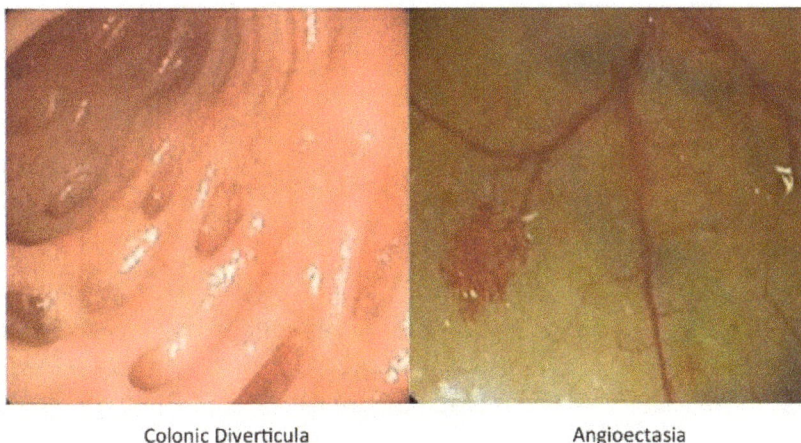

Colonic Diverticula   Angioectasia

Figure 16. Colonic diverticula and an angioectasia seen endoscopically.

6. Hemorrhoids and anal fissures

Hemorrhoids are vascular structures in the anal canal that act as cushions to help with stool control [103]. When they become swollen or inflamed, internal hemorrhoids (above the dentate line) can present as painless rectal bleeding. External hemorrhoids can result in pain when thrombosed, or painful bleeding if ulceration occurs from pressure necrosis [103]. Skin tags may be evidence of prior thrombosed external hemorrhoids.

An anal fissure is a linear tear or crack in the distal anal canal. It often presents as painful defecation. Initially it usually involves only the epithelium and progresses to include the full thickness of the anal mucosa. Figure 17 is an example of an internal hemorrhoid, external hemorrhoid, skin tag, and an anal fissure.

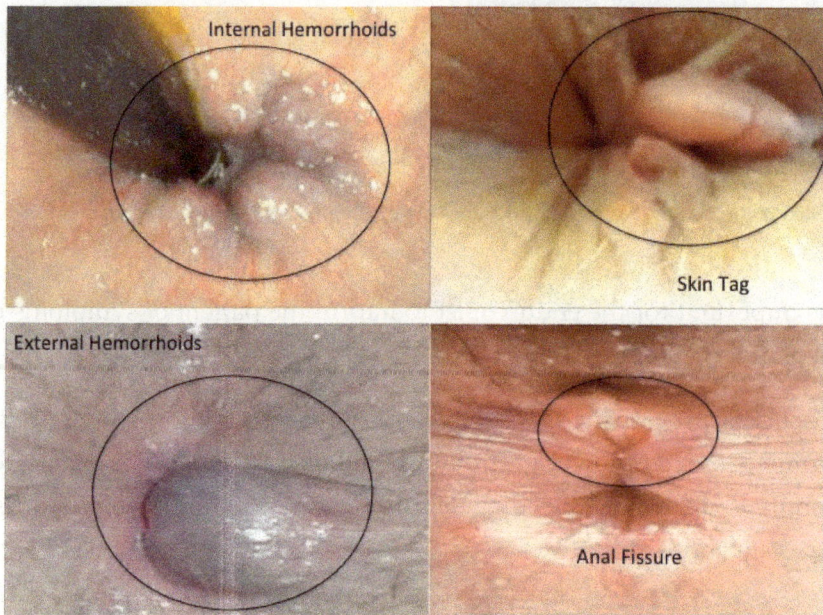

Figure 17. Internal hemorrhoid, external hemorrhoid, skin tag, and an anal fissure.

7. Conclusion

Colonoscopy is important in the diagnosis and therapeutic management of several disease states. To date, colonoscopy remains the gold standard in colorectal cancer prevention. It is the cornerstone in the diagnosis and therapeutic management of IBD, particularly with the recent paradigm shift in the therapeutic management of IBD stressing the importance of endoscopic remission in addition to symptomatic remission. In addition, a thorough colonoscopic exam can aid in the diagnosis of other non-IBD colitides. In the acute setting, findings during colonoscopy are not only crucial in diagnosing the underlying etiology but also driving therapeutic management. As technology evolves and indications for colonoscopy expand, it becomes increasingly more crucial for the clinical endoscopist to be knowledgeable of normal and pathologic findings during colonoscopy.

Author details

Parth J. Parekh and Sanjay K. Sikka*

*Address all correspondence to: ssikka2@tulane.edu

Department of Internal Medicine, Division of Gastroenterology and Hepatology, Tulane University, New Orleans, LA, USA

References

[1] Wolff WI. Colonoscopy: History and development. Am J Gastroenterol. 1989;84(9): 1017-25.

[2] Rex DK, Rahmani EY, Haseman JH, Lemmel GT, Kaster S, Buckley JS. Relative sensitivity of colonoscopy and barium enema for detection of colorectal cancer in clinical practice. Gastroenterology. 1997;112(1):17-23.

[3] Winawer SJ, Zauber AG, Fletcher RH, et al. Guidelines for colonoscopy surveillance after polypectomy: A consensus update by the US Multi-Society Task Force on Colorectal Cancer and the American Cancer Society. CA Cancer J Clin. 2006;56(3):143-59.

[4] Siegel R, Desantis C, Jemal A. Colorectal cancer statistics, 2014. CA Cancer J Clin. 2014;64(2):104-17.

[5] Torre LA, Bray F, Siegel RL, Ferlay J, Lortet-tieulent J, Jemal A. Global cancer statistics, 2012. CA Cancer J Clin. 2015;65(2):87-108.

[6] Winawer SJ, Zauber AG, Ho MN, et al. Prevention of colorectal cancer by colonoscopic polypectomy. The National Polyp Study Workgroup. N Engl J Med. 1993;329(27):1977-81.

[7] Zauber AG, Winawer SJ, O'brien MJ, et al. Colonoscopic polypectomy and long-term prevention of colorectal-cancer deaths. N Engl J Med. 2012;366(8):687-96.

[8] Bressler B, Paszat LF, Chen Z, Rothwell DM, Vinden C, Rabeneck L. Rates of new or missed colorectal cancers after colonoscopy and their risk factors: a population-based analysis. Gastroenterology. 2007;132(1):96-102.

[9]   Pickhardt PJ, Nugent PA, Mysliwiec PA, Choi JR, Schindler WR. Location of adenomas missed by optical colonoscopy. Ann Intern Med. 2004;141(5):352-9.

[10] Van gelder RE, Nio CY, Florie J, et al. Computed tomographic colonography compared with colonoscopy in patients at increased risk for colorectal cancer. Gastroenterology. 2004;127(1):41-8.

[11] Lieberman DA, Weiss DG, Harford WV, et al. Five-year colon surveillance after screening colonoscopy. Gastroenterology. 2007;133(4):1077-85.

[12] Martínez ME, Baron JA, Lieberman DA, et al. A pooled analysis of advanced colorectal neoplasia diagnoses after colonoscopic polypectomy. Gastroenterology. 2009;136(3):832-41.

[13] Pancione M, Remo A, Colantuoni V. Genetic and epigenetic events generate multiple pathways in colorectal cancer progression. Patholog Res Int. 2012;2012:509348.

[14] Luo Y, Wong CJ, Kaz AM, et al. Differences in DNA methylation signatures reveal multiple pathways of progression from adenoma to colorectal cancer. Gastroenterology. 2014;147(2):418-29.e8.

[15] The Paris endoscopic classification of superficial neoplastic lesions: esophagus, stomach, and colon: November 30 to December 1, 2002. Gastrointest Endosc. 2003;58(6 Suppl):S3-43.

[16] O'brien MJ, Winawer SJ, Zauber AG, et al. The National Polyp Study. Patient and polyp characteristics associated with high-grade dysplasia in colorectal adenomas. Gastroenterology. 1990;98(2):371-9.

[17] Binmoeller KF, Bohnacker S, Seifert H, Thonke F, Valdeyar H, Soehendra N. Endoscopic snare excision of "giant" colorectal polyps. Gastrointest Endosc. 1996;43(3): 183-8.

[18] Lieberman D, Moravec M, Holub J, Michaels L, Eisen G. Polyp size and advanced histology in patients undergoing colonoscopy screening: Implications for CT colonography. Gastroenterology. 2008;135(4):1100-5.

[19] Van doorn SC, Hazewinkel Y, East JE, et al. Polyp morphology: An interobserver evaluation for the Paris classification among international experts. Am J Gastroenterol. 2015;110(1):180-7.

[20] Leung WK, Lo OS, Liu KS, et al. Detection of colorectal adenoma by narrow band imaging (HQ190) vs. high-definition white light colonoscopy: A randomized controlled trial. Am J Gastroenterol. 2014;109(6):855-63.

[21] Jin XF, Chai TH, Shi JW, Yang XC, Sun QY. Meta-analysis for evaluating the accuracy of endoscopy with narrow band imaging in detecting colorectal adenomas. J Gastroenterol Hepatol. 2012;27(5):882-7.

[22] East JE, Ignjatovic A, Suzuki N, et al. A randomized, controlled trial of narrow-band imaging vs. high-definition white light for adenoma detection in patients at high risk of adenomas. Colorectal Dis. 2012;14(11):e771-8.

[23] Mizuno K, Kudo SE, Ohtsuka K, et al. Narrow-banding images and structures of microvessels of colonic lesions. Dig Dis Sci. 2011;56(6):1811-7.

[24] Winawer SJ, Zauber AG. The advanced adenoma as the primary target of screening. Gastrointest Endosc Clin N Am. 2002;12(1):1-9, v.

[25] Mattar M, Frankel P, David D, et al. Clinicopathologic significance of synchronous and metachronous adenomas in colorectal cancer. Clin Colorectal Cancer. 2005;5(4): 274-8.

[26] Karlitz JJ, Hsieh MC, Liu Y, et al. Population-based lynch syndrome screening by microsatellite instability in patients ≤50: Prevalence, testing determinants, and result availability prior to colon surgery. Am J Gastroenterol. 2015.

[27] Worthley DL, Leggett BA. Colorectal cancer: Molecular features and clinical opportunities. Clin Biochem Rev. 2010;31(2):31-8.

[28] Kakar S, Deng G, Cun L, Sahai V, Kim YS. CpG island methylation is frequently present in tubulovillous and villous adenomas and correlates with size, site, and villous component. Hum Pathol. 2008;39(1):30-6.

[29] Rosty C, Hewett DG, Brown IS, Leggett BA, Whitehall VL. Serrated polyps of the large intestine: current understanding of diagnosis, pathogenesis, and clinical management. J Gastroenterol. 2013;48(3):287-302.

[30] Rex DK, Ahnen DJ, Baron JA, et al. Serrated lesions of the colorectum: Review and recommendations from an expert panel. Am J Gastroenterol. 2012;107(9):1315-29.

[31] Spring KJ, Zhao ZZ, Karamatic R, et al. High prevalence of sessile serrated adenomas with BRAF mutations: A prospective study of patients undergoing colonoscopy. Gastroenterology. 2006;131(5):1400-7.

[32] Sweetser S, Smyrk TC, Sinicrope FA. Serrated colon polyps as precursors to colorectal cancer. Clin Gastroenterol Hepatol. 2013;11(7):760-7.

[33] Anderson JC. Pathogenesis and management of serrated polyps: Current status and future directions. Gut Liver. 2014;8(6):582-9.

[34] Weston AP, Campbell DR. Diminutive colonic polyps: Histopathology, spatial distribution, concomitant significant lesions, and treatment complications. Am J Gastroenterol. 1995;90(1):24-8.

[35] Butterly L, Robinson CM, Anderson JC, et al. Serrated and adenomatous polyp detection increases with longer withdrawal time: Results from the New Hampshire Colonoscopy Registry. Am J Gastroenterol. 2014;109(3):417-26.

[36] Anderson JC, Butterly LF, Goodrich M, Robinson CM, Weiss JE. Differences in detection rates of adenomas and serrated polyps in screening versus surveillance colonoscopies, based on the new hampshire colonoscopy registry. Clin Gastroenterol Hepatol. 2013;11(10):1308-12.

[37] Tadepalli US, Feihel D, Miller KM, et al. A morphologic analysis of sessile serrated polyps observed during routine colonoscopy (with video). Gastrointest Endosc. 2011;74(6):1360-8.

[38] Higuchi T, Sugihara K, Jass JR. Demographic and pathological characteristics of serrated polyps of colorectum. Histopathology. 2005;47(1):32-40.

[39] Provenzale D, Garrett JW, Condon SE, Sandler RS. Risk for colon adenomas in patients with rectosigmoid hyperplastic polyps. Ann Intern Med. 1990;113(10):760-3.

[40] Dave S, Hui S, Kroenke K, Imperiale TF. Is the distal hyperplastic polyp a marker for proximal neoplasia? J Gen Intern Med. 2003;18(2):128-37.

[41] Rex DK, Smith JJ, Ulbright TM, Lehman GA. Distal colonic hyperplastic polyps do not predict proximal adenomas in asymptomatic average-risk subjects. Gastroenterology. 1992;102(1):317-9.

[42] Lin OS, Schembre DB, Mccormick SE, et al. Risk of proximal colorectal neoplasia among asymptomatic patients with distal hyperplastic polyps. Am J Med. 2005;118(10):1113-9.

[43] Weston AP, Campbell DR. Diminutive colonic polyps: Histopathology, spatial distribution, concomitant significant lesions, and treatment complications. Am J Gastroenterol. 1995;90(1):24-8.

[44] Calva D, Howe JR. Hamartomatous polyposis syndromes. Surg Clin North Am. 2008;88(4):779-817, vii.

[45] Choi YS, Suh JP, Lee IT, et al. Regression of giant pseudopolyps in inflammatory bowel disease. J Crohns Colitis. 2012;6(2):240-3.

[46] Maldonado TS, Firoozi B, Stone D, Hiotis K. Colocolonic intussusception of a giant pseudopolyp in a patient with ulcerative colitis: a case report and review of the literature. Inflamm Bowel Dis. 2004;10(1):41-4.

[47] Wyse J, Lamoureux E, Gordon PH, Bitton A. Occult dysplasia in a localized giant pseudopolyp in Crohn's colitis: A case report. Can J Gastroenterol. 2009;23(7):477-8.

[48] Popiolek DA, Kahn E, Procaccino JA, Markowitz J. Nodular neuronal hyperplasia: A distinct morphologic type of pseudopolyp in inflammatory bowel disease. Arch Pathol Lab Med. 1998;122(2):194-6.

[49] Leighton JA, Shen B, Baron TH, et al. ASGE guideline: Endoscopy in the diagnosis and treatment of inflammatory bowel disease. Gastrointest Endosc. 2006;63(4):558-65.

[50] Sulz MC, Bertolini R, Frei R, Semadeni GM, Borovicka J, Meyenberger C. Multipurpose use of the over-the-scope-clip system ("Bear claw") in the gastrointestinal tract: Swiss experience in a tertiary center. World J Gastroenterol. 2014;20(43):16287-92.

[51] Fefferman DS, Farrell RJ. Endoscopy in inflammatory bowel disease: Indications, surveillance, and use in clinical practice. Clin Gastroenterol Hepatol. 2005;3(1):11-24.

[52] Chatzicostas C, Koutroubakis IE, Tzardi M, Roussomoustakaki M, Prassopoulos P, Kouroumalis EA. Colonic tuberculosis mimicking Crohn's disease: Case report. BMC Gastroenterol. 2002;2(1):10.

[53] Lee SK, Kim BK, Kim TI, Kim WH. Differential diagnosis of intestinal Behçet's disease and Crohn's disease by colonoscopic findings. Endoscopy. 2009;41(1):9-16.

[54] Del val JH. Old-age inflammatory bowel disease onset: A different problem? World J Gastroenterol. 2011;17(22):2734-9.

[55] Rameshshanker R, Arebi N. Endoscopy in inflammatory bowel disease when and why. World J Gastrointest Endosc. 2012;4(6):201-11.

[56] Kim B, Barnett JL, Kleer CG, Appelman HD. Endoscopic and histological patchiness in treated ulcerative colitis. Am J Gastroenterol. 1999;94(11):3258-62.

[57] Bernstein CN, Shanahan F, Anton PA, Weinstein WM. Patchiness of mucosal inflammation in treated ulcerative colitis: A prospective study. Gastrointest Endosc. 1995;42(3):232-7.

[58] Jevon GP, Madhur R. Endoscopic and histologic findings in pediatric inflammatory bowel disease. Gastroenterol Hepatol (N Y). 2010;6(3):174-80.

[59] Tontini GE, Vecchi M, Pastorelli L, Neurath MF, Neumann H. Differential diagnosis in inflammatory bowel disease colitis: State of the art and future perspectives. World J Gastroenterol. 2015;21(1):21-46.

[60] Lemmens B, Arijs I, Van assche G, et al. Correlation between the endoscopic and histologic score in assessing the activity of ulcerative colitis. Inflamm Bowel Dis. 2013;19(6):1194-201.

[61] Freeman HJ. Natural history and clinical behavior of Crohn's disease extending beyond two decades. J Clin Gastroenterol. 2003;37(3):216-9.

[62] Nikolaus S, Schreiber S. Diagnostics of inflammatory bowel disease. Gastroenterology. 2007;133(5):1670-89.

[63] Kaiser AM. Discussion of "Backwash ileitis is strongly associated with colorectal carcinoma in ulcerative colitis". Gastroenterology. 2002;122(1):245-6.

[64] Haskell H, Andrews CW, Reddy SI, et al. Pathologic features and clinical significance of "backwash" ileitis in ulcerative colitis. Am J Surg Pathol. 2005;29(11):1472-81.

[65] Daperno M, D'haens G, Van assche G, et al. Development and validation of a new, simplified endoscopic activity score for Crohn's disease: The SES-CD. Gastrointest Endosc. 2004;60(4):505-12.

[66] Ferrante M, Colombel JF, Sandborn WJ, et al. Validation of endoscopic activity scores in patients with Crohn's disease based on a post hoc analysis of data from SONIC. Gastroenterology. 2013;145(5):978-986.e5.

[67] Khanna R, Bouguen G, Feagan BG, et al. A systematic review of measurement of endoscopic disease activity and mucosal healing in Crohn's disease: Recommendations for clinical trial design. Inflamm Bowel Dis. 2014;20(10):1850-61.

[68] Park HS, Han DS, Ro YO, Eun CS, Yoo KS. Does lymphocytic colitis always present with normal endoscopic findings? Gut Liver. 2015;9(2):197-201.

[69] Nomura E, Kagaya H, Uchimi K, et al. Linear mucosal defects: a characteristic endoscopic finding of lansoprazole-associated collagenous colitis. Endoscopy. 2010;42 Suppl 2:E9-10.

[70] Couto G, Bispo M, Barreiro P, Monteiro L, Matos L. Unique endoscopy findings in collagenous colitis. Gastrointest Endosc. 2009;69(6):1186-8.

[71] Sato S, Matsui T, Tsuda S, et al. Endosocopic abnormalities in a Japanese patient with collagenous colitis. J Gastroenterol. 2003;38(8):812-3.

[72] Giardiello FM, Bayless TM, Yardley JH. Collagenous colitis. Compr Ther. 1989;15(2): 49-54.

[73] Pardi DS, Smyrk TC, Tremaine WJ, Sandborn WJ. Microscopic colitis: A review. Am J Gastroenterol. 2002;97(4):794-802.

[74] Alfadda AA, Storr MA, Shaffer EA. Eosinophilic colitis: Epidemiology, clinical features, and current management. Therap Adv Gastroenterol. 2011;4(5):301-9.

[75] Al samman M, Haque S, Long JD. Strongyloidiasis colitis: A case report and review of the literature. J Clin Gastroenterol. 1999;28(1):77-80.

[76] Liu LX, Chi J, Upton MP, Ash LR. Eosinophilic colitis associated with larvae of the pinworm Enterobius vermicularis. Lancet. 1995;346(8972):410-2.

[77] Chandrasekhara V, Arslanlar S, Sreenarasimhaiah J. Whipworm infection resulting in eosinophilic colitis with occult intestinal bleeding. Gastrointest Endosc. 2007;65(4): 709-10.

[78] Friedberg JW, Frankenburg FR, Burk J, Johnson W. Clozapine-caused eosinophilic colitis. Ann Clin Psychiatry. 1995;7(2):97-8.

[79] Anttila VJ, Valtonen M. Carbamazepine-induced eosinophilic colitis. Epilepsia. 1992;33(1):119-21.

[80] Lange P, Oun H, Fuller S, Turney JH. Eosinophilic colitis due to rifampicin. Lancet. 1994;344(8932):1296-7.

[81] Bridges AJ, Marshall JB, Diaz-arias AA. Acute eosinophilic colitis and hypersensitivity reaction associated with naproxen therapy. Am J Med. 1990;89(4):526-7.

[82] Jiménez-sáenz M, González-cámpora R, Linares-santiago E, Herrerías-gutiérrez JM. Bleeding colonic ulcer and eosinophilic colitis: a rare complication of nonsteroidal anti-inflammatory drugs. J Clin Gastroenterol. 2006;40(1):84-5.

[83] Saeed SA, Integlia MJ, Pleskow RG, et al. Tacrolimus-associated eosinophilic gastroenterocolitis in pediatric liver transplant recipients: role of potential food allergies in pathogenesis. Pediatr Transplant. 2006;10(6):730-5.

[84] Martin DM, Goldman JA, Gilliam J, Nasrallah SM. Gold-induced eosinophilic enterocolitis: Response to oral cromolyn sodium. Gastroenterology. 1981;80(6):1567-70.

[85] Clouse RE, Alpers DH, Hockenbery DM, Deschryver-kecskemeti K. Pericrypt eosinophilic enterocolitis and chronic diarrhea. Gastroenterology. 1992;103(1):168-76.

[86] Barbie DA, Mangi AA, Lauwers GY. Eosinophilic gastroenteritis associated with systemic lupus erythematosus. J Clin Gastroenterol. 2004;38(10):883-6.

[87] Ahmad M, Soetikno RM, Ahmed A. The differential diagnosis of eosinophilic esophagitis. J Clin Gastroenterol. 2000;30(3):242-4.

[88] Avgerinos A, Bourikas L, Tzardi M, Koutroubakis IE. Eosinophilic gastroenteritis associated with Churg-Strauss syndrome. Ann Gastroenterol. 2012;25(2):164.

[89] Huguier M, Barrier A, Boelle PY, Houry S, Lacaine F. Ischemic colitis. Am J Surg. 2006;192(5):679-84.

[90] Church J, Kao J. Bedside colonoscopy in intensive care units: indications, techniques, and outcomes. Surg Endosc. 2014;28(9):2679-82.

[91] Zuckerman GR, Prakash C, Merriman RB, Sawhney MS, Deschryver-kecskemeti K, Clouse RE. The colon single-stripe sign and its relationship to ischemic colitis. Am J Gastroenterol. 2003;98(9):2018-22.

[92] Zou X, Cao J, Yao Y, Liu W, Chen L. Endoscopic findings and clinicopathologic characteristics of ischemic colitis: A report of 85 cases. Dig Dis Sci. 2009;54(9):2009-15.

[93] Sultan M, Ramprasad J, Jensen MK, Margolis D, Werlin S. Endoscopic diagnosis of pediatric acute gastrointestinal graft-versus-host disease. J Pediatr Gastroenterol Nutr. 2012;55(4):417-20.

[94] Aslanian H, Chander B, Robert M, et al. Prospective evaluation of acute graft-versus-host disease. Dig Dis Sci. 2012;57(3):720-5.

[95] Crowell KR, Patel RA, Fluchel M, Lowichik A, Bryson S, Pohl JF. Endoscopy in the diagnosis of intestinal graft-versus-host disease: Is lower endoscopy with biopsy as

effective in diagnosis as upper endoscopy combined with lower endoscopy? Pediatr Blood Cancer. 2013;60(11):1798-800.

[96] Xu CF, Zhu LX, Xu XM, Chen WC, Wu DP. Endoscopic diagnosis of gastrointestinal graft-versus-host disease. World J Gastroenterol. 2008;14(14):2262-7.

[97] Strate LL, Ayanian JZ, Kotler G, Syngal S. Risk factors for mortality in lower intestinal bleeding. Clin Gastroenterol Hepatol. 2008;6(9):1004-10.

[98] Chait MM. Lower gastrointestinal bleeding in the elderly. World J Gastrointest Endosc. 2010;2(5):147-54.

[99] Farrell JJ, Friedman LS. Review article: The management of lower gastrointestinal bleeding. Aliment Pharmacol Ther. 2005;21(11):1281-98.

[100] Parekh PJ, Buerlein RC, Shams R, Vingan H, Johnson DA. Evaluation of gastrointestinal bleeding: Update of current radiologic strategies. World J Gastrointest Pharmacol Ther. 2014;5(4):200-8.

[101] Comparato G, Pilotto A, Franzè A, Franceschi M, Di mario F. Diverticular disease in the elderly. Dig Dis. 2007;25(2):151-9.

[102] Management of gastrointestinal angiodysplastic lesions (GIADs): A systematic review and meta-analysis. The American Journal of Gastroenterology. 2014;109(4):474.

[103] Sanchez C, Chinn BT. Hemorrhoids. Clin Colon Rectal Surg. 2011;24(1):5-13.

Permissions

The contributors of this book come from diverse backgrounds, making this book a truly international effort. This book will bring forth new frontiers with its revolutionizing research information and detailed analysis of the nascent developments around the world.

We would like to thank all the contributing authors for lending their expertise to make the book truly unique. They have played a crucial role in the development of this book. Without their invaluable contributions this book wouldn't have been possible. They have made vital efforts to compile up to date information on the varied aspects of this subject to make this book a valuable addition to the collection of many professionals and students.

This book was conceptualized with the vision of imparting up-to-date information and advanced data in this field. To ensure the same, a matchless editorial board was set up. Every individual on the board went through rigorous rounds of assessment to prove their worth. After which they invested a large part of their time researching and compiling the most relevant data for our readers.

The editorial board has been involved in producing this book since its inception. They have spent rigorous hours researching and exploring the diverse topics which have resulted in the successful publishing of this book. They have passed on their knowledge of decades through this book. To expedite this challenging task, the publisher supported the team at every step. A small team of assistant editors was also appointed to further simplify the editing procedure and attain best results for the readers.

Apart from the editorial board, the designing team has also invested a significant amount of their time in understanding the subject and creating the most relevant covers. They scrutinized every image to scout for the most suitable representation of the subject and create an appropriate cover for the book.

The publishing team has been an ardent support to the editorial, designing and production team. Their endless efforts to recruit the best for this project, has resulted in the accomplishment of this book. They are a veteran in the field of academics and their pool of knowledge is as vast as their experience in printing. Their expertise and guidance has proved useful at every step. Their uncompromising quality standards have made this book an exceptional effort. Their encouragement from time to time has been an inspiration for everyone.

The publisher and the editorial board hope that this book will prove to be a valuable piece of knowledge for researchers, students, practitioners and scholars across the globe.

List of Contributors

Jigar Bhagatwala, Arpit Singhal, Summer Aldrugh, Muhammed Sherid, Humberto Sifuentes and Subbaramiah Sridhar
Georgia Regents University, Augusta, GA, USA

David J. Harrison
School of Medicine, University of St Andrews, Fife, United Kingdom

Romina Briffa
School of Medicine, University of St Andrews, Fife, United Kingdom
Department of Pathology, Faculty of Medicine and Surgery, University of Malta, Msida, Malta

Godfrey Grech
Department of Pathology, Faculty of Medicine and Surgery, University of Malta, Msida, Malta

Simon P. Langdon
Cancer Research UK Edinburgh Centre and Division of Pathology Laboratory, Institute of Genetics and Molecular Medicine, University of Edinburgh, Edinburgh, United Kingdom

Jorge Bernal and F. Javier Sánchez
Computer Science Department at Universitat Autònoma de Barcelona and Computer Vision Center, Barcelona, Spain

Cristina Rodríguez de Miguel and Gloria Fernández-Esparrach
Endoscopy Unit, Gastroenterology Department, Hospital Clínic, IDIBAPS, CIBEREHD, University of Barcelona, Barcelona, Spain

Racho Ribarov
Faculty of Public Health, Medical University – Sofia, Sofia, Bulgaria

Rotimi R. Ayoola, Hamza Abdulla, Evan K. Brady, Muhammed Sherid and Humberto Sifuentes
Georgia Regents University, Augusta, GA, USA

Octav Ginghina
Department of Surgery, "Sf. Ioan" Emergency Clinical Hospital, Bucharest, Romania
Department II, Faculty of Dental Medicine, "Carol Davila" University of Medicine and Pharmacy Bucharest, Bucharest, Romania

Cornelia Nitipir
Department of Clinical Oncology, Elias Emergency Clinical Hospital, "Carol Davila" University of Medicine and Pharmacy, Bucharest, Romania

Camille Thélin and Sanjay Sikka
Department of Internal Medicine, Division of Gastroenterology and Hepatology, Tulane University, New Orleans, LA, United States

Hamid Elia Daaboul and Mirvat El-Sibai
Department of Natural Sciences, School of Arts and Sciences, Lebanese American University, Byblos, Lebanon

Parth J. Parekh and Sanjay K. Sikka
Department of Internal Medicine, Division of Gastroenterology and Hepatology, Tulane University, New Orleans, LA, USA

Index